Manual of
Otolaryngology

A Symptom-Oriented Text

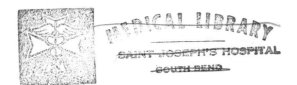

Manual of Otolaryngology

A Symptom-Oriented Text

Edited by:

Raymond P. Wood II, M.D.
Associate Professor and Vice Chairman
Department of Otolaryngology
University of Colorado Medical Center
Denver, Colorado

Jerry L. Northern, Ph.D.
Professor, Head of Audiology
Department of Otolaryngology
University of Colorado Medical Center
Denver, Colorado

Consulting Editor:

Bruce W. Jafek, M.D.
Professor and Chairman
Department of Otolaryngology
University of Colorado Medical Center
Denver, Colorado

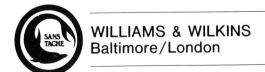

WILLIAMS & WILKINS
Baltimore/London

421

Copyright ©, 1979
The Williams & Wilkins Company
428 E. Preston Street
Baltimore, Md 21202, U.S.A.

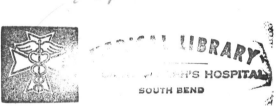

Made in the United States of America

Library of Congress Cataloging in Publication Data

Main entry under title:

Manual of otolaryngology.

  Includes index.
  1. Otolaryngology. I. Wood, Raymond P. II. Northern, Jerry L. III. Jafek, Bruce W. [DNLM: 1. Otorhinolar-
yngologic diseases. WV100.3 W878m]
RF46.M34   616.2′1   78-31442
ISBN 0-683-09252-9

Composed and printed at the
Waverly Press, Inc.
Mt. Royal and Guilford Aves.
Baltimore, Md 21202 U.S.A.

Acknowledgment

This book is dedicated to those who have taught us. Especially we would like to acknowledge the contributions of Dr. John R. Lindsay, Dr. William G. Hemenway, and Dr. Paul H. Ward, leaders in academic otolaryngology.

> "One can not *teach* anything to another person.
> One can only provide an environment in which
> another can *learn*."

421

Contributors

BRUCE B. BAKER, M.D.
Department of Otolaryngology
University Hospital
Boston University Medical Center
Boston, Massachusetts

THOMAS BALKANY, M.D.
Assistant Professor
Department of Otolaryngology
University of Colorado Medical Center
Denver, Colorado

RICHARD CUNDY, M.D.
Assistant Clinical Professor
Department of Otolaryngology
University of Colorado Medical Center
Denver, Colorado

MARION P. DOWNS, M.A.
Associate Professor, Audiology
Department of Otolaryngology
University of Colorado Medical Center
Denver, Colorado

GERALD M. ENGLISH, M.D.
Assistant Clinical Professor
Department of Otolaryngology
University of Colorado Medical Center
Denver, Colorado

DENNIS GREENE, M.D.
Associate Clinical Professor
Department of Otolaryngology
University of Colorado Medical Center
Denver, Colorado

ROBERT O. GREER, D.D.S.
Associate Professor and Chairman
University of Colorado Medical Center
School of Dentistry
Denver, Colorado

BRUCE W. JAFEK, M.D.
Professor and Chairman
Department of Otolaryngology
University of Colorado Medical Center
Denver, Colorado

ARLEN MEYERS, M.D.
Assistant Professor
Department of Otolaryngology
University of Colorado Medical Center
Denver, Colorado

ROBERT E. MISCHKE, M.D.
Assistant Professor
Department of Otolaryngology
University of Colorado Medical Center
Denver, Colorado

JAMES R. TABOR, M.D.
Associate Clinical Professor
Department of Otolaryngology
University of Colorado Medical Center
Denver, Colorado

MATTHEW L. WONG, M.D.
Assistant Professor
Department of Otolaryngology
University of Colorado Medical Center
Denver, Colorado

DARREL L. TETER, Ph.D.
Clinical Instructor
Department of Otolaryngology
University of Colorado Medical Center
Denver, Colorado

RAYMOND P. WOOD II, M.D.
Associate Professor and Vice Chairman
Department of Otolaryngology
University of Colorado Medical Center
Denver, Colorado

MARLIN E. WEAVER, M.D.
Associate Clinical Professor
Department of Otolaryngology
University of Colorado Medical Center
Denver, Colorado

JANET M. ZARNOCH, M.A.
Instructor, Audiology
Department of Otolaryngology
University of Colorado Medical Center
Denver, Colorado

W. BRUCE WILSON, M.D.
Department of Ophthalmology
University of Colorado Medical Center
Denver, Colorado

Contents

Introduction

Otorhinolaryngology (ORL), the science of diseases of the ear, nose, and throat, includes conditions requiring both surgical and medical management. ORL problems account for approximately 25% of the visits to the primary care physician; however, the amount of time devoted to ORL in the medical school curriculum averages less than two weeks of clinical experience; it may be only an elective. Internal medicine residencies rarely include additional training in ORL and, when they do, it is usually in the form of an elective. Even family practice and pediatric residencies often lack the additional necessary training in this area. The goal of this text is, therefore, to provide supplementary instructions on common otolaryngologic complaints, organized in problem-oriented format.

The development of the problem-oriented approach to medical problems by Lawrence Weed in the late 1950's and its gradual introduction into the medical record system of many medical centers offers an opportunity to alter the traditional organ system-oriented thinking and practice. Certain of the specialities, ORL being one, have been slow to accept and utilize this new method; it seems, however, superbly applicable to this field. The problem-oriented approach does not alter the final goal, to make a correct diagnosis. It only gives a more orderly approach to accomplishing this goal and gives a more lucid picture of the pattern, from presenting symptom to final diagnosis and therapy, a process which in the traditional system of history taking and examination sometimes becomes hopelessly complicated.

It is with this simplification in mind that we have chosen to present the diseases of the head and neck region in a problem-oriented format. The authors hope that this book will serve the needs of the medical student, internist, pediatrician, family physician, and emergency room physician. It is not intended to replace the many fine traditional textbooks which are necessary reference books, but to serve as an adjunct to them.

Raymond P. Wood II, M.D.

Jerry L. Northern, Ph.D.

Chapter 1

History Taking in Otorhinolaryngology

Raymond P. Wood II

In order to conform with the problem-oriented system, the subjective complaints of the patient must be evaluated to determine if they form a system complex (e.g., hearing loss, tinnitus, and vertigo in Meniere's disease) or if in fact they are separate symptoms (e.g., hearing loss, gradual or longstanding, and an ulcerative lesion of the tongue), in which case they will be treated under separate subjective complaint headings. We find it advantageous always to take the history and do the physical examination in the same order (e.g., ears, nose, throat) so as not to leave out any part.

SUBJECTIVE COMPLAINTS

Ears

Hearing—Normal or Abnormal

Symmetrical.
If loss, gradual or sudden onset.
Better ear?
Ear used with telephone.
Hear but not understand.
Worse in crowds or noise?
Loss, constant or fluctuating.
Previous use of hearing aid.
Associated symptoms: tinnitus (ringing or buzzing), dizziness, drainage from ear, fullness in ear.
Past medical history.
Head: trauma, unconsciousness.
Previous surgery.
Ear infections.
Noise exposure: occupational, military gunfire, tractors, airplanes, explosions, heavy equipment.
Drugs: aminoglycosides (injections, wound irrigations), diuretics.
Family history: hearing loss, ear surgery, hearing aids, dizziness, renal disease, congenital anomalies (von Recklinghousen's disease, low-set ears, Waardenburg syndrome, etc.).

Tinnitus

Bilateral or unilateral.
High-pitched ringing or buzzing.
Continuous, intermittent, pulsatile.
Longstanding or recent onset.
Altered by head position.

Altered by pressure on neck.
Associated symptoms: hearing loss, fullness or pressure in ears, dizziness.
Drugs: aspirin, quinine.

Discharge

Unilateral, bilateral.
Continuous, intermittent.
Odorless, foul.
Colored (yellow, green), clear, watery, bloody.
Painful, painless.
Associated symptoms: hearing loss, fever, dizziness, headache, upper respiratory infection (URI), facial weakness.
Past medical history: diabetes, head trauma, loss of consciousness, ear surgery, ear trauma.

Pain

Duration.
Continuous, intermittent.
Location (deep, superficial, circumaural).
Nature (sharp, dull, etc.).
Associated symptoms: drainage, hearing loss, tinnitus, dizziness, odynophagia, dysphagia, and sore throat.

Pinna Deformity

Acquired: traumatic, recent, old.
No trauma—other cartilaginous structures affected.
Congenital: bilateral, unilateral.
Other members of family affected.
    Hearing loss?
    Renal disease: patient, other family members

Nose

Epistaxis

Unilateral, bilateral.
Spontaneous, post-traumatic (nose picking, fracture, etc.).
Duration.
Intensity (increasing with attacks).
Associated problems: anticoagulants (including acetylsalicylic acid, ASA) easy bruising, other bleeding, hypertension, renal disease, nasal obstruction.

Obstruction and Rhinorrhea

Unilateral, bilateral (constant or alternating with position change).
Constant, intermittent (seasonal).
Pain.
Rhinorrhea: clear, bloody, green or yellow pus.
Spontaneous, post-traumatic.
Associated problems: drug use (nose drops, antihypertensives, cocaine, tranquilizers, hormones).
Facial pain, hyperesthesia (especially infraorbital).
Asthma, ASA sensitivity, allergies, itching and burning of eyes, itching of palate.

Nasal Deformity

Congenital (familial characteristic).
Recent or old trauma.
Associated problems: nasal obstruction, epistaxis.

Mouth

Oral Ulcerations

Location: constant, variable, in crops.
Duration.
Painful, nonpainful (acid foods).
Enlargement.
Associated problems: fever, malaise, other mucosal ulcerations (vaginal, urethral, anal), lip ulcerations.
Immunosuppressive drugs, sexual habits, venereal disease.

Intraoral Mass Lesions

Location.
Duration.
Enlargement.
Painful, nonpainful (acid foods).
Trismus.
Odynophagia, dysphagia.

Malocclusion

Congenital.
Acquired.
Post-traumatic.
Associated problems: trismus, pain, hypesthesia, ear pain.

Xerostomia

Associated problems: xerophthalmia, joint pain, skin rash, medications (tranquilizers, etc.).

Alterations in Taste

Dysgeusia (gasoline, garbage, etc.).
Hypogeusia.
Ageusia.
Recent, longstanding.
Associated problems: dysosmia, hyposmia, anosmia, nasal obstruction, medications, head injury, ear surgery, headache, visual disturbances, facial pain.

Hypopharynx—Larynx

Odynophagia

Duration.
Location—referral to ear?
Exacerbated by acid foods, solids, liquids.
Associated problems: hoarseness, dysphagia, stridor.

Dysphagia

Duration.
Localized to?
Occurs with: liquids, solids, tablets.
Associated with: hoarseness, stridor, odynophagia.

Airway Obstruction (Lower)—Stridor

Duration.
Location.
Exercise tolerance.
Nature: inspiratory stridor, expiratory stridor, both.
Exacerbated by: sleep, exercise.
Relieved by: opening mouth, protruding tongue, head positions.
Associated with: recent viral infection (URI?).
Pain, hoarseness, trauma to neck, neck or chest surgery, medications.

Hoarseness

Duration (congenital, acquired).
Stable, worsening.

Pattern (time of day worst).

Voice use (public speaking, singing, etc.).

Environment (high background noise, chemical exposure).

Stridor.

Pain.

Associated problems: smoking, alcohol, recent URI, cough, neck or chest surgery, thyroid status, trauma to neck, anesthetic intubation.

Salivary Glands (Parotid and Submaxillary Glands)

Discrete Swelling

Duration.

Pain.

Facial nerve function.

Constant or intermittent.

Associated with: pigmented skin lesions, bleeding lesions of skin and scalp, infection of external ear canal, recent URI.

Diffuse Swelling

Duration.

Uniglandular, multiglandular.

Painful, nonpainful.

Exacerbation with eating.

Previous history of mumps or vaccinations.

Associated problems: xerostomia, xerophthalmia, alcohol intake, starvation, iodides, bromides, antihypertensives, tranquilizers, joint pain, skin rashes, fever.

Lump in the Neck

Location.

Duration.

Size: stable, growing, alternating.

Single, multiple.

Tender, nontender.

Discrete, multiple, confluent.

Pulsatile.

Erythematous.

Associated problems: fever, chills, weight loss, positive tuberculin, nasal obstruction, serosanguineous discharge, hoarseness, odynophagia, dysphagia, intraoral lesions, pigmented skin lesions, ear pain.

Vertigo

Describe exact symptoms.

Motion: whirling, horizontal or vertical perception of movement.

Time of day of attack, relation to eating.

Duration.

Frequency.

Severity: increased or decreased with repetitive assumption of onset position.

Episodes, attacks.

Position of head during attack: ear down?

Neck rotation.

Position of body during attack: standing, lying, rolling over—what direction?

What makes attack better? Worse?

Attack worse with eyes open or closed?

Asymptomatic between attacks?

Onset with straining, increased intracranial or intrathoracic pressure.

Associated problems: neurologic disorders (loss of consciousness, diplopia, dysarthria, headache), head injury, whiplash, childhood motion sickness, tinnitus, hearing loss (sudden or longstanding), fluctuating hearing loss, loss of discrimination (understanding), diabetes mellitus, thyroid dysfunction, hypertension, hyperlipidemia, drug use, ototoxic drugs, nausea, vomiting epilepsy.

Chapter 2
Neurotology

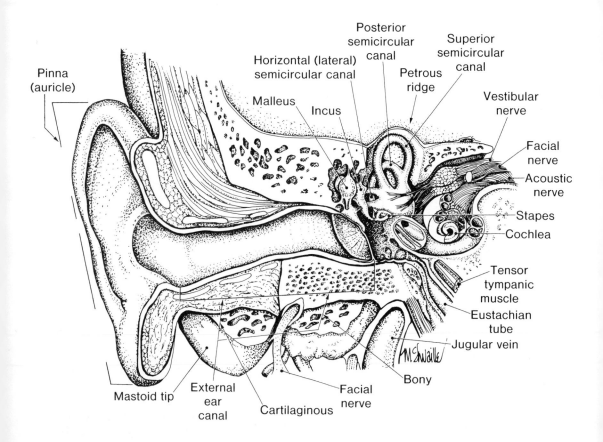

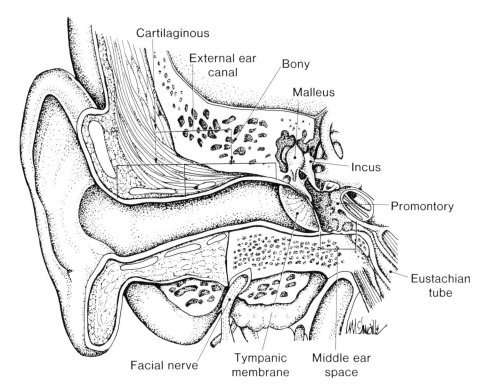

Cartilaginous

External ear canal

Bony

Malleus

Incus

Promontory

Eustachian tube

Facial nerve

Tympanic membrane

Middle ear space

Chapter 2.1

Sensorineural Hearing Loss

Marion P. Downs
Marlin E. Weaver

The term "sensorineural" hearing loss is a composite of words representing two different sites of lesion: A *sensory loss* is a reduction in hearing due to damage, degeneration, or failure to develop of the hair cells in the organ of Corti, in the basilar membrane, or any of the structures within the cochlear scalae. The hair cells are the end organs of hearing, and all lesions affecting their function result in a sensory loss.

A *neural loss* is a reduction in hearing due to damage, degeneration, or failure to develop of any of the neural structures central to the cochlear scalae and up to and including the cochlear nuclei of the brainstem. The nerve fibers and spiral ganglia within the helicotrema, plus the nerve fibers in the internal auditory meatus, constitute the neural transmission system.

Unless a definite diagnosis can be made of the site of lesion in such a hearing loss, it is not possible to identify the loss as *sensory,* or as *neural.* Therefore the term *sensorineural* is used to cover either possibility.

The lack of some hair cells or neural fibers in a sensorineural loss results in reduced clarity of reception. Speech sounds mildly to severely distorted. Part of the distortion may be caused by a differential hearing loss, where the low frequencies are heard better than the high tones—a common feature in sensorineural hearing losses (Fig. 2.1.1). The result is a lack of high fidelity reception of sound, with a breakdown in discrimination for speech sounds. This differential hearing loss is also responsible for poor hearing in the presence of background noise (such as cocktail parties). The ambient noise is always in the low pitches—an area where the individual with sensorineural loss may be dependent upon to hear. The low pitches are then masked out and the high frequencies are not heard well enough for speech to be understood. These phenomena are responsible for the subjective complaints one hears such as: "People mumble", "I can hear but can't understand"; "Can't hear in noisy places"; "Can only hear when someone's facing me"; "Don't shout—I can hear if you'll talk plainly." Complaints like these are almost always diagnostic of a sensorineural loss.

The reduced discrimination for speech is the greatest problem for those who suffer such losses. Hearing aids may not improve their potential understanding of speech, despite the fact that the amplification will make the sound louder. Yet these individuals must wear hearing aids in order to hear normal conversational speech. Training in using a hearing aid is often necessary for them because the unaccustomed sound a hearing aid brings requires a great deal of practice in listening. Such training, in an audiologic center, is usually highly successful and permits individuals with sensorineural losses to wear hearing aids with great benefit.

Most sensorineural losses are untreatable medically or surgically. But when they can be treated it is of the utmost urgency that they be identified and brought to proper management because their etiologies may be progressive or malignant.

Operationally a sensorineural hearing loss is defined by an audiogram showing identity between air conduction and bone conduction thresholds. The contour of the audiogram is sometimes suggestive of the etiology of the loss, but a great deal of variation exists in these losses.

Another prerequisite to identifying a sensorineural loss is a positive Rinne test. That is, when the tuning fork is placed first behind the ear on the mastoid process and then in front of the concha, it will be heard louder in front than in back. On the Weber test the fork may be heard at the midline, or it may be heard louder on one side if that side has the better sensorineural hearing.

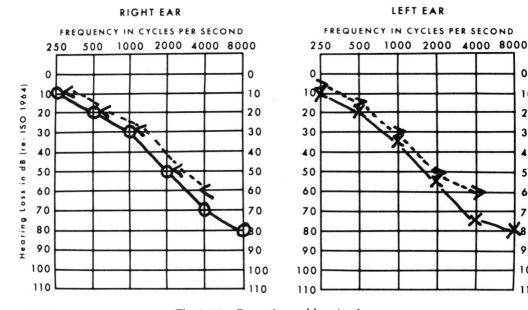

Fig. 2.1.1. Sensorineural hearing loss.

It is estimated that 14 million people in the U.S. have a hearing problem of some degree. Probably 80% of this number have sensorineural losses, most commonly due to presbycusis—the hearing loss that occurs with advancing age. The accompanying debilities of age make the problems of distortion in the speech signal and the difficulty of understanding in the presence of background noise particularly troublesome to this group. These problems will comprise the largest number of hearing problems seen in the physician's office.

SUDDEN SENSORINEURAL HEARING LOSS

Subjective Complaints

The object of a case history in sensorineural losses is to determine whether or not treatment will be beneficial, and whether certain elaborate tests should be performed. The most important condition to eliminate is an VIIIth nerve tumor. When diagnosed such a tumor must be treated surgically. When a sudden or gradual unilateral hearing loss is present without known cause it is obligatory to suspect an VIIIth nerve tumor. Other than this and in Meniere's syndrome indications, sensorineural losses from other causes are considered benign, albeit troublesome.

1. Loss of hearing: sometimes described as feeling that the ear is plugged; ear may feel "numb."
2. Unilateral or bilateral?
3. Nature of onset: occurring over few seconds, few minutes, or 1–2 hours; noted on arising in a.m.
4. Popping sensation with onset?
5. Related symptoms such as tinnitus or vertigo.
6. Coincident viral infection, head injury, noise exposure.

Objective Findings

1. Weber test lateralizes to better ear if unilateral.
2. Rinne test positive (air conduction better than bone conduction) in both ears.
3. Tympanic membrane normal: normal movement with pneumatic otoscopy.
4. Possible nystagmus.

5. Evidence of dysequilibration: Romberg tandem walk, etc.
6. Audiometric pure tone tests: sensorineural hearing loss >25 dB average; air and bone thresholds are equal.

Assessment

The etiologic diagnosis in sudden sensorineural hearing loss can sometimes be established by medical history. Below are listed some of the common etiologies of sudden loss with notes on pathogenesis and medical history.

1. Viral infection may be bloodborne to the inner ear: frequent history of coincident upper respiratory infection, sometimes associated with vertigo; hearing loss developed over several hours.
2. Ischemia of cochlea due to occlusion of labyrinthine vessels: loss may occur over few minutes or during sleep; usually there is no vertigo; pathogenesis may be related to vasospastic effects of caffeine or nicotine.
3. Membrane rupture, i.e., oval window or round window: onset in seconds and usually associated with popping sound; increased cerebrospinal fluid (CSF) pressure transmitted to perilymph causing rupture; occurs with pressure change (SCUBA diving et al.) or with heavy physical extention; vertigo sometimes present.
4. Trauma to the head may cause sudden loss if a fracture line involves the labyrinth or in the absence of a fracture if edema fluid accumulates in cochlea (concussion): loss usually immediate but may not be noted due to other more serious considerations; vertigo usually occurs.
5. Acoustic neurinoma usually causes a progressive hearing loss, but 10–15% of acoustic tumors cause a sudden hearing loss: loss is due to compression of the cochlear nerve by the neurilemoma of the vestibular nerve within the internal auditory canal; the sudden nature of the loss when it occurs is unexplainable.
6. Meniere's syndrome causes an increase in the amount of endolymph within the cochlea: when the membrane separating endolymph from perilymph ruptures there is sudden vertigo and sudden loss of hearing due to abnormal electrolytes bathing the hair cells; when the membrane heals some of the lost hearing returns.

7. Mumps can cause a sudden unilateral deafness, irreversible and profound—usually occurring in childhood.

Plan

1. If a history suggesting membrane rupture is elicited the patient must immediately be referred to an otologist for consideration of exploration of the middle ear and closure of a fistula. If this procedure is done early, further loss can usually be prevented and the existing impairment may be corrected. The remaining etiologies may be investigated in a more leisurely way.

2. Audiometry: site of lesion testing including (a) pure tone—air and bone; (b) discrimination—list of one-syllable words; (c) tone decay test—test of abnormal adaptation; (d) tests of recruitment. This testing is done by a qualified audiologist selected by the otologist.

3. Vestibular testing—electronystagmography to assess vestibular function.

4. Petrous pyramid polytomography for identification of a widened internal auditory canal or a possible skull fracture involving cochlear structure.

5. Treatment for viral and ischemic disease, Meniere's syndrome, and concussion is controversial. Some people feel that no treatment is of benefit. Others use vasodilating medications such as papaverine, nylidrin, intravenous histamine, etc. Such therapy should be undertaken by an otologist.

The primary concern in sudden hearing loss is the prospect for recovery of the hearing. If complete recovery is to occur in the viral or ischemic etiologies, it will usually occur within a few days after onset. Some people feel that medical therapy is of no benefit. The other four etiologies require further investigation.

GRADUAL (PROGRESSIVE) HEARING LOSS

Subjective Complaints

1. Loss of hearing: described as lack of understanding of speech; "people mumble"; "trouble in crowds"; may hear all right on telephone if mild; hears men better than women.

2. Unilateral or bilateral?

3. Nature of onset: over how many years; what age first noticed; first one ear and then the other?

4. Tinnitus: intermittent or constant; what pitch and intensity; how bothersome?

5. Related causes: diabetes, syphilis, head trauma.

6. Noise exposure: gunfire, tractors, explosions, airplanes, military, occupational?

7. Ototoxic drugs: aminoglycosides, diuretics, aspirin?

8. Family history of hearing loss?

9. Vertigo? Connected with position; while supine; rotary?

10. Age >60 years.

Objective Findings

1. Rinne test positive (air better than bone) and Weber may be midline if both ears are the same; otherwise it lateralizes to the best ear.

2. Tympanic membrane normal: normal movement with otoscopy; no cerumen occluding canal.

3. Possible nystagmus.

4. Audiometric tests: sensorineural hearing loss (air and bone thresholds equal); discrimination <90%, usually a bilateral loss >25 dB.

5. Other findings related to congenital deafness:

a. Craniofacial and skeletal: fused vertebrae, syndactyly, flexion contractures of digits, cleidocranial dysostosis, atresia, cleft palate, cleft lip, submucous cleft.

b. Integumentary and pigmentary: short nails, dry brittle hair, white forelock, lateral displacement of medial canthi, heterchromia of irides, lentigines, albinism.

c. Eye disorders: retinitis pigmentosa, congenital severe myopia, optic atrophy.

d. Nervous system: muscular dystrophy, cerebral palsy, ataxia and muscle wasting.

e. Cardiovascular system: episodes of syncope, prolonged Q-T interval on electrocardiogram (EKG).

f. Endocrine and metabolic system: goiter in adolescence or early infancy, hyperprolinemia, high protein-bound iodine level.

g. Chromosomal: trisomy 13–15, 18; multiple congenital anomalies.

Assessment

Presbycusis
1. Hears worse: in noise, when women talk, from distances, high bells.
2. Hears better: close, face-to-face, men.
3. Reduced hearing on audiogram: flat, sloping, or rapidly falling contour.
4. Starting by 60 years of age.
5. Usually cochlear indications on special audiometric tests.
6. May have familial history of same symptoms beginning at the same age.
7. Reduced discrimination: 20–80% (can be very low, indicating central effect of age).

Noise-Induced Hearing Loss
1. Reduced hearing, worse at 4000 Hz.
2. Reduced discrimination: 50–90%.
3. Tinnitus: usually matched at 4000 Hz.
4. History of noise exposure: explosion, industrial noise, gun fire, tractors.
5. Poor understanding in noisy situations.

Ototoxicity
1. Reduced hearing; may be total deafness.
2. Poor discrimination, 0–80%.
3. Tinnitus.
4. Cochlear findings on special tests.
5. Usually bilateral, but may be worse in one ear.

Meniere's Syndrome
1. Feeling of "fullness" in ear (usually unilateral).
2. Tinnitus intermittent or constant, sometimes high-pitched during attacks, low-pitched at other times.
3. Reduced hearing, usually unilateral and worse in low pitches.
4. Vertigo. (Symptoms 2, 3, and 4 comprise the triad of Meniere's syndrome. However, any one or two of them may result from endolymphatic hydrops.)
5. Cochlear findings on special audiometric tests.
6. Discrimination reduced, 40–80%.
7. Diplacusis.

VIIIth Nerve Tumor
1. Reduced hearing most commonly in one ear, or one ear worse than the other.

(Hearing can be normal.)
2. Reduced discrimination: 0–20%.
3. Tinnitus.
4. Vertigo.
5. Retrocochlear indications on audiometric tests.
6. Other cranial nerve signs: (a) polytomography; (b) computerized axial tomography (CAT) scan.

Syphilis
1. Rapidly progressing hearing loss.
2. Reduced discrimination: 0–20%.
3. Venereal Disease Research Laboratories (VDRL) test positive.

Hereditary Factors
1. Presence of some hearing loss prior to episode.
2. Family history of hearing loss, recessive in nature.
3. May be unilateral.

Associated with Chronic Otitis Media
1. History of chronic otitis (perforated tympanum with drainage).
2. Conductive loss with some degree of sensorineural loss (mixed loss).
3. May have some reduced discrimination: 50–90%.

Associated with Otosclerosis
1. Long-term otosclerosis may be associated with sensorineural loss, resulting in a mixed loss.

Plan

The treatment of sensorineural hearing loss ranges from simple reassurance to complex surgery for acoustic neuromas. The only proven treatments are: surgery for neuromas, drug treatment for syphilis, and surgery for the intractable vertigo of Meniere's syndrome. (Empirical treatments are in some general use for Meniere's syndrome and for sudden deafness of vascular or viral origin, but no studies have proved them to be valid treatments and they are herein described as empirical only.) When medical treatment cannot improve the condition, habilitative treatment should be advised. Such procedures, also called aural rehabilitation, are described at the end of this section.

Occasionally a hearing loss may fluctuate; i.e., it may become better and then worse, and continue to go up and down. Such fluctuations are infrequent, but are found in Meniere's syndrome and during treatment for syphilis. Eighth nerve neuromas may also fluctuate, as may sensorineural hearing loss associated with multiple sclerosis.

Presbycusis

1. Monitor hearing.
2. Give hearing conservation counseling.
3. Reassure that loss is benign but nontreatable.
4. Refer for hearing aid (H/A) and habilitative treatment if loss is significant (>30 dB average, 500–2000 Hz).

Noise-Induced Hearing Loss

1. Eliminate noise exposure by (a) removal from noise, or (b) recommending earplugs and/or ear muffs.
2. Refer for hearing aid and aural rehabilitation if loss is >25 dB average.

Ototoxicity

1. Remove drug if possible.
2. Monitor hearing.
3. Advise hearing aid and aural rehabilitation if loss becomes significant in speech frequencies.

Hereditary Factors. Refer for habilitative treatment.

Associated with Otitis Media

1. Treat ear appropriately for otitis media.
2. Refer for aural rehabilitation if loss is significant, 500–2000 Hz.

Meniere's Syndrome

1. Reassurance.
2. Empirical treatment by otologist: vasodilating medications such as papaverine, nylidrin, intravenous histamine, etc.
3. Advise hearing aid if loss is bilaterally greater than 25 dB.

VIIIth Nerve Tumor. Surgical removal.

Syphilis. Treat appropriately; monitor hearing; advise hearing aid use if loss is significant.

Congenital Factors

1. Refer for appropriate aural rehabilitation program.
2. Monitor ears and hearing: (a) every 6 months in young child; (b) every year after 12 years of age.

Habilitative Treatment (Aural Rehabilitation). If hearing level is bilaterally greater than 25 dB in young adults, 30 dB in older people, 15 dB in children (average of 500–2000 Hz):

1. Advise evaluation for hearing aid use by audiology center.
2. In case of borderline loss, advise a month's trial with an aid
3. Refer for aural rehabilitation by audiology center. (In adults: auditory training and lip reading. In children: auditory training, lip reading, speech training, educational techniques.)

NONPROGRESSIVE HEARING LOSS

Subjective Complaints

Congenital Factors

1. No speech by 2 years of age.
2. Faulty speech.
3. Language deficiency.
4. Voice quality strident or high-pitched.
5. Any of the following: (a) history of maternal rubella; (b) family history of early hearing loss; (c) blood incompatibility; (d) prematurity; (e) associated defects (eye, renal, endocrine, head and neck, skeletal, central nervous system, pigmentary); (f) ear infections.

Objective Findings

1. Audiologic tests show bilateral hearing loss >15 dB average in a child; air and bone conduction thresholds identical; speech discrimination reduced.
2. Associated at birth with: (a) asphyxia; (b) low birth weight; (c) blood incompatibility; (d) history of maternal rubella; (e)

any of the associated defects listed under Progressive Hearing Loss, Congenital.

3. Any of the following: (a) head trauma; (b) high fever; (c) meningitis, encephalitis; (d) measles.

Assessment

1. Hereditary if history of familial deafness, or accompanying other hereditary defect comprising deafness syndrome.

2. Acquired if associated with known disease or condition related to hearing loss.

Plan

1. Refer for appropriate aural rehabilitation program.

2. Monitor hearing and otologic status: (a) every 6 months in young child; (b) every year after 12 years of age.

Bibliography

1. English, G. (Ed.). *Otolaryngology.* Harper & Row, Publishers, New York, 1976.
2. Graham, B. (Ed.). *Sensorineural Hearing Processes and Disorders.* Little, Brown and Co., Boston, 1967.
3. Katz, J. (Ed.). *Handbook of Clinical Audiology,* ed. 2. The Williams & Wilkins Co., Baltimore, 1978.
4. Paparella, M. *Biochemical Mechanisms in Hearing and Deafness.* Charles C Thomas, Springfield, Ill., 1971.
5. Shambaugh, G. E., and Shea, M. D. (Eds.). *Proceedings of the Shambaugh Fifth International Workshop on Middle Ear Microsurgery and Fluctuant Hearing Loss.* The Strode Publishers, Inc., Huntsville, Ala., 1977.

Chapter 2.2

Conductive Hearing Loss

James R. Tabor

THE ANATOMY OF THE CONDUCTIVE MECHANISM OF THE EAR

(Refer to chapter opening figures.)

External Ear

The external ear is that portion of the ear external to the tympanic membrane. It consists of the auricle and the external auditory canal leading to the tympanic membrane. The outer one-third of the external canal consists of cartilage and the inner two-thirds consists of a bony canal covered by skin. The external meatus is approximately 3.5 cm in length. As it desquamates the keratin layer of the epithelium migrates to the external orifice, automatically cleansing the ear.

Tympanic Membrane

The tympanic membrane consists of three layers: the squamous outer layer, the fibrous middle layer, and the inner mucous membrane layer. The fibers of the middle layer insert into the handle (manubrium) of the malleus. When viewing the tympanic membrane, the manubrium of the malleus is visible; its superior limit is marked by the short process of the malleus which is a thumblike projection directed laterally. At the periphery of the tympanic membrane, the fibrous layer thickens, inserts into the sulcus of the temporal bone, and coalesces to form the tympanic annulus. The portion of the tympanic membrane superior to the short process of the malleus is called the pars flaccida (Shrapnell's membrane).

Middle Ear

The middle ear consists of space between the tympanic membrane and the otic capsule of the inner ear. The hypotympanum is a shallow space lying inferior to the tympanic membrane, and the epitympanum is that space of the middle ear situated above the upper extent of the tympanic membrane. The eustachian tube enters from the nasopharynx into the anterior wall of the middle ear, whereas the middle ear enters the mastoid air cell system at the superior-posterior wall. The medial wall of the middle ear consists of the bony otic capsule of the inner ear (the promontory), the oval window into which the stapes is situated, and the round window inferiorly and posteriorly. The heads of the malleus and incus are situated for the most part in the epitympanic portion of the middle ear.

Auditory Ossicles

The auditory ossicles form a system of bony levers and columns which transmit vibratory air-conducted sound energy from the tympanic membrane to the inner ear fluids, thereby stimulating the auditory nerve. The system is composed of the malleus, the incus, and the stapes. The malleus and incus operate largely as one unit, rotating in response to movements of the drum through a common axis, thereby vibrating the stapes, which is situated in the oval window. This rotation of movement is transferred into the stapes as a piston-like action. The stapes is shaped like a stirrup, consisting of a head, neck, anterior and posterior crura, and a base or footplate. The head of the stapes articulates to the long process of the incus. The footplate of the stapes is oval in shape and fits into the oval window of the inner ear, and the edge of the footplate is attached to the edge of the oval window by means of an annular ligament of fibrous tissue.

There are two muscles which attach to the ossicular chain. The tensor tympani arises from the semicanal of the middle ear and inserts by means of a tendon into the neck of the malleus. The stapedius muscle arises in its canal from the posterior wall of the middle ear and by means of the stapedius tendon inserts into the posterior aspect of the neck of the stapes.

PHYSIOLOGY OF THE CONDUCTIVE MECHANISM OF THE EAR

The fundamental purpose of the external and middle ear is to collect airborne sound and to convert it into sound vibrations in the inner ear fluids. The vibrations set up in the inner ear fluids activate the nerve endings of the auditory nerve, which in turn transfer the signals to the central nervous system. The external and middle ear, with their tympanic membrane and ossicular chain, act as a transformer between air-conducted sound and sound vibrations of the inner ear fluids.

External Ear

The external ear plays a small part in collecting airborne sound and directing it to the external ear canal and the tympanic membrane. Sound enters the external ear canal, reaching and vibrating the tympanic membrane.

Tympanic Membrane

Airborne sound sets the tympanic membrane into vibration which in turn vibrates the ossicular chain. The normal tympanic membrane has a relatively stiff surface and when vibrated moves in unison and acts as a piston on the ossicular chain.

Ossicular Chain

Since the fluids of the inner ear offer a much greater acoustic resistance than air, the function of the tympanic membrane on the ossicular chain is to overcome this impedance difference.

The ossicular chain participates in a piston-like function of the tympanic membrane in that air-conducted sound is collected on the relatively large surface of the tympanic membrane and the ossicular chain converts this energy to a relatively small surface area representing the stapedial footplate in the oval window. The lever mechanism of the ossicular chain is of lesser importance. Although the true function of the middle ear muscles is not known, most workers concede that the tensor tympani muscle does have some function in maintaining tension of the ossicular chain and the tympanic membrane. The contraction of the stapedius muscle on the stapes does change the frequency characteristics of the ossicular chain and contracts when the ear is exposed to excessive sound to reduce the amplitude of the vibrating ossicular chain.

METHODS OF TESTING HEARING

The minimal routine hearing tests needed for office diagnosis of ear diseases are:

1. Pure Tone Air and Bone Conduction Audiograms. The purpose of the audiogram is to provide a graphic plot of the patient's loss in threshold sensitivity at each test frequency. Frequencies are tested from 128 cycles per second (Hz) through 8000 cycles per second. The loss of hearing is plotted on a decibel scale for each frequency. The purpose of air conduction audiometry is to measure the sensitivity of the entire hearing mechanism: the external ear, the middle ear, and sensorineural mechanism of the cochlea and the auditory nerve for each frequency tested. The air conduction audiogram is obtained by presenting the tone through earphones placed on the patient. The purpose of bone conduction audiometry is to measure the sensitivity of the sensorineural mechanism only. The bone conduction audiogram is obtained by presenting the test tones directly to the patient's skull by means of a bone conductive vibrator held on the mastoid process for each test frequency.

2. Rinne and Weber Tuning Fork Tests. In certain cases, these should be added: (a) speech reception threshold tests; (b) speech discrimination score.

Interpretation of the Air Conduction Curve

The pure tone air curve by itself cannot be used to diagnose the type of hearing loss; that is, whether it is conductive or sensorineural in type. A greater loss for low frequency occurs in many conductive hearing losses; however, it may also occur in Meniere's syndrome, which is a pure cochlear type of loss. By the same token, a greater loss for high frequencies which is so characteristic of a sensorineural hearing loss occurs in the pure conductive hearing loss of serous otitis media. The pure tone air curve average for 500, 1000, and 2000 cycles per second (Hz), is a reasonably accurate measure of the practical hearing difficulty for speech in purely conductive hearing losses. A bone conduction curve by audiometric testing is necessary, therefore, to determine the type of hearing loss exhibited by the patient.

A patient is felt to have serviceable hearing if a loss by air conduction is no greater than an average of 40 dB for the three speech frequencies.

Interpretation of the Bone Conduction Curve by Audiometry

The bone conduction audiogram is a measure of the sensorineural hearing loss in the ear under test. This includes the central auditory pathways of the auditory nerve as well as the cochlear end organ. Since the limit of loudness produced by the bone receiver is about 60 dB above the threshold in the speech frequencies, when the sensorineural hearing loss is greater than 60 dB there will be no bone response by this method of testing.

Interpretation of the Air-Bone Gap

The air-bone gap is a measure of the integrity of the conductive mechanism of the ear. The air-bone gap is the difference between the air conduction tests (usually only for speech frequencies) and the average bone conduction loss for the speech frequencies. In normal hearing and in pure sensorineural hearing losses, the air and bone conduction curves should superimpose upon each other. One may allow a 10-dB variation inherent in air and bone conduction audiometry; therefore, any greater difference than a 10-dB average for speech frequencies between air conduction and bone conduction signifies a significant air-bone gap (therefore, a conductive hearing loss in the ear under test).

An air-bone gap of 20–30 dB indicates a

mild or very early conductive hearing loss. An air-bone gap of 30–45 dB indicates a moderate conductive hearing loss, and an air-bone gap of 45–60 dB indicates a maximum conductive hearing loss, such as is produced by interruption of the ossicular chain or by complete otosclerotic ankylosis of the stapes.

Technique for Tuning Fork Tests

Rinne Test. In cases of patients with a pure conductive hearing loss or a combined conductive hearing loss or a combined conductive and sensorineural hearing loss, tuning forks are a valuable adjunct to pure tone audiometry.

The Rinne test may be made with the 256-, 512-, or 1020-Hz tuning forks. The usual method for performing the Rinne test is alternately to place the stem of the fork on the patient's mastoid process, posteriorly to the auricle and superiorly on the on the mastoid process and then ½ inch away from the external meatus until the patient no longers hears it in one of these positions. The result is expressed as "Rinne positive" when heard longer by air, "Rinne equal" when heard the same by air as by bone, and "Rinne negative" when heard longer by bone. The Rinne test is negative at the 256 and the 512 forks in the case of a moderate conductive hearing loss. A negative Rinne test also for the 1024 fork indicates a more significant conductive hearing loss. It is to be remembered that the opposite ear must be masked by a noise maker when the Rinne test is done.

Weber Test. The Weber test is made by placing the tuning fork on the vertex or the middle line of the forehead and noting whether the sound is heard in the midline, expressed as "Weber negative," or whether it is referred to one ear or the other ear, expressed as "Weber right" or "Weber left." If there is more of a hearing loss in one ear than the other, the Weber test can be of value. The Weber is referred to the "bad ear" if the hearing loss in that ear is of a conductive type. The Weber refers to the "good ear" when the worse ear has a sensorineural hearing loss.

Speech Reception Threshold Test

The speech reception threshold is obtained by use of the live voice of a trained examiner or by means of a phonograph audiometer with records or tape. The decibel intensity at which 50% of spondee words are repeated correctly by the patient is his speech reception threshold (SRT). Spondee words are common English words of two syllables with equal accent on each syllable, such as "baseball." The average pure tone loss for speech frequencies (500, 1000, and 2000 cycles per second (Hz)) equals the SRT in fewer conductive hearing losses and in certain mixed losses (conductive and sensorineural loss combined).

Speech Discrimination Test

The ability to discriminate between single-syllable words selected to represent the phonetic composition of the English language may be measured by presenting these words to the patient 25 dB above his SRT. A live monitored voice or a phonograph audiometer may be used. The percentage of these words, termed phonetically balanced (PB), that the patient repeats correctly is his discrimination or PB score. A discrimination or PB score of 90–100% is obtained with normal hearing or in fewer conductive hearing losses. Certain mixed losses or a few sensorineural hearing losses may also show a score this high. When the PB score is poor, this usually indicates distortion caused by cochlear or auditory nerve disease.

Auditory Testing in Children

Neonatal Period. In the first months of life the patient responds to high intensity tones or noise by Moro response, blink, crying, or body movement. These responses may be observed or recorded. Electroencephalographic response audiometry may also record hearing loss in the newborn.

Infancy. Response of the infant to loud noise or tones may be discerned in eye movement, attention responses, and localization attempts.

Electroencephalographic response audiometry may also be used. During this age and older, impedance audiometry may be used, recording the stapedial reflex contraction in response to a tone as a measure of the extent of hearing loss.

Childhood. Beyond infancy hearing is

measured by play audiometry, speech audiometry, and conventional audiometric tests. The child may be induced to respond to pure tones or speech by numerous methods of play audiometry. Bone conduction responses may be obtained in the same way; however, it must be remembered that masking should be used frequently since lateralization may be quite unreliable in childhood testing.

Electroencephalographic response audiometry may also be used in questionable cases. In addition, impedance audiometry may be employed, recording stapedius muscle contraction in response to stimulus by means of tones or noise. Impedance audiometry may suggest the presence of middle ear fluid by alterations of the compliance of the tympanic membrane.

MECHANICS OF SOUND CONDUCTION IN THE DISEASED EAR

It has been the contention in the past that the low frequencies are impaired more than the high frequencies in lesions of the sound-conducting system, whereas the high frequencies are impaired more in diseases of the sensorineural portions of the inner ear. This general concept is not true, for in certain pure conductive hearing losses the impairment is primarily for high tones, whereas in some inner ear diseases, the loss may be greater for low tones than high tones.

Wax resting on the tympanic membrane causes a hearing loss for all tones, but somewhat greater for lower tones. In the case of a child with middle ear fluid due to serous or mucoid otitis, or chronic otitis media, the hearing loss is more for high tones than for low tones. With occlusion of the outer portion of the external auditory meatus, the loss is more for higher tones than lower tones. Hearing loss can be due to the external meatus being occluded by a large osteoma.

Occlusion of the ear canal by cerumen or foreign bodies usually shows no more than a 25- to 30-dB air-bone gap; however, in the case of an acquired fibrous external auditory meatus atresia, the air-bone gap may be approximately 40 dB due to the complete closure of the ear canal. Complete bony atresia with an air-bone gap of approximately 60 dB is usually thought to be the maximum extent of a conductive hearing loss.

Perforations of the tympanic membrane cause varying degrees of conductive hearing losses, depending upon the extent and location of the perforation. The mechanism of hearing impairment in simple perforation of the tympanic membrane is twofold. First, the loss due to a reduced surface upon which the sound pressure is exerted; and second, the effect due to sound reaching the round window directly which tends to cancel the vibrations mediated through the stapedial footplate. Small perforations usually show more of a loss of low tones, whereas total perforations show almost equal losses of low tones, whereas total perforations show almost equal losses for all tones and sometimes somewhat greater for high tones. Perforations of the anterior tympanic membrane usually show less of a hearing loss than perforations posteriorly which are situated directly over the round window. A conductive hearing loss due only to a tympanic membrane perforation is rarely over 40 dB, even though it may be a total perforation.

Interruption of the ossicular chain is usually due to chronic otitis media with a loss of the long process of the incus at the incudal stapedial joint. If there is a total interruption of the ossicular chain with an intact tympanic membrane, the conductive hearing loss is approximately 60 dB, or maximum. In most instances interruption of the ossicular chain is found in conjunction with a tympanic membrane perforation; therefore, interruption of the ossicular chain with a small perforation may show a large conductive hearing loss. Even with large perforations associated with interruption of the ossicular chain, the conductive hearing loss is never greater than 60 dB, however.

Occlusion of the eustachian tube in the first stages causes a negative intratympanic pressure with retraction of the tympanic membrane and increased stiffness of the conductive mechanism resulting in a greater loss of low tones. After some time the negative pressure results in a serous otitis media with fluid filling the middle ear and a conductive hearing loss more equal for all frequencies. With diminution of the negative pressure, there is a thickening of the fluid frequently so that a mucoid type of a fluid fills the middle ear, showing more of a conductive hearing loss than for high frequencies.

Otosclerosis is the most common cause of the isolated lesion fixing the stapes footplate. In rare cases fixation of the footplate may occur as a congenital anomaly involving the stapes. There also may be scar tissue and adhesions in the middle ear causing reduced vibratory freedom of the stapes. Also tympanosclerosis, a bony deposit secondary to chronic otitis media, may cause fixation of the stapes. In the earliest stages of otosclerosis, the fixation usually causes a conductive hearing loss more for low tones. As the fixation of the footplate increases, the conductive hearing loss assumes a flat configuration on the audiogram. When advanced involvement of the footplate with otosclerotic bone obtains, the conductive hearing loss is then maximum at approximately 60 dB.

CAUSES OF CONDUCTIVE HEARING LOSS

External Auditory Canal

1. Cerumen.
2. Foreign bodies.
3. External otitis.
4. Chronic stenosing external otitis.
5. Keratosis obturans.
6. Benign tumors of the external canal: fibroma; papilloma; cylindroma; osteoma; and exostosis; adenoma.
7. Malignant tumors of the external canal: epidermoid carcinoma; basal cell carcinoma; adenoid cystic epithelioma; sarcomas; malignant melanoma.
8. Congenital atresia of the external auditory canal.
9. Trauma.
10. Collapsed external canals.

Diseases of the Tympanic Membrane

1. Perforations: central; marginal; epitympanic; traumatic (slag, blowout, puncture, lightning).

2. Tympanosclerotic calcification.
3. Myringitis bullosa.
4. Chronic adhesive otitis media.

Eustachian Tube Dysfunction

Acute
1. Acute otitis media: serosanguineous stage; purulent stage; serous or mucoid stage.
2. Upper respiratory infection.
3. Allergic rhinitis:
a. Inhalants.
b. Foods: *Children:* milk, etc. *Adults:* caffeine, etc.; may be unilateral.
d. Acute adenotonsillitis.
e. Aerotitis and barotrauma.
f. Basilar skull fracture.

Chronic or Recurrent
1. Chronic obstructive hyperplasia of the adenoids.
2. Chronic sinusitis.
3. Chronic allergic rhinitis.
4. Cleft palate.
5. Stenosis of the bony portion of the eustachian tube.
6. Tumor of the nasopharynx: (a) angiofibroma; (b) carcinoma—adult male, unilateral, smoker.
7. Blue ear.

DIAGNOSIS AND TREATMENT OF CONDUCTIVE HEARING LOSSES (SYMPTOMS, FINDINGS, AND TREATMENT)

A general outline of the treatment for conductive hearing loss is given below, under External Auditory Canal. The treatment is discussed in general terms because medications change and newer drugs may be developed that have greater efficacy for specific diseases. It is not within the realm of this section to discuss the specific details of reconstructive surgical operations.

External Auditory Canal

Impacted cerumen usually has a history of intermittent hearing loss or pressure. Usually it is most noticeable upon arising in the morning and gradually clears intermittently during the day. The removal is best facilitated by small hooks or curettes if the cerumen is hard, but in the case of very soft cerumen irrigation with water provides the best chance to remove the inspissated cerumen in its entirety. If the cerumen has been impacted for some period of time it may be necessary to soften it with an oily otic drop.

Most foreign bodies can be removed with small hooks or curettes, or with irrigation. If the foreign body is vegetable in nature, such as a seed, there may be considerable external ear canal reaction or inflammation surrounding it, and the foreign body may have swollen due to its hydroscopic nature. In this case, it may even be necessary to use general anesthesia in order to remove the foreign body with small instruments.

External otitis causes a conductive hearing loss which is directly related to the amount of external ear canal edema. The conductive hearing loss reverts to normal after the external otitis is treated by removal of debris from the ear canal and administration of local or systemic antibiotics. If the external otitis is chronic and has caused a stenosis of the ear canal, this must be treated by surgical reconstruction of the ear canal to eliminate the conductive hearing loss associated with the stenosis. Keratosis obturans, or cholesteatoma of the ear canal, can be definitively treated only with surgical reconstruction. Most cases of keratosis obturans, however, are successfully controlled by repeated cleaning of the external ear canal to avoid obstruction of the ear canal by desquamative tissue.

Any tumor which occludes the external ear canal will cause a conductive hearing loss which is mild or moderate in severity. Removal of any such neoplasm relieves this type of hearing loss. Osteomas and exostoses are usually not severe enough to warrant removal because they rarely completely close the external ear canal. Malignant tumors of the external ear canal introduce the additional dimension of a life-threatening situation and complete removal of the tumor takes precedence over any attempt to relieve the conductive hearing loss.

Congenital atresia of the external ear canal causes a severe conductive hearing loss, usually 60 dB. This hearing loss is corrected by surgical reconstruction of the ear canal, tympanic membrane, and ossicular chain.

Trauma to the ear canals may cause soft tissue closure of the canal and is relieved by reconstruction of the cartilaginous portion of the external ear canal.

Collapsed ear canals as a cause for hearing loss during testing do not usually require treatment. The collapse of the canal is caused by pressure from the earphones and is rarely severe enough to cause a hearing loss otherwise.

Diseases of the Tympanic Membrane

Almost any disease of the tympanic membrane will cause some sort of conductive hearing loss. Perforations usually cause a hearing loss which may be very slight in small perforations, to a moderate hearing loss in complete absence of the tympanic membrane. One must remember if there is a total hearing loss in an ear associated with a large tympanic membrane perforation, then there is an additional cause for the hearing loss. Perforations are usually the result of recurrent acute or chronic otitis media, although they may be due to numerous types of trauma. Treatment of the conductive hearing loss is by means of tympanic membrane grafting or reconstruction.

Tympanosclerotic plaques, or calcifications of the tympanic membrane, are due to previous otitis media, usually in childhood. It is rare for tympanosclerotic plaques to cause a conductive hearing loss; however, in severe cases it may be present. If the conductive loss is due to such a calcification of the tympanic membrane, relief is obtained only through removal of the abnormal tympanic membrane and reconstruction by means of grafting. If a conductive hearing loss is discernible by testing, and the tympanic membrane shows calcific plaques, one must first suspect that there is a problem with the ossicular chain rather than the tympanic membrane, because tympanosclerosis commonly affects the ossicular chain rather than the tympanic membrane.

Myringitis bullosa, a rather common viral infection of the external ear canal and tympanic membrane, will cause a conductive hearing loss due to edema and bleb formation on the outer surface of the tympanic membrane. This conductive hearing loss reverts to normal after the infection has subsided. One must also remember that a sensorineural hearing loss is not uncommon with myringitis bullosa, and this hearing loss may be permanent, even after the external ear canal and tympanic membrane are healed. Therefore, in the case of a severe hearing loss associated with myringitis bullosa, the prognosis must be guarded since the sensorineural hearing loss component does not always revert to normal.

Chronic adhesive otitis media implies retraction of a very thin, diseased tympanic membrane to the medial wall of the middle ear. There may be enough of an air space so that the conductive component associated with this condition is only mild. However, if the tympanic membrane is retracted over the round window and stapes, the conductive loss may be quite severe. The cause of the condition is chronic eustachian tube dysfunction in childhood and this may continue throughout adulthood. However, if the eustachian tube in adulthood functions normally, the tympanic membrane can be surgically reconstructed to correct the conductive hearing loss.

Eustachian Tube Dysfunction

Eustachian tube dysfunction implies an impairment to the free flow of air from the nasopharynx to the middle ear space. This may result in a vacuum of the middle ear space with retraction of the ear drum, fluid in the middle ear, or eventual chronic otitis media. All of these conditions may result in varying degrees of conductive hearing loss.

In acute otitis media, there is usually complete closure of the eustachian tube which results in a fluid-filled middle ear space. Fluid in the middle ear may cause a mild to a moderate conductive hearing loss, and after treatment of such a condition the hearing will revert to normal. Antibiotics are the initial approach to treatment of acute otitis media. If there is no response, a myringotomy with drainage of the middle ear fluid may be necessary.

Allergic rhinitis and upper respiratory infections may cause eustachian tube dysfunction with resultant middle ear fluid.

The usual approach to this problem is systemic decongestants and antihistamines. Acute adenotonsillitis also may be the sole cause of eustachian tube dysfunction and is relieved after treatment of the infection. Aerotitis during flying and barotrauma during diving may result in closure of the eustachian tube with resultant retraction of the tympanic membrane and middle ear fluid. Here again, the treatment is decongestants and possible myringotomy for drainage purposes.

Basal skull fractures may result in edema, swelling, and trauma to the eustachian tube with resultant temporary eustachian tube dysfunction and middle ear fluid. Time will usually clear the fluid and correct any conductive hearing loss from middle ear fluid. Rarely, the basal skull fracture may be severe enough to completely close the eustachian tube and permanently impair its function. In this condition, reconstructive surgery of the eustachian tube is the only means of therapy.

Tumors of the nasopharynx may contribute to eustachian tube dysfunction, and examination of the nasopharynx must always be done in the adult patient. The adult male with chronic serous otitis media unilaterally and a history of cigarette smoking may have a nasopharyngeal carcinoma causing the eustachian tube dysfunction. Indirect nasopharyngoscopy must be done with a mirror to determine if the nasopharyngeal portion of the eustachian tube is normal.

Chronic eustachian tube dysfunction is common in children and may be aggravated by large tonsils or adenoids, allergic rhinitis, or cleft palate. In most cases, the eustachian tube dysfunction corrects itself as the child gains in physical stature and size. During the interim, it may be necessary to treat such a patient periodically with decongestants and antibiotics if recurrent acute otitis is part of the symptom complex. Frequently it is necessary to perform myringotomies, aspirate the middle ear fluid, and place a temporary aeration tube in the tympanic membrane. This procedure allows the middle ear to remain dry for a long period of time, providing normal hearing to the child, and eliminating most bouts of acute otitis media. These aeration tubes usually extrude to the external ear canal in time, allowing the tympanic membrane to heal spontaneously. The clinician then determines whether eustachian tube dysfunction has reverted to normal.

Control of allergic rhinitis may significantly benefit eustachian dysfunction in childhood. Adenoidectomy and adenotonsillectomy may be necessary to eliminate recurrent infections in the region of the nasopharynx.

There is a special type of mucoid otitis media designated as the "blue ear." Examination of the tympanic membrane in this condition reveals a deep blue cast to the tympanic membrane and the fluid in the middle ear due to old blood pigments in the mucoid fluid. This condition is no different than chronic mucoid otitis media, indicating chronic eustachian type dysfunction, except that in the case of this type of mucoid otitis media the eustachian tube dysfunction is quite severe. Decongestants are of little help, and it is usually necessary to perform a myringotomy, aspirate the fluid, and place an aeration tube to correct the conductive hearing loss.

Bibliography

1. Carhart, R. The clinical application of bone conduction audiometry. *Arch. Otolaryngol. 51:* 798, 1950.
2. English, G. M. *Otolaryngology: A Textbook.* Harper & Row Publishers, New York, 1976.
3. Kobrak, H. G. Physiology of the ear. In *Otolaryngology,* vol. 1, edited by G. M. Coates *et al.,* W. F. Prior Co., Hagerstown, Md., 1955.
4. Kobrak, H. The physiology of sound conduction. *Ann. Otol. Rhinol. Laryngol. 47:* 166, 1938.
5. Shambaugh, G. *Surgery of the Ear,* ed. 2. W. B. Saunders, Philadelphia, 1967.
6. Weaver, E. G., Lawrence, M., and Smith, K. R. The middle ear in sound conduction. *Arch. Otolaryngol. 48:* 19, 1948.

Chapter 2.3
Otorrhea

James R. Tabor

DEFINITION

Otorrhea is defined as the drainage of fluid from the external auditory canal. One may express otorrhea as either a symptom or a sign elicited in the course of recording an otologic history or found during the otologic examination. In either case, all characteristics of the otorrhea are important for the determination of the diagnosis and treatment of the condition.

Otorrhea may be the presenting symptom of ear disease. It may be the only symptom of some otologic diseases or it may be part of a symptom complex providing clues to the exact diagnosis. By obtaining an accurate history of the duration, constancy, nature, consistency, color, odor, and concomitancy with other symptoms, the physician may be provided with clues of its origin. Similarly, examination of the discharge with the help of laboratory evaluation by the microscope, culture, and chemical analysis not only specifies the appropriate treatment but may imply the etiology.

In general, there is usually nothing pathognomonic about the different aspects of otorrhea in a specific otologic disease process. Accurate diagnosis comes through a thorough evaluation of the component parts of the ear and, at times, even the patient's general health and incidental diseases.

Knowledge of otorrhea and its numerous characteristics will, however, provide the physician with the information to proceed more directly to the diagnosis and appropriate treatment of those otologic conditions exhibiting otorrhea.

The physician must remember that the symptom or sign of otorrhea introduces the possibilities of many types of ear diseases and includes all parts of the ear, namely, the external ear canal, the middle ear, and even the inner ear, as potential sources of otorrhea. Contiguous structures to these parts of the ear and the temporal bone also have the potential to become diseased and expel a discharge into the ear with eventual drainage to the external ear canal. An example might be metastatic neoplasm to the dura of the middle cranial fossa causing erosion of the bony roof of the middle ear and bony external auditory canal with fistulization of the subarachnoid space and subsequent cerebral spinal fluid drainage to the outer ear.

EVALUATION OF THE SYMPTOM OF OTORRHEA (CLINICAL FEATURES)

Observation of drainage from the ear by the patient must be initiated by proper questioning. Reporting of this symptom by the patient frequently includes many inaccuracies, and the physician must insist upon detailed information when taking the medical history. A light bit of cerumen on the end of a cotton-tipped applicator may take on an inordinately abnormal significance to some patients; whereas profuse, purulent drainage by another patient may scarcely be acknowledged. When estimating the amount of otorrhea at any specific time, the physician must ask specifically how the discharge is noticed: Is it cleaned from the ear with cotton-tipped applicators? Is it wiped from the outer ear or is a cotton pledget worn in the concha continuously? If so, how often is it changed? It is important to know how much drainage is noticed at night, and whether cotton is worn in the ear, since the ear may be dry until the head is placed in a dependent position.

Duration of the otorrhea holds special diagnostic relevance. Although the discharge may be present at the time of the examination, one must probe into the history for years and even into childhood to discern the complete picture. Many patients may forget that some 20 years ago the same ear drained for a time. Whether the discharge is recent, acute, intermittent, or constant is to be noted.

The nature of the otorrhea is also of importance but not diagnostic in any way. For example, the drainage may well change in consistency and composition from the site of origin to its expulsion from the external canal. In point, a concomitant external otitis may change an original serosanguineous fluid from a middle ear tumor to a purulent discharge. In addition, it is well worth noting any change in the nature of the otorrhea over a period of time as related by the patient. In years past the drainage may have been clear and intermittent, but then changing to a constant purulent type indicating more underlying chronicity of the basic disease.

Although it is more of a gross clue, the presence or absence of an odor to the discharge still provides the practitioner with a strong suggestion of the general class of etiologic organisms.

ETIOLOGY

External Ear Diseases

1. Acute circumscribed external otitis (furunculosis): (a) diffuse otitis—bacterial.

2. Chronic simple external otitis: diffuse—bacterial; fungal; allergic.

3. Malignant external otitis (acute necrotizing external otitis): a special type of external otitis seen usually in the elderly diabetic, caused by *Pseudomonas aeruginosa* and accompanied by high morbidity and mortality.

4. Myringitis bullosa: a viral external otitis mainly affecting the tympanic membrane and exhibiting blood-filled blebs.

5. Herpes zoster oticus (Ramsay Hunt symdrome): a herpes zoster (shingles) of the external auditory meatus.

6. Dermatitis of the external auditory

canal: a manifestation of a general dermatologic problem.

7. Neoplasms of the external auditory canal: (a) epidermoid carcinoma; (b) basal cell carcinoma; (c) other benign and malignant tumors.

8. Keratosis obturans: an accumulation of desquamative debris forming a thick crust in the external bony ear canal.

9. Perichondritis.

10. Foreign body of the external auditory canal.

Middle Ear Diseases

1. Acute otitis media with tympanic membrane perforation.

2. Chronic otitis media with tympanic membrane perforation (cholesteatoma absent).

3. Chronic otitis media with tympanic membrane perforation with cholesteatoma.

4. Mastoiditis.

5. Complications of otitis media: (a) labyrinthitis; (b) Bezold's abscess; (c) subperiosteal abscess; (d) extradural abscess; (e) subdural abscess; (f) brain abscess; (g) meningitis; (h) lateral sinus thrombosis.

6. Previous surgery.

7. Neoplasms of the middle ear: (a) carcinoma; (b) glomus jugulare; (c) childhood tumors (embryonal cell myoblastoma; eosinophilic granuloma; Letterer-Siwe disease); (d) metastatic neoplasms; (e) neoplasms from contiguous structures.

8. Wegener's granulomatosis.

Diseases of Contiguous and Associated Structures

1. Cerebral spinal fluid otorrhea: (a) spontaneous; (b) temporal bone fractures.

HISTORY

Pain

The pain related to diseases causing otorrhea is not in any way diagnostic. Characteristically the pain of an acute otitis media as well as an acute external otitis may be severe. If severe pain accompanies the onset of otorrhea, and over a period of weeks or months a purulent otorrhea continues in the absence of pain, this does suggest development of chronic otitis media as a result of tympanic perforation due to an acute bout of otitis media. Immediate pain after exposure to water or swimming suggests a perforation of the tympanic membrane whereas development of pain 24 hours after exposure to water or swimming suggests the onset of acute diffuse external otitis. It is characteristic for there to be noticeable absence of pain with otorrhea in the case of chronic otitis media. The pain is acutely severe with myringitis bullosa and, on the other hand, characteristically chronic, deep, and boring in the case of epidermoid carcinoma of the external ear canal, middle ear, and temporal bone. There is a surprising absence of pain with other neoplasms of the middle ear such as the glomus jugulare tumor. Children, for example, do not complain of pain with neoplasms such as embryonal cell myoblastoma and eosinophilic granuloma.

Tenderness

Tenderness as related by the patient in the course of history taking may give the practitioner further clues to a cause of recurrent otorrhea. If he complains of tenderness upon movement of the pinna or pressure on the outer ear, this does suggest external otitis as a cause for the otorrhea. There is usually no tenderness upon movement of the pinna in recurrent acute or chronic otitis media.

Duration

Longstanding otorrhea, especially of the purulent type, is highly suggestive of chronic otitis media. If this same type of drainage is related to a foul odor noticed by the patient, one should think of the possibility of a cholesteatoma as a cause for the chronic, persistent otitis media. Even if the drainage is intermittent, one still may be dealing with recurrent otitis media or recurrent external otitis. The constancy or intermittence of otorrhea is not diagnostic for differentiating chronic otitis media as a cause of neoplasms of the external or middle ear. Most generally, neoplasms in the region of the ear become infected and the frequency or duration of the otorrhea may mimic a chronic otitis media.

Type and Amount of Otorrhea

One cannot place undue importance upon the type of discharge noted by the patient because reporting by the patient can be quite inaccurate. Frequently the patient will report small amounts of yellow, rather liquid wax as a purulent drainage, therefore the amount of the drainage is important to denote. Frank bleeding from the ear in the absence of pain suggests neoplasm; however, bleeding from polyps secondary to chronic otitis media and external otitis is not uncommon. Serosanguineous drainage associated with pain is quite characteristic of the drainage associated with perforation of the tympanic membrane during the course of an acute otitis media. Intermittent chronic external otitis usually exhibits small amounts of purulent drainage, whereas chronic otitis media more commonly exhibits a rather profuse purulent drainage. On the other hand, it is not uncommon for chronic otitis media associated with cholesteatoma to infrequently discharge in small amounts of purulent material. If the patient relates that a "cheesy" type of material is associated with the drainage, this may suggest a cholesteatoma associated with chronic otitis media. In the case of myringitis bullosa, the initial drainage may be dark, serosanguineous, consisting of old blood resulting from the fluid draining from blood-filled blebs found on the external surface of the tympanic membrane and adjacent bony ear canal skin. Other causes of otorrhea such as neoplasms, dermatitis, and herpes zoster may cause serous, serosanguineous, or purulent drainage and have no diagnostic characteristics. Clear, watery drainage from the ear is, of course, quite characteristic of cerebral spinal fluid otorrhea, which may occur spontaneously. This type of drainage subsequent to a head injury or basilar skull fracture points to the diagnosis.

Hearing Loss

A hearing loss may be present with any type of disease causing otorrhea. The mere fact that there is fluid draining from, partially filling, or completely filling the external ear canal will cause a hearing loss.

The hearing loss related to an acute otitis media is usually mild to moderate and conductive in nature. When chronic otitis media establishes itself, the hearing loss is usually conductive, progressive, and may be quite severe. If complications occur from a chronic otitis media, namely, labyrinthitis, there may also be an associated sensorineural hearing loss. These same rules of hearing loss related to chronic otitis media apply to the progressive nature of a hearing loss due to neoplasms of the middle ear. The hearing loss related to temporal bone fracture and cerebral spinal fluid otorrhea is sudden in onset and may be conductive or sensorineural in type.

Vertigo

Vertigo is usually not associated with otorrhea if the disease is in the external ear canal. When vertigo is associated with middle ear disease it indicates inflammation of the labyrinth due to a chronic otitis media, especially if associated with a cholesteatoma. Neoplasms of the middle ear may also erode into the inner ear and cause vertigo by affecting the vestibular labyrinth.

Vertigo associated with otorrhea is a danger signal preceding frank labyrinthitis and possible complete sensorineural hearing loss of the ear.

Tinnitus

Tinnitus in the ear associated with otorrhea varies in severity with direct relationship to the amount of hearing loss, whether it be conductive in nature or sensorineural. The type of tinnitus, whether it be low-pitched ringing or an indescribable noise, is not diagnostic in any way.

Associated Factors

Associated factors may be a cause for or an aggravation of a discharging ear.

Exposure to water, for example, will prolong otorrhea related to external otitis and will, in fact, cause an otitis media if a perforation of the tympanic membrane is present. Instrumentation of the external ear may increase the amount of external otitis and thus start a discharge. History for foreign body in the external canal is also important, for many foreign bodies will cause otorrhea by local irritation and infection.

Associated infections, such as upper respiratory infections and pharyngitis, may cause the onset of recurrent otorrhea if chronic otitis media with a perforation of the tympanic membrane is present. The same is true with allergic rhinitis. Direct injury to the ear, of course, may cause perforations of the tympanic membrane and resultant otorrhea. Injury from lightning and concussive blasts will also cause perforations of the tympanic membranes, resulting in possible chronic otitis media with otorrhea. Head injury with skull fracture may result in either perforations of the tympanic membranes or cerebral spinal fluid otorrhea.

Associated Diseases

There are certain general conditions or additional diseases which may be associated with ear disease resulting in otorrhea.

The patient should be quizzed regarding other dermatologic problems if there are symptoms of external otitis. Seborrheic dermatitis, psoriasis, impetigo, and recurrent staphylococcal skin infections may be related to the external otitis.

Diabetics and those people ingesting unusual amounts of yeast in their diet tend to be more susceptible to the development of an external otitis. Previous otologic surgical procedures, such as mastoidectomy operations and fenestration operations, may well leave the mastoid cavity open to the external canal, with the possibility of this cavity as the source of the otorrhea.

LABORATORY DATA

The following is a list of laboratory data important to obtain in diagnosis of the cause of otorrhea.

1. Culture and sensitivity.
2. Chemical tests.
3. Tissue examination.
4. Hearing tests, including tuning fork and audiometric examinations.
5. Vestibular tests
6. X-ray examination.

DIAGNOSTIC APPROACH AND TREATMENT

External Auditory Canal Diseases

Acute External Otitis

When the physician first examines the patient exhibiting otorrhea, it should be noted whether there is tenderness at any point on the auricle or outer canal. Tenderness with movement of the auricle or pinna, or with pressure upon the tragus, indicates an acute external otitis, whereas otorrhea with no tenderness of pinna, auricle movement, or tragal pressure usually indicates that the drainage is arising from the middle ear region.

Most cases of external otitis are idiopathic; however, acute bouts may be brought about by exposure to water, insertion of a foreign body, use of a hearing aid mold or protective external ear canal plugs and instrumentation by the patient.

The next step in the examination is to gently cleanse or suction the ear canal as far as possible in order to view the skin on the ear canal both in its cartilaginous and bony portion and also to view the tympanic membrane, if possible. Guidelines as to the differentiation between acute external otitis and acute otitis media are listed in Table 2.3.1. If the ear canal is relatively normal after cleansing with a small suction and a perforation is seen in the tympanic membrane with discharge from the perforation, then a diagnosis of acute otitis media with perforation of the tympanic membrane can be made.

A polyp filling the ear canal in its most medial portion will obscure the diagnosis many times since one cannot tell whether the polyp originates from mucous membrane of the middle ear or from the ear

Table 2.3.1

Differentiation of Acute External Otitis and Acute Otitis Media

Sign and Symptoms	Acute External Otitis	Acute Otitis Media
Pressure on tragus or pinna	Painful	No pain
Lymphadenopathy	Frequent	Absent
Mastoid x-rays	Clear	Usually cloudy
Deep pain	Present	Present
Ear canal	Edematous	Normal
Season	Summer	Winter
Tympanic membrane	Normal	Perforation
Fever	Yes	Yes
Hearing loss	Slightly decreased or normal	Decreased

canal itself. By frequently cleaning such an ear and using combinations of hydrocortisone with antibiotics (colistin, neomycin, or polymyxin B), the inflammatory polyp may gradually disappear and a definite origin of the otorrhea can then be determined.

If such a polyp, whether it be on the wall of the external ear canal or originating from the middle ear through a perforation present in the tympanic membrane, does not show a reduction in size and disappear promptly with proper cleansing and use of antibiotic otic drops, then neoplasms must be suspected and biopsy must be entertained to make certain that a tumor of the middle ear or external canal is not present.

As far as physical examination is concerned, there are few typical appearances which would allow the physician to differentiate between inflammatory polyps or early neoplasm. Even granulation tissue of the external canal with ulceration and exposure to bone may be neoplastic or inflammatory. The special appearances of basal cell carcinoma of the external canal skin must be remembered, since a tiny ulceration with "rolled" edges may be the only sign of a rather extensive basal cell carcinoma, and these lesions must be biopsied if prompt healing is not witnessed with antibiotic treatment.

Edema, erythema, and cellulitis of the auricle and external canal are quite characteristic of acute external otitis. These findings are not present in uncomplicated acute otitis media. If acute mastoiditis develops secondary to acute otitis media, there may be edema and erythema postauricularly on the mastoid planum, and especially over the antrum of the mastoid in the superior postauricular region. There may be point tenderness in this region, denoting mastoiditis rather than external otitis media. There may also be displacement of the auricle anteriorly in the case of acute mastoiditis, especially in children.

Tender lymphadenopathy of the cervical chain is quite characteristic of acute external otitis but not found in uncomplicated acute otitis media or mastoiditis. One must remember that there may also be cervical lymphadenopathy with neoplasms of the ear.

In treatment of acute external otitis, it is important to clean the ear canal as much as possible. Instructions to the patient to stop any instrumentation or exposure to water are important. Local treatment with antibiotic drops in combination with hydrocortisone should be started and the general use of antibiotics should be instituted according to the severity of the symptoms and findings. If cellulitis, tenderness and lymphadenopathy, and fever are present, systemic antibiotics should always be used. In cases with these severe symptoms, culture and sensitivity studies should be done. It is important to examine the head and neck region for regional infections of the skin which might be related to an external otitis. Since infections of this nature are more common in the diabetic, when such infections are found, appropriate tests for diabetes should be made. Treatment depends upon the specific bacteria involved.

Chronic External Otitis

Examination in the case of chronic otitis externa shows edema of the ear canal with thickening, slight erythema, and no tenderness. The drainage from this condition is usually intermittent, small in amount, and either serous or purulent in nature. The drainage may be only enough to result in a crusting at the meatus of the external canal. The main symptom is itching, and persistence of the condition may be aggravated by instrumentation and water irrigation by the patient. In cases which are recalcitrant to treatment, diabetes must be considered. People who ingest an unusual amount of yeast in their diet seem to have a propensity for persistent chronic external otitis. Chronic fungal infections must also be a consideration in the condition of chronic external otitis, and if a typical black or white growth is seen in association with this condition, treatment should be altered accordingly.

At times a small abscess or isolated furuncle is seen as a cause for the so-called "circumscribed" external otitis. These infections are usually caused by Staphylococcus and any significant abscess formation should be incised and drained. One must remember that recurrent staphylococcal infections of the external canal may be associated with a chronic vestibulitis of the nose due to Staphylococcus. Other bacterial infections associated with the external canal may be related to impetigo.

In chronic otitis externa, one must also in the examination make certain that there are no associated dermatologic problems such as seborrheic dermatitis, psoriasis, etc., because treatment of the external otitis then becomes part of the dermatologic treatment.

Malignant External Otitis (Progressive Necrotizing Otitis)

This serious type of external otitis is found in the elderly diabetic and has a high morbidity and mortality. It is usually caused by *Pseudomonas aeruginosa*, but occasionally by *Staphylococcus aureus* and by Proteus.

The external ear canal exhibits edema, cellulitis, and necrosis. The infection spreads to the mastoid process and may involve the region of the jugular bulb with paralysis of cranial nerves IX, X, and XI. It is not unusual for there to be a nerve VII paralysis. Early signs accompanying the external otitis are pain, edema, purulent discharge, and persistent granulation tissue in the floor of the external auditory canal. Dysphasia, hoarseness, aspiration, and facial paralysis may accompany the paresis of the cranial nerve VII, IX, X, or XI.

Local antibiotic ear drops with anti-inflammatory agents such as cortisone should be started. Systemic antibiotics, namely gentamicin and carbenicillin, may be the most efficacious combination.

Fungal External Otitis

Common pathogens of fungal external otitis are Mucor, Aspergillus, and *Candida albicans*. A curious type of chronic external otitis may be aggravated by an allergic response in people who ingest an unusual amount of yeast in their diet. The symptoms of fungal external otitis may vary from acute otitis to chronic external otitis.

In treatment of chronic fungal infections of the external ear canal, cleansing is most important. Antifungal medications such as nystatin may be effective. Painting the ear canal with gentian violet is also effective in many cases. General treatment with antibiotics is indicated if the particular fungus is sensitive to antibiotics. For example, actinomycosis has been recorded as causing a chronic and subacute external otitis and fungal cultures should be taken along with bacterial cultures if simple methods of treatment do not result in a response.

Myringitis Bullosa

This virus infection causes almost pathognomonic findings in the external ear canal, namely blood-filled blebs in the skin of the external surface of the tympanic membrane and adjacent bony canal wall. There is considerable pain associated with the infection and some tenderness of the external canal. The type of otorrhea is typically serosanguineous and occurs when the blebs spontaneously burst. The hearing loss associated with the infection is usually conductive in nature due to the infection of the tympanic membrane and occasional serous otitis. There may be, however, a sensorineural hearing loss with the infection which may be permanent. Commonly, this infection is seen associated with an epidemic of influenza. Vertigo may be present if the vestibular nerve is involved and facial paralysis also may occur if the facial nerve is affected. These symptoms and signs are usually reversible.

Treatment is symptomatic for the pain. Local treatment is given for any superimposed bacterial infection in the way of antibiotic otic drops. Broad spectrum antibiotics may be given if the symptoms are severe and fever is present. If there is no immediate response, culture and sensitivity for a bacterial overgrowth is indicated.

Herpes Zoster Oticus (Ramsay Hunt Syndrome)

In this condition, typical blebs with the dermatitis seen in herpes zoster (shingles) are present over the posterior external ear canal and conchal region. A neuritic type of pain lasting longer than the dermatitis is typical. Frequently there is an associated facial nerve paralysis which almost always clears spontaneously. Occasionally associated with the conductive hearing loss due to regional edema is a sensorineural hearing loss due to a transitory neuronitis of the cochlear nerve. There may also be a labyrinthitis causing vertigo during the early stages.

Treatment is for symptomatic relief and local or general antibiotics for any superimposed infection.

Dermatitis of the External Ear Canal

A subacute or chronic external otitis may be a manifestation of general derma-

tologic problems. The most common of these are seborrheic dermatitis and psoriasis.

When external otitis is seen, it is important to quiz the patient regarding other dermatologic diseases and to examine the head and neck region for evidence of a general dermatologic problem. Treatment is directed along dermatologic lines when the external otitis is found as a manifestation of a dermatologic disease.

One of the prevalent dermatologic problems in external otitis is contact allergy. Most generally, this type of external otitis is a contact allergy to some type of cosmetic or soap; however, it may involve any chemical carried to the external ear canals by the hands. It is best treated by restriction of cosmetics and quizzing the patient regarding possible allergens. Initially, treatment is with a cortisone solution or ointment applied locally to the external canal and auricle. This type of chronic external otitis involves none of the bony external canal and only the most exterior portion of the cartilaginous canal. This dermatitis is most evident over the conchal portion of the auricle, but it may also involve all of the auricle.

Neoplasms of the External Ear Canal

Neoplasms of the external ear canal may be malignant or benign. Malignant tumors usually fall into the category of squamous cell carcinoma or basal cell carcinoma. Other malignant tumors are more rare. Benign tumors usually are those of skin appendages and may present themselves as polypoid in nature.

Squamous cell carcinoma occurs most often in the 50-year age group and 90% are female. Initial symptoms are usually pruritus and pain with later purulent otorrhea. Many of these patients have had chronic otorrhea due to chronic otitis media for some time and the majority have had symptoms for at least 2 years. Facial paralysis usually occurs early in the disease. Examination shows friable ulcerated granulation tissue of the external ear canal bathed in purulent exudate. There may be granular polyps of the external ear canal and the ulceration may expose bone. A significant number of people have regional lymphadenopathy and metastasis. There is frequently extension of the neoplasm to the parotid gland. Treatment is by radical surgical excision and/or radiation therapy.

Basal cell carcinoma of the external ear canal is similar in nature to basal cell carcinoma in the head and neck region. The ulceration may be quite small with a subepithelial extension of the basal cell carcinoma beyond the lesion for a number of millimeters. Rolled edges characteristic of this tumor are also seen in the external ear canal and any small ulcerations which do not heal should be biopsied to rule out this lesion.

Perichondritis

Perichondritis is limited to the external auricle but may extend to the cartilage of the external ear canal. This infection may be nonspecific as far as bacterial etiology is concerned or culture may show one etiologic agent such as *Pseudomonas aeruginosa*. The auricle usually becomes edematous and erythematous with a thickening of the skin over the auricle. There may be multiple fistulas with purulent drainage from the auricle, conchal region, or external ear canal.

Antibiotic therapy is best instituted after culture and sensitivity tests have been acquired.

Foreign Body of the External Ear Canal

Foreign bodies may be removed by irrigating fluid or instrumentation. One must remember upon removing foreign bodies that it is very easy to impact the foreign body in the medial-most portion of the osseous external ear canal against the tympanic membrane, unless appropriate small instruments and hooks are used.

Inanimate foreign bodies usually cause little in the way of tissue reactions; however, foreign bodies from plant life, such as seeds, will frequently, after a period of time, cause considerable tissue reaction and infection with otorrhea. Therefore, without properly cleansing of the external ear canal, active otorrhea may hide the foreign body, therefore obscuring the cause of the otorrhea.

Middle Ear Diseases

Acute Otitis Media with Perforation of the Tympanic Membrane

Spontaneous perforation of the tympanic membrane during the course of an acute otitis media is quite common. Otorrhea from this type of perforation is usually serosanguineous in nature when it first occurs. It may then turn serous or mucoid in nature and finally to a purulent otorrhea if bacterial infection complicates the viral infection in the middle ear.

Pain usually subsides after otorrhea commences in the case of acute otitis media, and there is little tenderness of the ear canal. Hearing loss is commensurate with the severity of the infection and of course temporary if resolution occurs. Tinnitus is not a prominent symptom.

Physical examination shows little tenderness of the ear canal, and a perforation of the tympanic membrane may be seen. Lymphadenitis of the cervical chain is usually not a part of the picture.

If the infection does not respond to appropriate antibiotics, culture and sensitivity should be taken to determine the specific etiologic bacteria. Audiometric tests usually show a mild to moderate conductive hearing loss. Otic drops locally to the ear canal usually are important for resolution of the otorrhea.

Chronic Otitis Media without Cholesteatoma

A chronic perforation of the tympanic membrane may be associated with intermittent otorrhea. This usually occurs in conjunction with an upper respiratory infection or after exposure to water through the external ear canal, such as swimming.

Most infections of this type will respond to an otic ear drop locally to the ear canal. At times, the infection may be severe enough to warrant general antibiotics.

As in the case of acute otitis media, it may be necessary to obtain culture and sensitivity for a specific antibiotic therapy.

X-ray evaluation of the middle ear and mastoid is usually not necessary in these cases.

Chronic Otitis Media with Tympanic Membrane Perforation and Cholesteatoma

Whenever a perforation of the tympanic membrane is seen and there is a history of intermittent otorrhea, one must suspect that a cholesteatoma might be associated with the tympanic membrane perforation. If the external ear canal and tympanic membrane perforation are visible after cleansing the ear, the white, desquamative debris of cholesteatoma in the middle ear may be seen. Here again, the otorrhea is usually not associated with tenderness or symptoms of external otitis. Commonly, a granulation tissue polyp may be associated with the cholesteatoma and usually these polyps arise from the mucous membrane of the middle ear and extend through the perforation into the external ear canal. The first course of treatment is by means of antibiotic otic drops locally to control the exacerbation of chronic otitis media. An otic drop containing cortisone will be helpful if granulation tissue polyps are present, because the cortisone will cause the inflammation resulting in the polyp to subside. If the polyps do not disappear with such treatment, neoplasm of the middle ear must be suspected. In association with treatment by antibiotic drops, one must make certain that the patient avoids all exposure to water, since this is a source of reinfection to such ears.

The hearing loss associated with cholesteatoma and chronic otitis media is usually conductive in nature; however, any recurrent labyrinthitis due to the cholesteatoma and recurrent bouts of chronic otitis media may cause a sensorineural hearing loss gradually over a period of years. If this be the case, tinnitus is usually a symptom associated with such a hearing loss.

Here again, it may be necessary to obtain culture and sensitivity of the otorrhea in order to institute the proper otic drops. It might be said systemic antibiotics are not very successful in treatment of chronic otitis media. A biopsy should be taken of polyps if they do not completely disappear with treatment.

Definitive treatment can be obtained only through surgical reconstruction of the middle ear and mastoid if an associated chronic mastoiditis is present. The basic tenet of surgical treatment is removal of all chronically infected tissue, including cholesteatoma of the middle ear and mastoid, and reconstruction of the tympanic membrane and ossicular chain.

X-ray examination may show clouding of the mastoid cavity, indicating a mastoiditis or fluid in the mastoid cavity. If sclerosis is seen by x-ray, the disease has been of long standing. Cholesteatoma may erode the middle ear and mastoid cavity in addition, and this may be seen on x-ray evaluation. Usually roentgenographic evaluation does not significantly alter the course of treatment in chronic otitis media with cholesteatoma.

Mastoiditis

The symptoms of mastoiditis are: dull, aching pain behind the ear, a low grade temperature, tenderness of the mastoid process, and tenderness of the mastoid planum superiorly and directly inferior to the auricle.

Chronic mastoiditis as associated with chronic otitis media is treated in the course of treating the chronic otitis media. Acute mastoiditis with an acute otitis media may require immediate operation; however, this is rare. Usually, the addition of antibiotics will clear the mastoiditis associated with acute otitis media.

Complications of Otitis Media (Table 2.3.2)

When otorrhea occurs in relationship to acute or chronic otitis media, one must always think of the possibility of a complication to otitis media. A diagnosis of complications of otitis media usually can be made by history, physical findings, and examination. In some cases, a complication of otitis media is not discerned until it is apparent at the time of surgery.

Table 2.3.2

Complications of Otitis Media (Acute or Chronic)

A. External ear
 1. External otitis (acute or chronic)
 2. Perichondritis
B. Inner ear
 1. Labyrinthitis
 2. Fistula formation
C. Intracranial
 1. Epidural abscess
 2. Subdural abscess
 3. Sigmoid sinus thrombosis
 4. Brain abscess
 5. Meningitis
D. Mastoid
 1. Acute mastoiditis
 2. Chronic mastoiditis
E. Facial nerve paralysis

Labyrinthitis. Labyrinthitis rarely occurs during the course of acute otitis media. With chronic otitis media and cholesteatoma it is rare, but at times a problem. The cardinal symptom of labyrinthitis is vertigo, which may vary from unsteadiness to the more severe cases as an acute rotatory vertiginous attack with nausea and vomiting. This may accompanied by spontaneous nystagmus to the side of the otitis media if the labyrinth is irritated only, and away from the side of the infection if the labyrinthitis has destroyed the inner ear. Associated with the dizziness frequently is a sensorineural hearing loss.

If these symptoms occur with otorrhea and chronic otitis media, it indicates that surgery should be done immediately to remove all infection from the mastoid cavity and middle ear. Also, culture and sensitivity should be sent and appropriate antibiotics should be given.

Bezold's Abscess. During the course of chronic otitis media and mastoiditis, the tip of the mastoid may be eroded so that infection within may form an abscess in the soft tissue space at the tip of the mastoid medial to the origin of the sternocleidal mastoid muscle. Deep tenderness, pain, and fever are present.

The treatment, of course, is drainage, appropriate antibiotic therapy, and tympanomastoid surgery.

Subperiosteal Abscess. Subperiosteal abscess may occur on the planum of the mastoid process and squamous bone.

The findings are typically a swelling over the region with tenderness and fluctuation.

Definitive treatment includes incision, drainage, appropriate antibiotic therapy, and tympanomastoid surgery.

Extradural and Subdural Abscesses. Abscesses in the region of the dura usually cause symptoms of deep pain, headaches, and recurrent fever as associated with otorrhea and chronic otitis media. These abscesses are usually associated with recurrent and chronic mastoiditis and otorrhea.

Then are frequently found incidentally in the course of mastoid surgery.

Brain Abscess. When in the course of chronic otitis media, especially with cholesteatoma, there is erosion of the bony plate between the middle or posterior cranial fossa, infection may extend from the mastoid cavity into brain tissue causing single or multiple abscesses.

The symptoms characteristically are recurrent, low grade temperature, alterations in the mental state, papilledema, hemiplegia, and convulsions.

As in the case of all complications of otitis media, treatment involves appropriate antibiotic therapy, culture and sensitivity of the otorrhea, and tympanomastoidectomy. In the case of brain abscesses, an appropriate neurosurgical drainage procedure must be done.

Sigmoid Sinus Thrombosis. If thrombosis occurs in the sigmoid sinus, there is usually in addition to otalgia, headache, otorrhea, evidence of chronic otitis media, and mastoiditis, a recurrent high grade fever which may reach 105°F at times. There may be tenderness of the jugular vein high in the neck.

Treatment is as for other intracranial complications of otitis media, but in addition, the jugular vein must be tied high in the neck and the sigmoid sinus must be packed superiorly so that the infected thrombus can be surgically removed during the course of tympanomastoid surgery.

Gradenigo's Syndrome. This syndrome is associated with chronic otitis media and otorrhea. It occurs when the infection from the chronic otitis media and mastoiditis extends medially to the petrous apex, causing symptoms by involvement of cranial nerves V and VI. This causes deep and unilateral pain medial to the ear and posterior to the eye, associated with paralysis of cranial nerve VI.

Treatment is by appropriate antibiotic therapy, culture and sensitivity, and tympanomastoid surgery with exposure of the petrous tip so that drainage may adequately be obtained for this area.

Meningitis. Otorrhea with chronic otitis media and mastoiditis may cause the complication of meningitis.

The typical symptoms of high grade fever, alterations in the mental state, and nuchal rigidity (Kernig's sign) are characteristic.

Treatment is by means of appropriate antibiotics, culture and sensitivity of the cerebral spinal fluid, and immediate tympanomastoid surgery.

Facial Nerve Paralysis. Facial nerve paralysis may occur as a complication of acute otitis media or chronic otitis media associated with mastoiditis.

In treatment of acute otitis media with otorrhea and facial nerve paralysis, appropriate systemic antibiotic therapy should be instituted and antibiotic otic drops should be added.

If facial nerve paralysis is associated with chronic otitis media and mastoiditis, an immediate mastoidectomy with appropriate reconstructive procedures should be done. In addition, a decompression of the facial nerve should be done in the fallopian canal.

Previous Surgery

Intermittent otorrhea may occur after mastoid surgery if a significant mastoid cavity is present which becomes intermittently infected.

Initially the otorrhea and mastoid cavity infection should be treated with antibiotic otic drops and cleansing of the mastoid bowl.

In the case of the mastoid bowl, it is important to instruct the patient on water avoidance because water to the mastoid bowl is the most common cause of recurrent otorrhea in these patients.

Neoplasms of the Middle Ear

Most importantly, one must suspect neoplasms of the middle ear as a cause for otorrhea when granulation tissue or polyps are present. This is especially true for carcinoma and childhood tumors. If granulations or polyps do not completely disappear with antibiotic otic drops in conjunction with hydrocortisone, a biopsy must be taken in order to discern the diagnosis.

If the tumor is extensive, there will be x-ray changes of the mastoid cavity and middle ear on mastoid x-rays or tomography of the middle ear.

Appropriate treatment is in accordance with the type of tumor present.

In the case of glomus jugulare tumors of the middle ear, they rarely erode the tympanic membrane causing recurrent otorrhea. The "cherry-red" globular formation of the tumor is quite characteristic and if infected with the perforation of the tympanic membrane the drainage is frequently serosanguineous due to the marked vascularity of the tumor. Here again, treatment is first by antibiotic control of the superimposed infection and then definitive treatment to the glomus jugulare tumor in the way of surgery or radiation therapy.

Wegener's Granulomatosis

Although rare, Wegener's granulomatosis of the middle ear causes extensive granulation tissue formation with frequent perforation of the tympanic membrane, mastoiditis, and superimposed infection. This infection will result in otorrhea which may be serosanguineous or purulent in nature.

This granulation tissue ordinarily does not respond to local treatment in the way of antibiotic otic drops; therefore, a tissue biopsy is necessary. Because Wegener's granulomatosis is usually a generalized disease, treatment depends upon the extent of involvement of other structures in the body.

Diseases of Contiguous and Associated Structures

Cerebral spinal fluid otorrhea may occur spontaneously, presumably due to congenital fissures and fistulas of the cranium resulting in cerebral spinal fluid gaining access to the middle ear and external canal. Diagnosis can usually be made by determining the sugar content of the fluid although, if there is superimposed infection, the exact cause of the otorrhea may initially be obscure. Treatment is by surgical repair of the dural defect.

Temporal bone fractures frequently cause cerebral spinal fluid otorrhea. Diag-

nosis again is made by a determination of the sugar content of the fluid. In the case of temporal fractures, there is usually spontaneous closure of the defect after the injury. If this does not obtain, then surgery repair is necessary.

Bibliography

1. Ballatyne, J., and Groves, J. *Diseases of the Ear, Nose and Throat*, ed. 3, vol. 2. J. B. Lippincott Co., Philadelphia, 1971.
2. Chandler, J. R. Malignant external otitis. *Laryngoscope 78*: 1259–1294, 1968.
3. Jerger, J. Studies in impedance audiometry. *Arch. Otolaryngol. 99*: 165–171, 1974.
4. Johns, M. E. Squamous cell carcinoma of the external ear canal. *Arch. Otolaryngol. 100*: 45–49, 1974.
5. Moore, G. R. *et al.* Chemodectomas of the middle ear. *Arch. Otlaryngol. 98*: 330–335, 1973.
6. Senturia, B. *Diseases of the External Ear*. Charles C Thomas, Springfield, Ill., 1957.

Chapter 2.4

Ear Pain

Marlin E. Weaver

Sensation to the ear is supplied by three cranial nerves and two cervical nerves. The characteristics of ear pain—location, duration, rapidity of onset, and intensity— are helpful in establishing an etiologic diagnosis.

These five nerves (V, IX, X, C2, and C3) also supply other areas of the head and neck. Pain referred to the ear may be the result of disease affecting nerve endings of any branch of the involved nerve. Table 2.4.1 lists (1) the nerves involved, (2) the portion of the ear supplied by the nerve, and (3) other sites supplied by the same nerve.

Ear pain is a prominent symptom in the illnesses described below. An outline for

establishing a diagnosis and for treatment is presented.

ACUTE OTITIS MEDIA

Subjective Complaints

1. Pain (starting as pressure sensation deep in the ear and evolving to excruciating pain over 30 minutes to several hours).
2. Hearing loss.
3. Fever.
4. Slight to moderate vertigo.
5. Purulent and bloody drainage (frequently preceded by "popping" sound and followed by relief of pain).

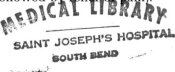

Table 2.4.1

Nerves Involved in Ear Pain

Nerves	Portion of Ear Supplied	Other Sites Supplied
V Mandibular division	1. Mastoid cells (spinous nerve arises before split into anterior-posterior division) 2. Anterior auricle and tragus (auriculotemporal n.) 3. Upper portion of the external auditory meatus (auriculotemporal n.) 4. Tympanic membrane (TM) (auriculotemporal n.)	1. Anterior two-thirds of the tongue (lingual n.) 2. Lower teeth (inferior alveolar n.) 3. Temporomandibular joint (articular branch of articulotemporal n.) 4. Parotid gland (auriculotemporal n.) 5. Skin of the temporal region (auriculotemporal n.) 6. Buccal mucosa (buccinator n.) 7. Tonsil (branch from lingual n.)
IX	1. Middle ear mucosa (tympanic branch; nerve of Jacobson) 2. Eustachian tube mucosa (tympanic plexus)	1. Pharyngeal mucosa (pharyngeal branch) 2. Part of soft palate (pharyngeal branch) 3. Tonsil (pharyngeal branch)
X	1. Posterior-inferior external auditory canal (auricular branch; nerve of Arnold) 2. Lower external surface of TM (auricular branch) 3. Posterior surface of auricle (auricular branch)	1. Dura in the area of the lateral sinus (meningeal branch) 2. Mucosa of both surfaces of the epiglottis (internal branch of the superior laryngeal n.) 3. Mucosa of the larynx (internal branch of superior laryngeal n.)
C2, C3	1. Upper portion of the posterior surface of the auricle (auricular branch of the small occipital n.) 2. Skin over the mastoid (mastoid branch of the small occipital n. and mastoid branch of the great auricular n.) 3. Midportion of the skin of the posterior surface of the auricle (auricular branch of the great auricular n.) 4. Lobule of the auricle (auricular branch of the great auricular n.)	1. Skin over the occiput (occipital branch of the small occipital n.) 2. Parotid gland (facial branch of the great auricular n.) 3. Skin of the neck (transverse branch of the cervical plexus) 4. Fascia and skin of the occiput (great occipital n.)

Objective Findings

1. Conductive hearing loss (Weber lateralized to the involved ear).
2. Tympanic membrane (TM) immobile.
3. TM opaque (incus not visible); bulging; surface slightly bluish with folded or ridged appearance of the skin.
4. TM amber; bulging.
5. Fever or afebrile.
6. Possible coincident upper respiratory infection.
7. Purulent discharge in external auditory canal.

Assessment

1. There is infection of the middle ear and mastoid spaces with pressure behind the TM and possible rupture of the TM.
2. If patient has received antibiotics, persistent infection suggests that the agent is not sensitive to the antibiotic or that the antibiotics are not reaching the involved tissues.
3. Concern is indicated regarding spread of infection beyond middle ear and mastoid to (a) meninges via bony suture lines or directly through demineralized eroded

bone of the tegmen tympani or mastoid, (b) invasion of sigmoid sinus, (c) spread to postauricular soft tissue by way of tympanomastoid fissure, or (d) spread to preauricular soft tissue via petrotympanic fissure.

Plan

1. Best available culture: otorrhea, nasophayrnx, or myringotomy knife.
2. Complete blood count (CBC).
3. Local treatment of pain: warm anesthetic ear drops (in the absence of purulent drainage): local heat.
4. Myringotomy (with severe bulging and pain): will relieve pressure, secure specimen for culture, and help prevent complications.
5. Antibiotics: ampicillin in small children; penicillin in older children and adults; erythromycin or cephalosporin with penicillin hypersensitivity.
6. Decongestants.
7. Analgesics.
8. Follow-up to be certain that middle ear fluid is evacuated (decongestant should be continued until fluid has cleared).
9. Referral to otolarynogologist if prompt response to therapy is not observed.

(If the mastoid portion of the infection does not respond to antibiotics and becomes sealed off from the middle ear by thickened mucosa in the epitympanic space, myringotomy will not provide adequate drainage. Pain and tenderness will persist despite treatment. In these cases incision and drainage by way of a simple mastoidectomy may be required. Mastoid x-rays are sometimes helpful in establishing the necessity for drainage.)

Serous Otitis Media

Subjective Complaints

1. Pain: sporadic; brief, lasting 20–30 minutes; mild to moderate severity.
2. Pain with nose blowing.
3. Hearing loss: mild to severe.
4. Vertigo: slight.
5. Antecedent ear infection.

Objective Findings

1. Conductive hearing loss: 10–40 dB.
2. TM dull (incus not visible); immobile to pneumatic otoscopy; possibly retracted (initially in the pars flaccida).
3. Eustachian tube obstruction by tumor, i.e., adenoid or neoplasm.

Assessment

1. Pain related to sporadic changes in middle ear pressure; pain following nose blowing due to increased pressure which may remain for several minutes.
2. Fluid in the middle ear and mastoid evidenced by conductive hearing loss and failure of TM to move on pneumatic otoscopy.
3. Concern when longstanding: (a) atrophic changes in the TM due to retraction, (b) possible cholesteatoma development if deep retraction pocket is present, (c) delayed development of speech and language in young children, (d) predisposition to recurrent purulent otitis media.
4. Fluid may remain following purulent otitis media due to inadequate decongestant therapy or to obstruction of eustachian tube by tumor, i.e., adenoid tissue or neoplasm.

Plan

1. Audiometry to help establish diagnosis and establish baseline for evaluating efficacy of treatment.
2. Impedence testing for the same two purposes.
3. Nasopharyngeal examination: mirror examination and/or nasopharyngoscopy to rule out tumor.
4. Decongestant treatment: pseudoepinephrine (sometimes causes irritability in small children).
5. Antihistamine/decongestant therapy: antihistamines may cause inspissation of middle ear fluid and/or sedation.
6. Topical decongestants: nose drops or nasal spray; value unpredictable.
7. Eliminate supine bottle feeding of infants; feeding in this posture causes direct irritation of the eustachian tube mucosa.
8. Referral to otolaryngologist if medical therapy fails. In case of unilateral serous

otitis in adults, nasopharynx must be biopsied to rule out nasopharyngeal tumor *even when no tumor is seen.*

(If middle ear fluid remains or severe retraction of the TM persists, tympanotomy with ventilation tube placement, adenoidectomy, or other surgery may be required.)

OTITIS EXTERNA, FURUNCLE, FOREIGN BODY

Subjective Complaints

1. Pain: superficial or deep.
2. Tenderness to manipulation of pinna.
3. Normal hearing or slight conductive impairment.
4. Drainage: usually minimal.
5. History of antecedent pruritus.

Objective Findings

1. Canal skin thick and erythematous; purulent exudate; fungal hyphae with wet, sometimes black, membranous exudate.
2. Canal may be occluded by thickened skin or furuncle.
3. Pain with manipulation of pinna.
4. Foreign body: insect, eraser, bead, bean, paper, cotton, etc.
5. Conductive hearing loss: usually mild unless canal is completely occluded.
6. Skin of the pinna, face, and neck may be involved.

Assessment

1. Protective mechanism of cerumen has given way to inflammation of canal skin.
2. Infectious etiology, including bacteria or fungus.
3. Noninfectious etiology, including trauma from attempts to clean external canal, chemical irritation from hair spray, proprietary cerumen-removal products, or foreign body.
4. Previous treatment failure: (a) inadequate debridement preventing topical medication from getting to the involved skin, (b) failure to recognize the presence of foreign body, (c) improper choice of topical medication, e.g., fungus infection, (d) diabetes.
5. Concern regarding progression of disease into "malignant" form, especially in diabetics. Possible development of stenosis of the external auditory canal.

Plan

1. Debridement with small (size 18 blunt needle) aspirating tip.
2. Burow's solution wick when canal is narrow; cotton wick in the external auditory canal; soak with Burow's solution (one packet of powder in a pint of water; mix fresh daily).
3. Topical liquid containing polymyxin B or colistin and a steroid: clear preparation is best when the skin is dry and scaly, whereas milky suspension is better when the skin is wet.
4. Fungus treated with solution containing Vioform, 1.0%; hydrocortisone, 1.0%; and nystatin, 500,000 units. The solution is prepared in propylene glycol.
5. Systemic antibiotics if regional lymph nodes are enlarged and tender.
6. Extraction of foreign body by forceps (insect, paper, cotton, etc.) or small, blunt Day hook for solid foreign bodies such as a bean or an eraser.
7. Incision and drainage of furuncle.
8. Wet soaks to the pinna and face: Burow's or Dalibour solution.
9. Referral to otolaryngologist in the event that prompt response to therapy has not occurred.

BULLOUS MYRINGITIS

Subjective Complaints

1. Excruciating ear pain: usually sudden onset; spontaneous relief associated with minimal serosanguineous drainage.
2. Hearing loss: mild to moderate.
3. Possible coincident symptoms suggesting mild pneumonia.

Objective Findings

1. Ear examination demonstrates multiple bullae involving the TM and adjacent canal wall skin.

2. Hearing may be normal to moderately impaired; conductive loss.

3. Usually afebrile and less toxic than with purulent otitis media.

4. Rales suggesting pneumonia.

Assessment

1. Ear findings are clearly diagnostic of bullous myringitis caused by *Mycoplasma pneumoniae*.

2. Spontaneous rupture of bullae gives less drainage than with purulent otitis media.

3. There may be coincident serous otitis media or pneumonia.

Plan

1. Perforation of bullae to relieve pain.

2. Lidosporin ear drops and local heat.

3. Examination of chest; possible chest x-ray if pneumonia is suspected.

4. Oral antibiotics to prevent bacterial complications such as acute otitis media; best choice is tetracycline in adults and erythromycin in children.

MASTOIDITIS, CHRONIC, WITH CHOLESTEATOMA

Subjective Complaints

1. Pain: deep constant pressure, gradually increasing over a period of days to weeks.

2. May or may not have history of antecedent purulent otitis media (note: mastoiditis associated with acute purulent otitis media predictably resolves as the purulent otitis media resolves); no significant otorrhea.

3. Hearing usually normal or slightly impaired.

4. Vertigo with head movement.

5. There may be a history of intermittent otorrhea *with* or *without* pain

Objective Findings

1. Small defect in the upper TM: may be obscured by overlying crust; keratin debris may be visible in defect.

2. Normal contour of the pars tensa.

3. Tenderness over the mastoid.

4. Mobility of TM *may* be normal on pneumatoscopy.

Assessment

1. Cholesteatoma has gradually enlarged beginning in the pars flaccida and extending into the mastoid; enlargement due to pressure caused by inexorable increase in keratin debris and by collagenolytic enzymes on the advancing surface of the cholesteatoma sac.

2. Diagnosis missed because there is no drainage. TM defect is quite small and the hearing may be near normal.

3. If untreated the sac will erode into (a) lateral semicircular canal, (b) middle or posterior fossa, (c) sigmoid sinus.

Plan

Refer to otolaryngologist for diagnosis and treatment.

PETROSITIS

Subjective Complaints

1. Pain: deep in the ear.

2. Longstanding otorrhea.

3. Diplopia on lateral gaze (Gradenigo's syndrome).

4. Hearing loss: conductive or sensorineural.

5. Possible vertigo.

Objective Findings

1. TM perforation; purulent discharge.

2. Ipsilateral VIth nerve palsy.

Assessment

1. Chronic otitis media with longstanding perforation of the TM is usually painless. In petrositis the mastoid cells which are deep to the labyrinth do not drain adequately. This causes infection which develops in a closed space. The infection may spread to create an extradural abscess causing ipsilateral VIth palsy (Gradenigo's syndrome).

Plan

Referral to otolaryngologist for diagnosis and treatment.

TEMPORAL BONE TUMOR, BENIGN OR MALIGNANT (PRIMARY OR SECONDARY)

Subjective Complaints

1. Pain: insidious beginning with pressure sensation and increase in severity.
2. May or may not have hearing loss, vertigo, or otorrhea, depending on the location.
3. Possible pulsatile tinnitus.

Objective Findings

1. Examination of the ear may be normal; possible serous fluid in the middle ear; possible pulsatile red mass behind the TM.
2. Hearing loss: conductive or sensorineural.
3. Other known malignant tumor, e.g., breast, kidney, lung, etc.

Assessment

1. Tumor pain results from compression or stretching of pain-sensitive tissues such as the eardrum, the middle ear, or mastoid mucosa.
2. Pulsatile red mass behind the TM is likely to be a glomus jugulare tumor.

Plan

Referral to otolaryngologist for diagnosis and treatment.

TEMPOROMANDIBULAR JOINT SYNDROME

Subjective Complaints

1. Pain: deep in the ear or just anterior to the ear; mild to very severe; may radiate to the temporal area.
2. Pain may be aggravated by chewing; may be worse at night.
3. Recent dental restoration or orthodontia.

4. History of mandibular trauma, bruxism, gum-chewing, etc.
5. No hearing loss or otorrhea.

Objective Findings

1. Hearing normal; external auditory canal and TM normal.
2. Tenderness of temporomandibular joint to gentle digital pressure during full excursion of mandible.
3. Palpable crepitance with mandibular excursion

Assessment

1. Arthritis in temporomandibular joint imitating auricular branch of auriculotemporal nerve, causing referred pain to the ear.
2. Arthritis due to joint trauma from bruxism, masticative abuse (gum-chewing, etc.), change in dental occlusion, mandibular trauma, or immobilization during dental restoration (infrequently related to rheumatoid arthritis).

Plan

1. Local heat and analgesics; occasionally muscle relaxant (Valium, 5 mg *q.i.d.*).
2. Restrict mastication.
3. Dolowitz mandibular exercises (see Facial Pain and Headache, Chapter 5).

PHARYNGEAL OR LARYNGEAL TUMOR

Subjective Complaints

1. "Ear" pain: usually described as "dull" and constant with gradual progression.
2. No hearing loss or otorrhea.
3. Possible hemoptysis, hoarseness, or sensation of a "lump" in throat on swallowing.
4. History of heavy smoking and alcohol intake.

Objective Findings

1. Ear examination normal.
2. Tumor mass visible by direct exami-

nation, mirror examination, or nasopharyngoscopy.

Assessment

Tumor compressing tissues supplied by nerves V, IX, or X, causing pain referred to ear.

Plan

Referral to otolaryngologist to confirm diagnosis of tumor or to rule out possibility of tumor if symptoms are present but tumor not identified.

Bibliography

1. Beddoe, G. H. M. Otalgia. *Am. Fam. Physician 11:* 108–110, 1975.
2. Kern, E. B. Referred pain to the ear. *Minn. Med.* 55: 896–898, 1972.
3. Schaeffer, J. P. *Morris' Human Anatomy.* Blakiston, Div. of McGraw-Hill, New York, 1951.
4. Stemmer, A. L. Dental otalgia. *Laryngoscope 77:* 1155–1167, 1967.

Chapter 2.5
Tinnitus Aurium

Dennis A. Greene

Subjective Complaints

Tinnitus, or "head noise," is an extremely common complaint, probably experienced by everyone at one time or another, usually after an upper respiratory infection or loud noise exposure. It is usually of very short duration. Persistent tinnitus may be associated with literally dozens of conditions that directly or indirectly affect the ear or auditory system. In this section we will discuss "pure" tinnitus. If the patient has the additional subjective complaint of hearing loss or vertigo, the reader should refer to either the introduction to Chapter 2.1, Sensorineural Hearing Loss, or Chapter 2.6, Disorders of Imbalance.

Tinnitus is a sound experience that is perceived by the patient, but which most often has no external source. It originates within the patient himself. It may be heard by the examiner, but this is not often the case.

One must not confuse tinnitus with auditory hallucinations. The latter are described as voices, bells, or other well-defined, complex, and recognizable sounds. They are symptoms of psychiatric disease.

Tinnitus is not well-defined or complex. It is a simple sound, such as buzzing, ringing, humming, roaring, blowing, clicking, or popping. It may be present in one or both ears, or may be impossible to localize. It may occur at certain times of day or with certain types of activity. It may be present constantly, or it may be intermittent in duration. It may have developed suddenly, or slowly, over a period of hours or days (Table 2.5.1).

Objective Findings

A well performed examination of the head and neck, including pneumatic otoscopy, nasopharyngeal examination, and auscultation of the neck, head, and ears should be done. Auscultation of the ears may be performed with a stethoscope or Toynbee tube. Certain types of continuous and pulsatile (or clicking) tinnitus may be heard by the examining physician (*objec-*

Table 2.5.1
Tinnitus Aurium: Subjective Complaints

Onset
  Sudden
  Progressive
Pattern
  Nonpulsatile (steady)
  Pulsatile (with heart beat)
  Clicking
  Blowing (with respiration)
Pitch
  High
  Low
Location
  Unilateral
  Bilateral
  Indeterminate (central)
Intensity
  Loud
  Soft
Presence
  Intermittent (regular or random)
  Continuous

tive tinnitus), a fortunate situation that often vastly simplifies the diagnostic evaluation. When the tinnitus is only *subjective* (heard by the patient alone), a clear description is essential, for the physical examination may be unrevealing.

Important positive physical findings in the following areas include:

Ears. Vascular lesions of the pinnae; obstructed external auditory canals; foreign body or insect; tympanic membrane erythema, vesiculation, perforation, or retraction; middle ear fluid; pulsatile mass in the middle ear; red or blue mass in the middle ear.

Nose and Nasopharynx. Mass in nose or nasopharynx; eustachian tubal swelling or obstruction; spastic or clonic palatal musculature.

Oropharynx. Spastic or clonic palatal musculature.

Head-Neck Vascular System. Thrills or bruits over named arteries; tinnitus may be altered by jugular or carotid compression.

Appraisal

Most patients should receive an audiogram (pure tone-air and bone conduction, speech reception threshold, and speech discrimination) and roentgenograms of the internal acoustic canals. Plain films in the transorbital and Stenver (oblique) views are usually adequate, but tomography may be necessary.

Audiometry may be normal or show a high frequency, neurosensory hearing loss. The patient will often state that the tinnitus corresponds with the 4000-Hz pure tone, especially if there is hearing loss in that frequency. This is most often seen in those who have been exposed to noise of traumatic intensity and duration.

The roentgenogram may be normal or may show lytic areas that correspond with cholesteatoma, vascular lesions, cerebellopontine angle tumors, cysts, or localized areas of infection. Tomograms may indicate areas of new bone formation in the cochlear capsule, indicative of cochlear otosclerosis (otospongiosis).

Patients with pulsatile tinnitus may be candidates for carotid arteriography or jugular venography, which may be diagnostic of an arterial or venous malformation or a glomus jugulare tumor.

Plan

Individuals with sensorineural hearing loss of whatever etiology so often have tinnitus that one is hard put to consider it an abnormality in these patients. Many of the conditions, referred to in Table 2.5.2 and causing acute tinnitus, will be readily noted and easily treated by the primary care physician. Most patients with pure, nonpulsatile tinnitus will recover spontaneously within 2 weeks. No medication has proved itself to be of any benefit at all in the treatment of idiopathic tinnitus. Nicotinic acid or papaverine, in flushing doses; histamine, intravenous, subcutaneous, or sublingual; and others have been used, but are not endorsed.

Patients whose tinnitus has persisted for longer than 2 weeks should be referred to an otorhinolaryngologist for diagnosis and management. Nonpulsatile tinnitus that produces severe anxiety may require that the patient be given tranquilizers for varying durations. That associated with coch-

Table 2.5.2
Tinnitus Aurium: Appraisal

	Pulsatile or Clicking or Blowing	Nonpulsatile
External ear	External otitis Bullous myringitis Foreign body (insect, etc.)	Cerumen Perforation of tympanic membrane Foreign body
Middle ear	Otitis media Eustachian tube dysfunction Vascular anomalies Neoplasm Muscular clonus or spasm	Otosclerosis Serous otitis
Inner ear	Vascular anomaly	Cochlear otosclerosis Meniere's disease Labyrinthitis Trauma Presbycusis Toxicity
Central nervous system	Vascular anomaly Hypertension	Cerebellopontine angle tumor Syphilis Degenerative CNS disease Cerebral atherosclerosis

lear otosclerosis (otospongiosis) may respond to sodium fluoride, 40–60 mg daily. Biofeedback training has shown itself to be helpful in many cases. Mechanical masking generators, some of which are miniaturized and may be worn in the ear, are often beneficial (available through the American Tinnitus Association, Portland, Oregon). A bedside clock or radio is helpful at night.

Pulsatile tinnitus that is proven to be caused by a vascular anomaly of the middle ear, such as a persistent stapedial artery, may respond to arterial ligation. Tumors of the glomus tympanicum or glomus jugulare are treated by excision and/or radiotherapy.

Clonus of the palatal, eustachian tubal, or middle ear muscles often responds to tranquilizers, muscle relaxants, or anticonvulsants, such as diphenylhydantoin. Surgical section of the involved muscle may be helpful if medication fails.

In summary, tinnitus aurium is a symptom that may reflect a great variety of possible pathologic conditions, many of which can be effectively diagnosed and treated, but some of which will remain occult until techniques of examination become much more precise. Most tinnitus is of short duration and may be adequately managed by the primary care physician. Patients with tinnitus of long duration should be referred to an otolaryngologist with special interest in this complaint.

Bibliography

1. Goodhill, V. The management of tinnitus. *Laryngoscope 60:* 448–450, 1950.
2. Graham, J. T. Tinnitus aurium. *Acta Otolaryngol.* Suppl. 202, 1965.
3. Parkin, J. L. Tinnitus evaluation. *Am. Fam. Physician 8:* 150–155, 1973.

Chapter 2.6

Disorders of Imbalance—Vertigo and Dizziness

Raymond P. Wood II

Vertigo may be defined as an abnormal perception of motion. Most physicians consider "true vertigo" to be a sensation of rotary movement, most often related to disorders of the vestibular portion of the inner ear. Other vertiginous sensations probably related to disorders of the utricular macula include sensations of continuing to fall when leaning forward or backward, continuing horizontal linear motion in an automobile when stopping, and continuing vertical motion when stopping from descent or ascent as in an elevator. The difference between subjective vertigo (patient spinning) and objective vertigo (room spinning) is of little importance, related to the eyes being open or closed.

Vertigo *excludes* "blacking out," loss of consciousness, light-headedness, and "unsteadiness," although unsteadiness may be present between attacks of vertigo. "Dizziness" which comes on *only* when arising from lying or sitting positions is usually *not* vertigo.

SUBJECTIVE SYMPTOMS

There are very few areas in medicine where the patient's subjective complaints and history are more important in making a diagnosis than in the evaluation of vertigo. In fact, if a fairly firm diagnostic impression is not formed on the basis of the history, the likelihood of ever making a positive diagnosis declines appreciably. In few areas of history taking is it more important to avoid suggestion to the patient in the description of his symptoms. For this reason, many physicians use a history form filled out by the patient.

The object of history taking is to determine whether the patient's complaint is vertigo or another form of imbalance or dizziness; if the vertigo is of vestibular origin; if the vertigo is related to the vestibular labyrinth alone or if there is associated cochlear dysfunction.

Present Illness

Onset: gradual; sudden.
Pattern: continuous; episodic.
Duration: attacks; episodes.
Frequency.
Duration of attacks: seconds, minutes, hours, days.
Intensity: mild, moderate, severe (unable to stand alone).
Accompanied by nausea and vomiting?
Temporal relationship: time of day of attack; awakening from sleep; relationship to meals.
Positional relationship: comes on while recumbent, sitting, standing, arising, turning head to one side, looking upward, with which ear down if lying down. Does vertigo come on immediately upon assuming a certain position? Is there a latency period?
What makes attack better? Worse?
Does any event precede attack?

Tinnitus

Unilateral; bilateral.
High-pitched; low-pitched.
Increase in intensity or change with attacks.
Pulsatile.
Change with head position.

Hearing

Loss in either ear; both ears.
Fluctuation in hearing with attacks.
Able to hear but not understand.
Sensitivity to loud sounds.

Ear

Pain.
Drainage.

Associated Symptoms

Headache.
Diplopia.
Dysarthria.
Unconsciousness.
Tendency to fall? To which side?
Loss of sensation.
Visual field cuts.
Grimacing.
Aura.
Postictal state.

OBJECTIVE FINDINGS

Ear

Tuning Fork Tests (512 and 1024 Hz)

Weber; Rinne; air conduction comparison; test for recruitment (compare two ears by air conduction while striking fork progressively harder).

Physical Examination

Pinna lesions: herpetic.
External ear canal: tumor, bleeding, irregularity of bony canal wall.
Tympanic membrane: Intact? Perforated? Drainage; tumor in middle ear; movement with pneumatic massage; cholesteatoma.
Fistula test: pressure with pneumatic otoscope or cupped hand over pinna produces deviation of eyes toward the affected side.

Eyes

Test with and without Frenzel glasses.
Spontaneous nystagmus: horizontal, vertical, or rotary; slow phase; fast phase or jerk.
Gaze nystagmus: deviate eyes 20° right or left.
Positional nystagmus: patient seated, supine, and head hanging right and left. To rule out effect of cervical torsion, when positional nystagmus is present, repeat with neck collar on patient and go from seated to right ear down and left ear down without neck torsion. Does nystagmus fatigue on assuming position repeatedly?
Eye tracking: evidence of eye tracking overshoot.
Caloric examination: head elevated 30° above supine; either irrigate with 5 ml of cool tap water or with 0.2-ml increments of ice water (Kobrak minimal calorics). Expected result, brisk nystagmus away from irrigated ear. Does it reproduce symptoms?
Fixation suppression: during maximum response to calorics, have patient focus on finger; nystagmus should diminish or stop, if not, "failure of fixation suppression" is present.

Neurologic Examination

Cranial nerves: special attention to cranial nerves V (corneal reflex) and VII (facial function, twitching of face).
Gait: normal or wide-based; heel to toe walking; tendency to fall right or left; finger to nose testing; heel to shin testing; past pointing; rapid alternating movements; Romberg.

General Examination

Blood pressure: lying and standing.
Stigmata of neurofibromas: café au lait spots.
Interstitial keratitis, Hutchinson's teeth, saber shins.

Special Testing

Audiometric Tests—Routine

Pure tone bone line and air line.
Speech discrimination tests.
Tone decay test, alternate binaural loudness balance (ABLB).

Uncomfortable loudness level (ULL), short increment sensitivity index (SISI).

Electronystagmography — Routine

In addition to eye tests above, electronystagmography (ENG) includes calibration tests and optokinetic drum testing.

X-ray Studies

Plain (Stenver's) views of internal auditory canals (IAC's) (routine).
Polytomography of IAC's (where indicated).
Computerized axial tomography (CAT) scan (where indicated).
Posterior fossa myelogram (where indicated).
Carotid arteriogram (where indicated).
Pneumoencephalogram (where indicated).

Spinal Fluid Tests (Where Indicated)

Protein.
Protein fractions (γ-globulins).
Fluorescent treponemal antibody (FTA).

Blood Tests

Complete blood count (CBC) (routine).
VDRL (routine).
Thyroxine (T_4), and T_4 normalized (routine).
Fasting blood sugar (FBS) and 2-hour postprandial blood sugar (PPBS) (routine).
FTA (where indicated).
Five-hour glucose tolerance test (GTT) (where indicated).

ASSESSMENT

Dizziness Other than True Vertigo

Initially, the evaluation of the problem entails deciding, on the basis of history, whether the patient is describing true vertigo or not. If there is not a sensation of whirling motion or perverted linear motion, the problem is not true vertigo.
Orthostatic hypotension may be differentiated by the fact that it never comes on while lying down or turning over. It is present only when sitting or standing up. The sensation is usually one of blacking out. The lying and standing blood pressure may be of value. Other tests are all normal.

Hypoglycemia has a definite temporal relationship with eating. It is usually not manifested by true vertigo, although it may be, and is usually accompanied by lightheadedness, sweating, and tremulousness. The 5-hour GTT will aid in the diagnosis. Other tests are normal.

Hyperventilation syndrome likewise is usually a sensation of lightheadedness and impending loss of consciousness or blacking out. It is associated with circumoral numbness and tingling, and tingling and drawing up of the hands and feet. Observation of the hyperventilation during the attack will confirm the diagnosis. The symptoms may be alleviated by having the patient rebreathe in a paper bag.

Disorders without Hearing Problems

There are three common disorders of vertigo which have some similarities. In the case of *epidemic vertigo* versus *viral or acute labyrinthitis*, the difference is whether several cases occur in temporal and geographic proximity (*epidemic vertigo*) or as an apparently isolated incident (*viral or acute labyrinthitis*). These disorders usually follow a typical upper respiratory infection (URI) by about 1 week. They are characterized by an acute onset of vertigo which is continuous and severe for 48–72 hours, then begins to get better and is usually much improved in 1 week. After the initial 2–3 days, the patient may have only positional vertigo. Nausea and vomiting may occur. Examination and tests reveal normal hearing, spontaneous nystagmus, and normal caloric examination. The nystagmus may initially be horizontal, vertical, or rotary. It then becomes horizontal. It resolves without any residual deficits. The etiology is said to be viral.

A similar disease which is sometimes confused with the above is *vestibular neuronitis*. In fact it is very different both in history and findings. The onset of vestibular neuronitis is usually acute. However, the acute episode is slow to resolve with the patient having persistent vertigo lasting up to several months. There may be a persistent positional vertigo which is permanent, or which improves over several months. On examination, the hearing is normal; spontaneous nystagmus is present initially, but after weeks to months is replaced by positional nystagmus. The caloric examination reveals a decreased or absent caloric response on the side of the lesion. This will persist as a canal paresis or paralysis permanently. There is evidence that the disorder is related to presumably viral damage to the vestibular (Scarpa's) ganglion.

Benign positional vertigo and its associated disorder, *cupulolithiasis*, are characterized by vertigo with direction-fixed nystagmus coming on in certain head positions. It may be either sudden in onset or come on insidiously. The most striking feature is its positional character. In the case of cupololithiasis, there may be a history of previous head injury. The nystagmus is present only with attacks and is horizontal. There is a period of latency between assuming the position and the onset of the vertigo, and the severity of the attacks tends to fatigue with repeated assumption of triggering position.

Cervical vertigo (post-whiplash vertigo) is characterized by the onset, immediate or delayed, of a positional vertigo after neck injury. Tinnitus may be associated. The nystagmus is usually horizontal. There may be mild unsteadiness between attacks. When seen late, there may be little *visible* nystagmus with the eyes open. Audiometric and other tests are normal except for the ENG. Here, a special position test is carried out, once with positions assumed with neck torsion, and then repeated with a cervical collar with whole body rotation. The nystagmus should be present with neck torsion but not with the cervical collar. The etiology is unknown but is assumed to be related to cervical kinesthetic afferent impulses.

Vertigo caused by central nervous system stimulants or depressants is difficult to diagnose as the symptoms are frequently vague and without fixed temporal or positional relationships. Other than the presence of spontaneous nystagmus, the tests usually show normal results. Only a careful history may bring out the diagnosis. This may be seen with almost any of sleeping medications (barbiturates, tranquilizers, etc.) The test is to stop the medication.

Vertigo caused by *vascular disease* usually presents without alterations in hearing. The three most common disorders are: *basilar artery insufficiency, Wallenberg's syndrome,* and the *subclavian steal syndrome.* The most important differentiating finding with these disorders is other neurologic signs. They are almost always accompanied by one of the *three D's*—diplopia, dysphagia, or dysarthria. The subclavian steal syndrome includes diminished pulse in the arm on the affected side and pulse lag.

Two uncommon forms of vertigo should be mentioned. These are *migrainous vertigo* and *vertiginous epilepsy.* The history is important in making the diagnosis. In the case of migrainous vertigo, the vertigo may accompany the classic migraine headache or may occur at other times. Vertiginous epilepsy may occur in patients with or without other epileptiform manifestations. The vertiginous attacks may be accompanied by an aura and postictal state. With both of these disorders, the only finding may be spontaneous nystagmus during the attacks. An electroencephalogram (EEG) may or may not be helpful in making the diagnosis.

Perversions of Linear Motion without Hearing Changes

Although not frequently diagnosed, disorders of the vestibular maculae cause perversion of perception of linear motion. In these disorders, there is no sense of rotary motion, but instead the patient reports either difficulty when ascending or descending in elevators, or the sense of continuing motion when bending over or when stopping in an automobile. In our experience, a common factor in the past history is the presence of motion sickness early in life and frequently, a strong family history of motion sickness. Current methods of vestibular testing in common use do not test this aspect of the system. Other tests are normal.

Table 2.6.1*

	Hearing Loss	Poor Discrimination	Tinnitus	Recruitment	Positional Vertigo	Decreased or Absent Calorics	Calibration Overshoot	Failure of Fixation Suppression	Other Neurologic Findings	X-ray Finding	Other
Epidemic vertigo; viral or acute labyrinthitis	−	−	−	−	±	−	−	−	−	−	
Vestibular neuronitis	−	−	−	−	±	++	−	−	−	−	
Benign positional vertigo	−	−	−	−	++	−	−	−	−	−	
Meniere's syndrome	+	±	++	++	−	+	−	−	−	−	
Syphilitic vertigo	+	+	+	+	−	+	−	−	−	−	Serum, CSF, FTA
Acoustic neuroma	+	++	+	−	−	+	−	−	+	±	
Cupulolithiasis	−	−	±	−	++	−	−	−	+	−	
Whiplash	−	−	±	−	++	−	−	−	−	−	
Labyrinthic fistula	+	+	+	−	−	+	−	−	+	−	
Vestibular granuloma	+	++	+	−	−	+	−	−	−	−	
Labyrinthic concussion	−	−	+	−	±	−	−	−	−	−	
Temporal bone fracture	±	±	+	−	±	±	−	−	±	−	Tomos
Basilar artery insufficiency	−	−	−	−	+	−	−	−	++	−	
Wallenberg's syndrome	−	−	−	−	−	−	−	−	++	−	
Multiple sclerosis	+	++	+	−	−	±	++	++	+	−	
Migrainous vertigo	−	−	−	−	−	−	−	−	−	−	Migraine headache
Vertiginous epilepsy	−	−	−	−	−	−	−	−	+	−	EEG

* Absent, −; sometimes present, ±; present, +; frequently present, ++.

Vertigo with Hearing Changes

The most common disorder in this group is *Meniere's syndrome*. It is characterized by *fluctuating hearing loss, tinnitus,* and *vertigo.* The syndrome may begin with any or all of the above symptoms. The true vertigo comes on suddenly, frequently accompanied by nausea and vomiting, and lasts minutes to hours. It may be relieved by vomiting, or by lying down quietly. The patient is usually asymptomatic between attacks. The attacks tend to come in a series (an *episode*). The patient complains of a "full" or "stuffy" feeling in one ear (about 15% is bilateral) which precedes or accompanies the attack. The hearing is diminished in the affected ear, especially in the low tones, and there may be a complaint of sensitivity to loud sounds (recruitment). Tinnitus, which may be low-pitched or roaring or occasionally high-pitched ringing, may precede or accompany the attack.

On physical examination during an attack, nystagmus will be present but may be obscured by fixation if Frenzel glasses are not used. The nystagmus may be either horizontal or rotary (especially early in the attack). There usually is not a positional component to the vertigo. The Weber test early in the course will usually refer to the good ear. The Rinne tests will show air conduction better than bone conduction. The comparison test will show the fork to be heard better by air conduction in the unaffected ear than the affected ear. However, recruitment will probably be present in the affected ear. An audiogram early in the course will show a small low tone conductive hearing loss in the affected ear. Later, the conductive loss may disappear and a *fluctuating sensorineural loss* may be present. During attacks, the speech discrimination score will be diminished. The ABLB and SISI tests will suggest recruitment, as will the uncomfortable loudness test. Between attacks the hearing may be normal or show only a mild to moderate sensorineural hearing loss. Electronystagmography will reveal a spontaneous nystagmus during the attack (occasionally between attacks). Early on, the caloric responses may be equal but, with time, the

caloric response in the affected ear will become weak or lost. The other tests on ENG are normal. X-rays of the inner ear are normal.

Despite reports of other authors, this author has not been able to demonstrate abnormalities of thyroid function, serum electrolyte imbalance, or abnormal glucose tolerance tests in patients with Meniere's syndrome. We have seen one case in which an allergic response to yeast products was involved in the etiology.

It must be noted here that although the older literature carefully differentiates the presenting history and physical findings and audiometric test results of Meniere's syndrome from those of acoustic neuroma, it is now well documented that they may present *exactly alike.* Consequently, a high index of suspicion and careful follow-up are needed. The *usual* findings are different, however. In acoustic neuromas, the patient may describe a mild unsteadiness rather than true vertigo. Decreased corneal response, facial paresis or paralysis, and headache are seen in late, large tumors only. A pure sensorineural hearing loss is usually present, although the earliest finding may be only a decreased discrimination score. The tests for recruitment are negative, but the tone decay test is positive (patient cannot continue to hear an ongoing pure tone signal). On ENG, nystagmus may or may not be present, but canal paresis or absent caloric response will be seen. On x-ray of the petrous pyramids, either widening or flaring of the internal auditory canal may be seen. In early tumors the bony canal will not be affected and a posterior fossa myelogram will be required to see tumor filling the IAC. The CAT scan will show extracanalicular tumors. Cerebrospinal fluid (CSF) examination (done early when there is no evidence of increased CSF pressure) will show an increase in protein only in the case of tumors larger than 1–2 cm in diameter.

Another disorder which may mimic Meniere's syndrome is *syphilis* of the inner ear. The symptoms may begin early in life (congenital syphilis) or later in life (acquired syphilis). It may be unilateral or bilateral. There may be an associated *sudden* sensorineural hearing loss. The important findings include a *fluctuating senso-rineural hearing loss*, poor discrimination score, sometimes spontaneous nystagmus, and decreased or absent caloric responses. On occasion the fistula test is positive (Henneber's sign). Most important is the presence of positive serologic test for syphilis. A positive VDRL should be confirmed by a fluorescent treponemal antibody-absorption (FTA-Abs) test. Further examination includes a CSF FTA-Abs.

Vertigo with Hearing Disorder following Head Trauma

Following head injury ranging from concussion to temporal bone fracture, vertigo and hearing problems may occur. These range from transient vertigo and tinnitus to severe vertigo with sensorineural hearing loss ranging from mild to complete. The history of the head trauma followed by the onset of vertigo establishes the diagnosis. Fracture of the temporal bone rarely, if ever, occurs without unconsciousness. Physical examination may reveal laceration or hematoma of the scalp. Battle's sign (postauricular hematoma) or bleeding from the external auditory canal are suggestive of fracture. The bleeding may come from an obviously disrupted external bony canal or from a laceration of the tympanic membrane. There may be CSF otorrhea. The Weber test may refer to the injured ear (where a conductive loss has resulted from middle ear trauma) and the Rinne may be either positive (AC > BC) in the case of a sensorineural loss or negative where a conductive loss results from middle ear damage. The ENG may show a spontaneous nystagmus, which several weeks after injury may not be visible with eyes open. Late in the course the nystagmus may be positional. The caloric responses range from equal to absent. Neck torsion tests will help to rule out cervical vertigo. Evaluation of the facial nerve function is important as the nerve may be avulsed or damaged by fractures which traverse the fallopian canal. In addition to standard skull x-rays, which often fail to reveal fractures of the temporal bone, polytomographic x-rays are needed.

Vertigo after Ear Surgery or Associated with Ear Infection

Vertigo which comes on after ear surgery in which the perilymph space has been deliberately entered (stapedectomy) or inadvertently entered, or vertigo which is associated with middle ear or mastoid infection or cholesteatoma, may be due to any one of these conditions: *serous labyrinthitis, suppurative labyrinthitis, perilymphatic fistula, or granuloma of the vestibule.*

Serous labyrinthitis is a transient disorder of mild vertigo accompanied by a mild sensorineural hearing loss and some decline in the speech discrimination score. A spontaneous nystagmus is present, but caloric tests may not be carried out in these ears. There may be complete resolution or persistence of the hearing loss and depressed caloric responses.

Suppurative labyrinthitis, which may be associated with surgery on the otic capsule, cholesteatoma erosion, or meningitis, produces profound vertigo and hearing loss. The inner ear may be completely destroyed. In this event, there is spontaneous nystagmus and no response to sound or to caloric stimulation of the ear.

Perilymphatic fistula has a presentation in which the vertigo may come on suddenly weeks to months or years after stapes surgery. It may follow a sudden change in middle ear or CSF pressure such as seen in diving, Valsalva maneuvers, coughing, and sneezing. There is usually a sudden onset of vertigo, tinnitus, and sensorineural hearing loss. The speech discrimination score usually falls precipitously to levels of less than 50%. The fistula test (apply pressure in the external ear canal and produce eye movement) may be positive. In the case of chronic ear disease and, in particular, attic cholesteatoma, the onset of symptoms may be gradual. Physical examination will reveal the typical retraction pocket or perforation in the posterior superior portion of the tympanic membrane.

Poststapedectomy granuloma is a condition which comes on days to weeks after stapedectomy. The symptoms and findings are similar except that the fistula test is usually negative.

Vertigo with or without Hearing Loss

Vertigo Associated with Multiple Sclerosis

One disorder which may present with variable findings ranging from unsteadiness or ataxia to true vertigo with or without hearing loss is multiple sclerosis. The young adult age of onset is typical. The hearing loss may be reported as only difficulty in understanding during noise. Physical examination may reveal overshoot of the eyes on gaze testing or diplopia. Nystagmus which is horizontal, vertical, or rotary may be present. Vertigo and nystagmus may be *worse with the eyes open*. Audiometric tests may show only a sensorineural loss or poor speech discrimination. The electronystagmogram will probably show calibration overshoots, poor optokinetic tracking, and failure of fixation supression. Examination of the spinal fluid for proteins and electrophoreis are very helpful. The overall picture is one of remission and exacerbation. Multiple sclerosis is one of perhaps only three diseases which show true *fluctuating sensorineural hearing loss* when followed over a period of time (the other two are syphilis and Meniere's).

Vertigo Caused by Ototoxic Drugs

Vertigo caused by ototoxic drugs, especially the aminoglycoside antibiotics, may or may not have associated hearing loss. Most of these drugs have a predilection for either the cochlea or the vestibular portion of the inner ear. In some cases, if a sufficient quantity of the drug is given, the other system will become involved also. Although the symptoms usually become apparent during the administration of the drug, the effects may be delayed. The effects are usually, but not always, present in both ears. The patient may complain more of severe unsteadiness than true vertigo, and the complaint is constant. These patients have difficulty walking in the dark. Examination may reveal normal hearing or sensorineural hearing loss ranging from mild to complete. They manifest ataxia in walking. Nystagmus may be present especially with the eyes closed. If a hearing loss is present, so may be recruitment.

PLAN

The treatment of vertigo ranges from no treatment at all to highly specialized otoneurosurgical resection of acoustic neuromas. Symptomatic drug therapy is confusing and bewildering because much of it is based upon both unproved assumptions as to the cause of the vertigo and unproved pharmacologic actions of the drugs. This section therefore reflects the author's assumptions and prejudices.

Epidemic vertigo, viral or acute labyrinthitis are benign, self-limited disorders which are generally better in 4 or 5 days. If the initial attack is disabling, symptomatic management such as Compazine suppositories, 25 mg every 8 hours, or droperidol, 1 ml intramuscularly (im) may be used to alleviate the symptoms.

Vestibular neuronitis is much slower to resolve. The acute attack may be treated as above and long-term management may require the use of an agent such as Antivert, 12.5 or 25 mg four times a day.

Benign positional vertigo or cupulolithiasis likewise may be benefited by the use of Antivert. In addition, conditioning exercises (Cawthorne's exercises) may be used to bring on the attack and thus "fatigue" the responses.

Cervical vertigo is usually treated by use of a cervical collar and muscle relaxants such as Valium, 5 mg four times a day.

Basilar artery insufficiency and Wallenberg's syndrome should be referred to a neurologist for management.

Subclavian steal syndrome should be referred to a vascular surgeon for correction.

Migrainous vertigo and vertiginous epilepsy should be treated by treating the underlying disorder.

Macular vertigo is difficult to manage. Antivert may be of some benefit as may treatment with Arlidin, 6 mg four times a day, and Butisol sodium (butabarbital), 15–30 mg four times a day.

Meniere's syndrome has more proposed treatments than any other of these disorders. They include such things as dietary control, salt-free diet and diuretics, anti-nausea drugs such as Antivert or Marezine, 25–50 mg four times a day, Arlidin and Butisol (as above), and for control of the severe acute attack, droperidol, 1 ml im. For intractable, disabling attacks, surgery must be considered. The procedures range from vestibular nerve section and endolymphatic sac operations to destructive labyrinthotomies, depending upon the status of the hearing.

Acoustic neuroma is treated by surgical resection.

Syphilitic vertigo should be managed in conjunction with specialists in infectious disease, utilizing appropriate high dose penicillin and steroids.

Head trauma with persistent vertigo usually improves slowly with time. It may be influenced by use of Antivert.

Serous labyrinthitis is usually self-limited. It has been treated with histamine injections, etc. Antibiotics and steroids are also used.

Suppurative labyrinthitis should be treated with appropriate antibiotics if due to meningitis. Otherwise, treatment should be with agents which are effective against *Haemophilus influenzae* as well as Pneumococcus.

Perilymphatic fistula and granuloma are treated by surgical exploration of the middle ear and correction. These are *surgical emergencies.*

Multiple sclerosis has no specific treatment. Although the underlying disease sometimes responds to steroids, the author is not convinced that this greatly affects the hearing loss and vertigo. Responses are difficult to ascertain because of the natural history of the disease.

The effects of ototoxic drugs are very difficult to treat. Young persons usually learn to compensate with proprioceptive and visual system clues. Older persons may be severely handicapped by the loss of vestibular responses. Physical therapy and careful conditioning combined with the use of canes or walkers may be required.

Bibliography

1. Beddoe, G. Vertigo in childhood. *Otolaryngol. Clin. North Am. 10:* 139–144, 1977.
2. English, G. M. (Ed.). Vestibular diseases. In *Otolaryngology*, pp. 98–115. Harper & Row, Hagerstown, Md., 1976.
3. Wolfson, R. J. (Ed.). Vertigo. *Otolaryngol. Clin. North Am. 6 (1):* 1973.

Chapter 2.7

Lesions of the Ear

Raymond P. Wood II

DIFFUSE LESIONS OF THE PINNA

Subjective Complaints. Diffuse lesions may present as swelling of a portion of the pinna or involve all of the pinna. They are usually painful but may be only pruritic. There may be a history of antecedent trauma to the ear. There may be a history of associated tenderness involving other cartilaginous structures (e.g., the nose or larynx).

Objective Findings. Inspection of the pinna will reveal loss of the normal contour of the pinna and anatomic landmarks. There may be marked erythema. The skin may be tense. The pinna should be palpated for fluctuance. If the lesion is pruritic, the lesion more likely will be scaly and eczematoid. If so, it may assume a pattern in the line of drainage from the ear canal.

Assessment. If there is a history of trauma to the ear (blunt or sharp), the three most common lesions are *cellulitis, hematoma, and subperichondrial abscess.* All three are painful, erythematous, and may be warm to the touch. They may be difficult to distinguish. Fluctuance is associated with abscess. The scaly eczematoid reaction may be dry or it may be wet, in which case it usually involves the lower pinna and is associated with pus drainage from the ear canal. Relapsing polychondritis usually involves other cartilages in the body.

Plan. Where trauma is involved, if there is marked swelling, hematoma or abscess should be suspected. The pinna is carefully cleansed with iodophor solution, and a sterile needle aspirate of the subperichondrial area is made. If blood is obtained, it is cultured. It may be necessary to incise to express any clot. The pinna is then packed with sterile cotton covered with antibiotic ointment to conform to the normal contours of the ear, and a mastoid dressing is placed. The patient is started on antibiotics such as erythromycin or ampicillin, 250 mg q.i.d., and the dressing is replaced after 2 days.

If pus is obtained, it is cultured for aerobic and anerobic organisms and treatment with a conforming dressing as above. The same antibiotics are used until the culture report is returned. The dressing is changed daily, however. If the lesion worsens, then surgical drainage and hospitalization are required. Cellulitis will usually respond to the antibiotics and dressing.

In the case of eczematoid lesions, any pus from the canal should be cultured for bacteria and fungi, as should any dry scales. If in the area of drainage of pus from the ear canal, the pinna lesion will usually respond to treatment of the external canal or middle ear infection with antibiotic-steroid ear drops (such as Cortisporin or Coly-Mycin). The dry eczematoid lesions may respond to the application of 1% hydrocortisone cream. Occasionally in patients using a neomycin-containing ear drop, an inflamed eczematoid reaction will develop in the area of drainage. The drops should be stopped and hydrocortisone cream applied.

Relapsing polychondritis may have associated erythrocyte sedimentation rate (ESR) elevation, positive serologic tests for collagen vascular disease, and other systemic manifestations. These patients should be referred to an internist for workup and steroid therapy.

LESIONS OF THE EAR LOBE

Subjective Complaints. These usually present as either a firm, slow-growing, nontender mass, commonly associated with ear piercing, or as small, sometimes tender nodules, frequently multiple beneath the skin. They may become larger or smaller with time.

Objective Findings. The former lesions are usually fixed to the skin and single. The latter are small, pea-sized, firm nodules which can be rolled between the fingers.

Assessment. Keloids are usually associated with ear piercing or trauma to the lobe. They are more common in Blacks. Inclusion cysts are of unknown etiology.

Plan. Keloids are treated by intralesional steroid injection, preferably using a hydrospray injection. If they do not respond, they should be excised and the area injected once a week for 3 weeks with steroids.

Inclusion cysts may be excised if troublesome or if they become infected after first treating the infection with systemic antibiotics. The incisions are placed behind the ear lobe. The cysts may recur.

DISCRETE LESIONS OF THE PINNA

Anterior Helix

Subjective Complaints. These usually present in association with a small pit or tract just above and anterior to the crus helicis. They are present in childhood. They may present as a painless swelling or become infected, painful, and erythematous and drain pus from a tract.

Objective Findings. The lesions, as above, are almost always only associated with the anterior helix.

Assessment. These are congenital anomalies, auricular pits and cysts.

Plan. Where a tract is found, it should

be injected with methylene blue and the tract and cyst excised. When carefully removed, they do not recur.

Pigmented Lesions

Subjective Complaints. Brown, black, or blue-black lesions may be asymptomatic or may be pruritic or associated with minor bleeding, especially if traumatized.

Objective Findings. The lesions should be examined carefully for satellite lesions. The areas of preauricular and postauricular lymph nodes should be carefully palpated, as should the cervical lymph nodes.

Assessment. Especially if the patient is fair-skinned with reddish hair, melanoma should be ruled out. Pigmented nevi of course also may appear similar.

Plan. The lesion must be biopsied. If it is a melanoma, a metastatic workup is carried out. Treatment is by excision, usually wide field, with lymph node dissection and frequently chemoimmunotherapy. Referral to a head and neck surgeon is mandatory.

Vesicular, Painful

Subjective Complaints. The patient may first present with lancinating pain in the distribution of the second and third divisions of the Vth cranial nerve. Discrete lesions which are first vesicular and then ulcerated, painful, or pruritic appear. There may be a complaint of intraoral painful lesions as well. In addition, the patient may complain of facial weakness or paralysis.

Objective Findings. As above. The vesicular lesions may come to involve the distribution of the second and third divisions of nerve V.

Assessment. This is a typical presentation of herpes zoster oticus (Ramsay Hunt syndrome).

Plan. If there is involvement of the first division of the Vth nerve, ophthalmologic consultation is required. Examination to rule out occult lymphoma or other debilitating disease is carried out. If the lesions are wet and weeping, a calamine shake lotion may be used. Although many treatments are advocated, their efficacy is not proven. Steroids may be used to lessen the symptoms but should not be used where there is eye involvement.

Helical Rim, Painful

Subjective Complaints. The patient complains of very tender, painful, slowly growing lesions of helical rim. They may make sleeping on the involved ear impossible.

Objective Findings. The firm, very tender lesions may be single or multiple. They are usually a few millimeters in diameter.

Assessment. About the only lesion which presents this way is *chondrodermatitis nodularis chronica helicis*. It is of unknown etiology.

Plan. These lesions may respond to intralesional injection of triamcinolone. If not, small lesions may be treated with electrodesiccation. Large lesions should be excised, removing a small portion of the underlying cartilage.

Nonpainful

Subjective Complaints. These usually present as slowly growing, nonpainful, occasionally pruritic lesions. They may be raised and umbilicated or flat and ulcerated. Frequently the complaint is that they crust over but fail to heal. They may be anywhere on the pinna.

Objective Findings. As above. Careful examination of the ear canal is carried out, as well as palpation of the pre- and post-auricular lymph nodes and the cervical lymph nodes.

Assessment. Although common lesions such as *senile keratosis* may present in this fashion, *squamous cell* and *basal cell carcinomas* must be ruled out.

Plan. These lesions must be biopsied. If the lesion extends to the external ear canal, tomographic x-rays of the bony external ear canal must be obtained in cases of carcinoma. The treatment of these lesions is surgical, with lymph node dissection and temporal bone dissection, sometimes combined with radiation therapy, where indicated. Basal cell carcinomas may usually be treated with surgical exci-

sion with a margin of normal tissue about the tumor. Cartilage must almost always be excised with the tumor.

Vascular, Nonpainful

Subjective Complaints. There are two relatively uncommon vascular lesions of the pinna—*hemangioma* and *arteriovenous malformations*. The former presents as a typical elevated bluish or red mass which may bleed if traumatized. They may also present as a flat "port wine stain." Arteriovenous anomalies more often present as varicosities covered by normal-appearing skin.

Objective Findings. As above.

Assessment. As above. Rarely are studies needed on these lesions. Only in the case of a very large arteriovenous malformation would arteriography be required.

Plan. When hemangiomas occur in infants, they should be watched, as they resolve with growth. If not, and the lesion grows, it should be treated. If bleeding is a problem, treatment is required. Most can be excised under local anesthesia (in adults) and the base electrocoagulated or treated with cryosurgery. Malignancy is very rare.

Arteriovenous malformations likewise may be observed. If growth occurs they should be treated by ligation of the vessels. They frequently recur, arising from the difficulty of locating all of the feeding vessels. Injection with sclerosing agents may be used.

Port wine stain capillary hemangiomas are more of a cosmetic problem than anything else. Application of cosmetics to cover the lesion or tattooing with skin-colored pigment may be used.

LESIONS OF THE EAR CANAL

(See also Chapters 2.3, Otorrhea; 2.4, Ear Pain; and 2.5, Tinnitus.)

Diffuse Lesions—Painful or Pruritic

Subjective Complaints. The patient may present with either pruritus or pain. There may be a complaint of drainage from the ear canal and sometimes reduced hearing. If there is drainage it may be yellow and foul-smelling or serosanguineous.

Objective Findings. Discharge may be visible in the canal and meatus. On pulling on the pinna to straighten the canal and insert the speculum, the patient may complain of *pain*. Often in external otitis the ear canal is swollen and red. If severe, it may be difficult to insert a speculum. In cases of fungal infections, white or black plaques of fungus with visible hyphae may be seen. In the case of pruritus without pain, the ear canal may be dry and scaly or appear normal.

Assessment. Where pus and debris are present, it is necessary to clean the ear canal to rule out a middle ear infection with perforation of the drum and drainage. Fungal plaques may occur in many ears with suppurative otitis due to bacterial infections as secondary (opportunistic) invaders. Fungal external otitis is common in humid climates but rare in dry climates. In patients with *diabetes mellitus, malignant external otitis* may occur. This is associated with severe pain, bony erosion, and sometimes *facial paralysis*.

Pruritic, scaly lesions are usually eczematoid, but occasionally fungal infections present this way. In the case of pruritus without visible lesions, sensitivity to soap may be involved.

Plan. In all of these disorders *aural hygiene* is required. This means keeping soap and water out of the ears, using cotton in the canals, and smearing Vaseline over the outside.

All pus and debris must be cleaned from the canal by using cotton applicators and suction.

In the case of pruritic lesions, aural hygiene may be all that is required. If not, an agent such as hydrocortisone cream, ½%, applied to the ear canal *b.i.d.* may be helpful.

In suppurative external otitis which is uncomplicated, if there is significant swelling of the canal, it should be dilated with a speculum. A ¼-inch selvage gauze is inserted down to the tympanic membrane. Either Domeboro otic solution or Cortisporin otic drops are used *q.i.d.* to moisten the wick.

If fungal infection is the etiology, a drop made up of Vioform-HC cream with 100,000 units of nystatin per 30 ml is diluted to ear drop consistency and used *q.i.d.*

We do not routinely culture uncomplicated external otitis because of the cost involved. If the infection does not respond to the above treatments (this will be rare), the drops are stopped and a culture is obtained for fungus and bacteria.

Patients with diabetes are routinely cultured. Those with family histories of diabetes have a fasting blood sugar and 2-hour postprandial blood sugar. Patients with facial paralysis are admitted to the hospital and tomograms of the external ear canal and mastoid carried out. They usually require surgical management along with intravenous antibiotics effective against Pseudomonas, Proteus, and Staphylococcus. All such patients should be referred to an otolaryngologist. There is a significant mortality among these patients from intracranial complications.

Otherwise uncomplicated suppurative external otitis occasionally will spread to produce a cellulitis of the pinna. When this occurs, erythromycin, 250 or 500 mg *q.i.d.*, plus hot packs to the pinna should be used. Failure to respond in 48–72 hours suggests that infection may be due to Pseudomonas or Proteus (usually mixed flora). Hospitalization, biopsy, and culture of the lesion are then indicated and the appropriate systemic antibiotics begun.

DISCRETE LESIONS OF THE EXTERNAL EAR CANAL

Asymptomatic

Subjective Complaints. These lesions are usually found during a routine examination. The two most common such lesions are *osteoma* of the external canal and *exostoses*. Exostoses are almost always seen in cold water swimmers.

Objective Findings. Osteoma of the external canal usually arises from the posterior canal wall and presents as a smooth, raised lesion covered by normal skin. It is hard to palpation and is single.

Exostoses may be single or multiple and

occur immediately lateral to the tympanic membrane. They are also covered by normal canal skin and are hard to palpation.

Assessment. As above.

Plan. Exostoses require no treatment. Osteomas should be worked up by x-ray of the external canal, usually by polytomography if there is doubt as to the diagnosis. Rarely, a tumor such as ceruminoma may appear like an osteoma. Further question can be resolved by biopsy under local anesthesia. Osteomas usually require no treatment unless they obstruct the canal and cause accumulation of debris next to the tympanic membrane. This may cause a conductive hearing loss or recurrent infection.

Foreign Body

Subjective Complaints. These usually occur in children but may be seen in adults. They may be accompanied by tinnitus (insects), pruritus, or drainage. They may be asymptomatic.

Objective Findings. The foreign body may be seen with an otoscope. Peas, beans, and beads are common in children. Ticks and other insects occur at any age.

Assessment. As above.

Plan. If a living insect is seen, it may be drowned by filling the canal with rubbing alcohol or ethyl alcohol and then retrieved with a forceps.

In children, the object may be wedged in the canal. A small amount of lidocaine, 2%, may be injected around the bony cartilaginous junction to provide anesthesia, and the object is removed.

After removal of the object, ear drops should be used for 3 or 4 days to prevent infection from the trauma.

Mild Discomfort

Subjective Complaints. The patient may complain of little or no pain but only of mild discomfort. Many times the lesions are discovered on physical examination and are without symptoms. Occasionally there is only minimal discharge from the ear. There may or may not be a mild conductive hearing loss.

Objective Findings. Examination of the ear canal will reveal either an ulcerated lesion or heaped-up lesion both with disruption of the normal epithelium and some degree of erythema. The lesion may be tender to palpation. They may occur in any part of the canal. Some lesions of this group may present as a swelling of the ear canal covered by normal canal skin.

Assessment. This group of lesions comprises the more common tumors of the ear canal. Those with epithelial disruption are usually squamous or basal cell carcinomas. Those with a normal epithelial covering are more likely cylindromas.

Plan. Examination of the preauricular, postauricular, and cervical lymph nodes is made to determine metastases. The lesion should be biopsied under local anesthesia as soon as possible. Polytomographic x-rays of the external ear canal, middle ear, and mastoid are carried out to determine the extent of the lesion. These should all be referred to an otolaryngologic head and neck surgeon. The treatment is wide surgical excision, sometimes including temporal bone resection and/or irradiation therapy.

In children there are rare tumors such as embryonal cell rhabdomyosarcomas. They are handled similarly, but with very poor prognosis.

Polypoid Lesions

Subjective Complaints. These lesions may be incidental findings or they may present with drainage or conductive hearing loss.

Objective Findings. Examination may demonstrate a mild conductive hearing loss. There may be clear or purulent drainage or debris in the ear canal. The lesions are usually on the lateral surface of the tympanic membrane or protruding through a posterior perforation of the membrane. The polypoid lesions are pale gray to beefy red in color.

Assessment. Most commonly these lesions are beefy red *aural polyps* extending through a perforation in the tympanic membrane and will be accompanied by a conductive hearing loss and infection. A much less common lesion will be the red or bluish red polypoid *chemodectoma* of the middle ear (glomus tympanicum or glomus jugulare). Rare indeed are the pale gray lesions of *rhabdomyosarcoma* or *histiocytosis* X, seen almost exclusively in children.

Plan. These lesions should all be referred for treatment. Biopsy must be carried out *very carefully*. In the case of benign aural polyps, the stalk may be intimately associated with the ossicles which could be avulsed. Biopsy of a chemodectoma can produce serious or fatal hemorrhage.

Aural polyps usually respond to treatment with a corticosteroid-antibiotic ear drop, but are not infrequently associated with cholesteatoma. Therefore, surgical repair of the membrane perforation with mastoid exploration may be required.

Where chemodectoma is suspected, tomograms to determine bony erosion, carotid arteriograms to determine extent of tumor, and feeding vessels and jugular venography should be done *before* biopsy. Biopsy is carried out in the operating room with preparations to control hemorrhage. Treatment is by surgical excision and/or irradiation.

Histocytosis X is treated with irradiation therapy after biopsy.

Rhabdomyosarcomas are now treated with surgery, irradiation, and chemotherapy. There are now some reported survivals in these cases.

Bibliography

1. Ash, J. E., and Raum, M. *An Atlas of Otolaryngic Pathology.* Armed Forces Institute of Pathology, Washington, D. C., 1949.
2. English, G. M. *Otolaryngology: A Textbook.* Harper & Row, Hagerstown, Md., 1976.
3. Paparella, M. M., and Shumrick, D. A. (Eds.). Otolaryngology. In *The Ear,* vol. 2. W. B. Saunders Co., Philadelphia, 1973.

Chapter 2.8

Interpretation of Test Results

Janet M. Zarnoch

Sound can be transmitted to the inner ear in two ways: through the air conduction (AC) pathway or the bone conduction (BC) pathway. Air conduction refers to airborne sounds which are funneled into the external ear canal, causing the eardrum to vibrate which in turn sets up vibrations in the ossicles so that the stapes begins to vibrate in the oval window, causing fluid waves within the cochlea. The fluid displacement within the cochlea causes a mechanical bending of the hair cells of the organ of Corti, which triggers the neural impulses of the auditory nerve at the peripheral level.

The bone conduction pathway, on the other hand, bypasses the conductive mechanism of the ear and stimulates the hair cells of the cochlea directly through the bones of the skull.

Hearing losses can be classified according to three main types: *conductive, sensorineural, and mixed hearing loss.*

1. Conductive hearing loss. As the word "conductive" implies, this type of hearing loss occurs when there is disease or obstruction involving the conductive mechanism of the ear. The conductive mechanism includes the external auditory canal, tympanic membrane, and the middle ear space and structures.

a. Common causes: see Chapter 2.2.

b. Manifestations: see Chapter 2.2.

2. Sensorineural hearing loss. A sensorineural hearing impairment occurs when there is damage to the sensory end organ, hair cells, or the auditory nerve.

a. Common causes: see Chapter 2.1.

b. Manifestations: see Chapter 2.1.

3. Mixed hearing loss. A mixed hearing loss has a conductive and sensorineural component. Thus, bone and air conduction thresholds are depressed (see Chapters 2.1 and 2.2 for detailed discussion).

TUNING FORKS

When a patient complains of a decrease in hearing sensitivity, either unilaterally or bilaterally, he is frequently referred to an otolaryngologist for an otologic evaluation, which usually includes a audiologic assessment. The audiologist utilizes an instrument known as an audiometer to obtain a precise, accurate view of a patient's hearing function over a specified frequency range. However, prior to discussing pure tone audiometry, we must discuss the traditional method of evaluating hearing function, namely, tuning forks. Tuning forks assist the physician in making a qualitative judgment of hearing, as well as confirming the pure tone audiogram. The two tuning forks most widely used are those with a frequency of 512 Hz and 1024 Hz. Lower frequency forks are not used because the vibrations are more often "felt" than heard. As for forks with a frequency above 1024 Hz, the vibrations decay too quickly and are therefore not as applicable as the 1024-Hz fork. Tuning forks are inexpensive, easy to use, and never malfunction. The findings, however, are subject to misinterpretation.

There are several standard tuning fork tests which are included in the otologic evaluation. A brief description of the test procedures, as well as interpretation of results, follows. The Weber and Rinne tuning fork tests work best when carried out at an intensity near the patient's threshold for hearing.

Weber Test

The Weber test detects any difference in hearing between the two ears.

Procedure

The 512-Hz tuning fork is struck once on the heel of the physician's shoe, or some equally firm surface. The overtones are dampened by touching the fork at its base with the finger, and placing the vibrating fork in the midline on the frontal bone. The patient is asked to lateralize the sound, *i.e.*, does he hear it in the right ear, left ear, or in the center of his head? Some patients may have difficulty determining where they hear the tone. In those cases, the vibrating fork may be placed directly on the patient's upper two front teeth, usually resulting in a definite response as to where they are hearing the tone. False teeth work just as well as real ones.

Interpretation

Weber Midline. A midline Weber indicates that the right and left ears hear *equally*, or are *symmetrical*. It does not necessarily mean that hearing is normal, as persons with symmetrical sensorineural losses, or symmetrical conductive losses, as well as normal-hearing persons, will demonstrate midline sensation of the sound.

Weber Lateralized to One Ear. A Weber which lateralizes to one ear may mean the following:

1. If the ear which hears the sound is the person's "poorer hearing ear," then this suggests a unilateral conductive loss in that ear, or a bilateral conductive or mixed loss which has a greater air-bone gap in the ear which is hearing the sound.

2. If the ear which hears the sound is the person's "better hearing ear" it is usually indicative of a unilateral sensorineural hearing loss in the opposite ear, or a bilateral asymmetrical sensorineural loss, where the ear hearing the tuning fork has the better hearing (or the least sensorineural impairment).

3. A person feigning a unilateral hearing impairment will also demonstrate lateralization of the vibrating fork to their "better or *only hearing ear.*" This Weber finding will agree with their complaint of a non-hearing or dead ear, but when the Rinne tuning fork test is administered, the malingerer will slip up and reveal the inorgan-

icity of his complaint. This will be discussed in the section on the Rinne test.

Weber Not Heard. The only instance when a tuning fork will not be heard is when a patient has a bilateral severe to profound hearing loss. If the *loss exceeds* the loudness level of the tuning fork, no sound will be heard. However, if the fork is struck with sufficient force, a louder sound will be emitted, which when placed on the forehead or teeth, may be "felt" rather than heard.

Rinne Test

The Rinne test is a test of air and bone conduction.

Procedure

The tuning fork is again struck lightly and the stem is placed firmly on the flat part of the mastoid bone just behind the upper portion of the pinna. When the patient no longer hears the fork, it is brought out and the tines of the fork held 2–3 inches lateral to the ear canal. It should now be heard fairly loudly. If air conduction is louder than bone conduction (AC > BC), the result is normal (positive Rinne). If bone conduction is louder than air conduction (BC > AC) (abnormal), the result is said to be a negative Rinne.

Interpretation

Positive Rinne (AC > BC). Normal-hearing persons as well as those with sensorineural loss will reveal a positive Rinne when they hear sounds longer by AC than by BC. The reason is that it takes considerably more energy to generate bone conducted sounds.

Negative Rinne (BC > AC). The only instance in which a patient will hear better by BC than AC is if a conductive component (air-bone gap) greater than 25–30 dB exists in the ear being tested. The reason for this is apparent; in the ear with a purely conductive hearing loss, hearing by air conduction is depressed, and bone conduction hearing is normal. In one instance, a false negative Rinne will result; when a dead ear (no useful hearing) is tested, the fork will actually be heard by bone conduction in the good ear. However, when the air conduction is tested, the fork will not be heard. The patient may be unaware of this crossing over.

On occasion a patient may state that he hears the AC and BC sounds equally loud. In that case, the patient may have a conductive element present but not of sufficient magnitude (25–30 dB) to hear better by BC. The Rinne results would be recorded as Rinne ±.

If a person is feigning a unilateral hearing loss, he will frequently report no response for that ear for AC as well as BC. This should alert the examiner immediately, as the patient should have reported hearing the BC sounds in his good ear. A bone conducting mechanism placed anywhere on the skull stimulates both cochleas almost simultaneously. Therefore, if a patient reports one good ear and one bad, then he should also legitimately report hearing the sound from the tuning fork placed on either mastoid, in the better hearing ear.

Schwabach Test

The Schwabach test is a test of bone conduction.

Procedure

The examiner strikes the tuning fork lightly and places the vibrating fork on the patient's mastoid. The patient is instructed to signal when he can no longer hear the tone. At that point the examiner places the fork on his own mastoid to see if he hears the fork.

Interpretation

If the examiner hears the tone from the vibrating fork after the patient has reportedly stopped hearing it, then a decrease in the patient's bone conduction sensitivity is present. If, however, the examiner also does not hear the tone from the tuning fork, then it can be said that sensitivity for bone conduction is normal. It is acceptable to record the Schwabach test results in terms of whether the patient's bone conduction was better, worse, or equal to the examiner's.

Test for Recruitment

Recruitment is the perception of an abnormal growth of loudness. It is seen in cases where there is hair cell damage (cochlear sensorineural hearing loss) as opposed to retrocochlear (VIIIth nerve hearing loss).

Procedure

Strike the tuning fork lightly and place it a few inches from the patient's ear, alternating back and forth between the right and left ear, continually asking the patient if the vibrating fork is of equal loudness or if it sounds louder on one side or the other. The fork is then struck successively harder to produce greater loudness as the test is repeated. This is usually, although not always, carried out when the one ear shows a greater sensorineural loss than the other.

Interpretation

1. No change in loudness between the two ears. This indicates that there is no recruitment and is a normal finding.

2. Heard *louder* in the poorer ear as intensity increases. This means that recruitment is present in the poorer ear.

In summary, tuning fork tests provide us with useful clinical information, but only in a qualitative sense. The Weber test tells us if there is a hearing impairment present, and if one ear is worse than the other. The Rinne test provides information on the type of impairment which is present. In addition, the tuning forks can be used to uncover a patient feigning a hearing impairment. It is important to note, however, that tuning forks do not give quantitative information, *i.e., how much* hearing loss is present. Only by utilizing an audiometer to assess hearing function can the degree and slope of hearing impairment be accurately determined.

PURE TONE AUDIOMETRY

The conventional audiologic assessment consists of obtaining pure tone thresholds across the frequency from 250 Hz to 8000 Hz, thresholds for speech reception, and speech discrimination scores. Each of these will be discussed separately in the following sections.

Some brief definitions of the basic physical principles underlying pure tone audiometry are supplied for better understanding of the subject.

Frequency. The number of vibrations of a sound wave. Traditionally frequency has been referred to as the number of cycles per second, but is now referred to as hertz (Hz). For example, if a sound wave has 1000 vibrations (1000 compressions and rarefactions), we say that it has a frequency of 1000 Hz. Pitch is the psychologic correlate of frequency and refers to a person perceiving a high frequency sound as having a high pitch, and a low frequency as having a low pitch.

Intensity. The intensity of sound is measured in logarithmic units, *decibels (dB)* which represent a ratio between the intensity of the sound measured and a reference level of intensity. Loudness is the psychologic correlate to intensity, and refers to a person's perception of a high intensity sound as being very loud, and a low intensity sound as being very soft.

The intensity scale we are concerned with in pure tone audiometry is the *Hearing Level (HL) scale*, or the *Hearing Threshold Level (HTL) scale*, which is a *relative* scale based on *averages of normal human hearing.* The HL scale ranges from 0 dB HL to 110 dB HL, with 0 dB HL being an extremely "soft sound," barely detectable by normal-hearing listeners, and 110 dB HL being a "very loud" sound to the normal ear. A jet engine has an intensity of approximately 110 dB HL. Normal conversational speech has an intensity of 40–50 dB HL.

Threshold. Threshold refers to the lowest intensity level at which a person can detect the presence of sound at least 50% of the time. The threshold for normal hearing is considered to be 0–15 dB HL. If a person demonstrates a threshold greater (worse) than 15 dB at any given frequency he is said to have a hearing loss at that frequency.

Pure Tone. A pure tone has only one frequency, with no overtones. The pure tones utilized in pure tone audiometric testing are 250 Hz, 500 Hz, 1000 Hz, 2000 Hz, 4000 Hz, and 8000 Hz. When a patient's hearing is evaluated with pure tone audiometry, the responses obtained at each frequency are referred to as "pure tone thresholds." The pure tone thresholds are plotted on a graph known as an audiogram, resulting in a graphic representation of hearing function for octave frequencies between 250 Hz and 8000 Hz.

Audiometer. The audiometer is an instrument used in pure tone audiometry to measure hearing sensitivity. It generates pure tones of various frequencies and ranges of intensities, which can be controlled to obtain precise, accurate, and reliable threshold responses from patients.

Air Conduction Testing

The patient is tested in a soundproof room using headphones. He is asked to respond when he hears a tone, even if it is very faint. Pure tone testing always begins at the frequency of 1000 Hz and at an intensity level above threshold, usually about 40 dB. In this way, the patient is certain to hear the tone, and understand the task clearly. The intensity is gradually decreased in 10-dB steps until the patient no longer responds. The intensity is then increased in 5-dB steps until a response is again noted. Once again, intensity is decreased by 10 dB and increased by 5 dB, until the patient responds at a particular level 50% of the time. This 50% point is considered the threshold of hearing for that pure tone and is plotted on the audiogram. The symbols used for threshold responses are 0's to depict right ear responses and X's to show left ear responses. This procedure of obtaining thresholds is repeated for 2000 Hz, 4000 Hz, 8000 Hz, 500 Hz, and 250 Hz, in that sequence, for both ears. Testing for bone conduction follows the air conduction test.

Bone Conduction Testing

The earphones used during air conduction testing are removed. A thin metal headband attached to a small bone conduction vibrator is now placed on the patient's head so that the vibrator portion (or oscillator) rests securely on the flat portion of the mastoid just behind the upper pinna. It is important to make sure that the oscillator is not touching the pinna, otherwise there may be contamination of the stimulus tones by air conduction. The patient is instructed to again listen for very soft tones and raise a hand every time one is heard.

If a patient has normal hearing by air conduction, it is not necessary to perform bone conduction testing, as bone conduction will also be normal. The audiometer is calibrated so that bone conduction thresholds can never be better than air conduction thresholds.

Masking

When there is a 40-dB or greater difference in hearing levels between the two ears, it is necessary to employ masking. This refers to keeping the good ear "busy" while the poorer ear is under test. If masking is not used and a sufficiently loud tone is presented to the "bad" ear, the tone "crosses over" to the "good" ear and results in an erroneous threshold. Masking is accomplished by putting noise into the better ear. With this method we are sure that we are testing each ear separately. Masking, when performed, will be clearly noted on the face of the audiogram.

Speech Audiometry

The evaluation of a patient's ability to hear and understand speech is a critical part of the audiologic evaluation. Speech audiometry consists of two separate testing procedures. The first is to obtain a *Speech Reception Threshold* (SRT), and the second to obtain a *Speech Discrimination Score* (SDS). Each of these procedures is discussed in the following sections.

Speech Reception Threshold (SRT). The SRT is the lowest intensity at which a patient can correctly repeat two-syllable words 50% of the time. The two-syllable words are called spondee words and include words such as baseball, ice cream, sidewalk, and hot dog. The main purpose for obtaining an SRT is to check the accuracy of the pure tone average (PTA), *i.e.*, the average of the thresholds for the speech frequencies of 500, 1000, and 2000 Hz. The SRT and PTA should agree with ±6 dB. If there is a disagreement greater than 6 dB, it will typically be that the SRT is "better" than the PTA, since speech "sounds louder" than pure tones of the same intensity. A disagreement between the SRT and PTA is an important clue to the audiologist that the patient may not be responding at his true level of hearing, and may in fact be feigning a hearing loss. The second purpose for obtaining an SRT is that it determines the level at which speech discrimination testing will be performed.

Speech   Discrimination   Test.   The speech discrimination test determines, in part, a patient's ability to *understand* speech. Unlike the test for SRT, the speech discrimination test utilizes phonetically balanced (PB) monosyllabic words such as tree, please, smile, etc. The problem with routine discrimination testing, however, is that is does not tell us how much difficulty a hearing-impaired patient is having in everyday   communicative   encounters. Thus, we must look at the speech discrimination scores as only part of a much broader picture of communication function.

It should be pointed out that speech discrimination scores are affected mainly in sensorineural type hearing losses, and not in conductive type losses. Usually, if speech is made sufficiently loud to overcome the degree of conductive loss, the patient will have normal discrimination scores (80–100%). The reason discrimination ability remains good in view of conductive losses is that the inner ear is functioning *normally*. However, this is not the case in sensorineural loss where there is damage to the hair cells and/or VIIIth nerve. This damage interferes with normal intelligibility of speech. Speech is no longer heard clearly, but becomes "distorted." In addition, for the patient with a sensorineural loss, making the speech louder very often does not make speech clearer, but creates more distortion of the sounds, especially if recruitment is present. Hence, we usually see a decrease in speech discrimination scores in persons with sensorineural hearing losses. The patient with a loss only at 4000 and 8000 Hz will probably notice some slight difficulty in differentiating between high frequency speech such as /p/ and /b/, /t/ and /d/, /f/ and /v/, etc. However, the person with the more extensive loss across the frequencies will confuse many more speech sounds and will need to rely more heavily on visual cues for the understanding of speech.

Auditory Evaluation of Infants and Children

Infants and young children cannot be expected to respond to the traditional hand-raising technique of hearing testing. However, through alternate methods of audiologic evaluation infants can be accurately and reliably tested. From birth through 2 years of age, every normal infant goes through a very definite sequence of auditory maturation. At 3 months of age, or 8 months of age, an infant can be expected to respond to auditory stimuli in a very predictable manner. It is precisely the sequence of auditory maturation which allows us to test the infant and obtain consistent,   repeatable   behavioral   responses to sound. Correlating the infant's response to the auditory stimulus with the normal response pattern for that age, enables the audiologist to make a judgment about how the infant is hearing.

Testing   the   Infant   from   Birth   to   4 Months. From birth to 4 months of age noisemakers are utilized to assess hearing, and reflexive responses to sound are observed, such as the Moro reflex to a very loud sound (65 dB or greater). An eye blink or a slight head turn may also be observed as a response. Earphones are not used at this young age. Sounds are introduced through speakers in a sound-treated room, thus each ear cannot be tested separately. However, if an infant responds normally to sound, the audiologist knows that he has at least one normal hearing ear which is responding to the auditory stimuli. Audiologic test results for the newborn are usually written on an audiogram in the following manner: "Responds normally to soft and loud noisemakers. Large startle reflex to a moderately loud bell."

Testing the Older Infant. By the age of 4 months the normal infant begins to demonstrate a rudimentary head turn toward the direction of the sound source. The infant will localize sound on either side of him by 7 months of age. It is not until 21-24 months of age that an infant can locate a sound source coming from any angle of the room.

At approximately 4-6 months, we begin utilizing *Behavioral Observation Audiometry (BOA)*, which simply means observing and recording the infant's behavioral response to sound. Speech stimuli or warbled pure tones are presented at carefully controlled intensity levels, always proceeding in an ascending manner. The point is to determine the softest intensity level at which the infant will respond to the auditory stimulus. As the infant grows older, less intensity is required to observe the appropriate response. One should always try to elicit a startle reflex at 65 dB HL, as its presence or absence will confirm the other behavioral responses. Results from BOA are usually recorded on an audiogram as follows: "Localization to speech at 10 dB to the right and 15 dB to the left. Large startle reflex to speech at 65 dB." For the older infant the auditory information is a bit more concrete as compared to the newborn. However, the two ears still have not been tested separately. By 2-3 years of age, however, the child will usually tolerate the placement of earphones, and techniques such as *Conditioned Play Audiometry* can be utilized. In most cases by the time a child is 4-5 years old, a conventional hand-raising response to pure tones can be used accurately and reliably.

High Risk Register. The High Risk Register is another method of identifying hearing loss in infants. If a newborn conforms to any one of the following categories, he is considered to be *AT RISK* for hearing loss and is placed on the High Risk Regis-ter. The categories are:

1. History of hereditary childhood deafness.

2. Rubella or other nonbacterial intrauterine fetal infection (e.g., cytomegalovirus infections, herpes infection).

3. Defects of the ear, nose, or throat: malformed, low-set, or absent pinnae; cleft lip or palate (including submucous cleft); any residual abnormality of the otorhinolaryngeal system.

4. Birth weight less than 1500 g.

5. Bilirubin level greater than 20 mg/100 ml of serum.

Any newborn who is placed on the register automatically receives a thorough audiologic evaluation within the first few months of life, and at regular intervals during the first few years. Many familial types of hearing loss are not present at birth but develop sometime afterward. Thus, it is critical that an infant be followed audiologically, even if the hearing appears normal at birth.

Special Auditory Testing (Site of Lesion Testing)

When a physician is uncertain of the etiology of a sensorineural hearing loss he/she may order a series of special auditory tests to aid in diagnosis of the site of lesion. These auditory tests, referred to as the *Site of Lesion Test Battery,* are useful in differentiating between cochlear and retrocochlear lesions. A brief description of some of the commonly used tests in the battery will be presented.

Short Increment Sensitivity Test (SISI)

Procedure. The SISI test is administered by presenting a constant pure tone, 20 dB above threshold, to one ear at a time. Every 5 seconds the tone is increased by 1 dB. A series of 20 1-dB increments ("pips") are presented, and the patient is asked to raise his index finger each time he hears a "pip." For each correct pip the patient responds to, a value of 5% is assigned. The SISI test is based on the fact that ears with lesions in the cochlea can perceive small changes in the intensity of a tone, in cases where persons with normal hearing, conductive losses, or retrocochlear lesions cannot.

Interpretation

SISI Test Score	Site of Lesion
55–100%	Cochlear
25–50%	Nonlocalizing
0–20%	Retrocochlear*

* Normal hearing ears as well as those with conductive losses will also hear only 0–20% of the increments.

Tone Decay Test

Procedure. The tone decay test is also administered at a suprathreshold level. A continuous pure tone, 5–10 dB above threshold, is presented. The patient is asked to keep his hand raised as long as he continues to hear the tone, and to drop his hand if he stops hearing it. The object of the tone decay test is to determine the intensity level at which the patient can "hold" (or hear) the tone for 1 full minute. Every time the patient drops his hand, indicating that he can no longer hear it, the tone is increased by 5 dB. This procedure continues until the tone no longer decays, and the patient hears it continually for 60 seconds. Retrocochlear lesions are associated with abnormally rapid decay of the tone.

Interpretation

Amount of Tone Decay	Site of Lesion
0–15 dB	Cochlear or normal*
15–30 dB	Cochlear
30 dB or greater	Retrocochlear

* Normal hearing ears as well as those with conductive losses will also show 0–15 dB of tone decay.

Alternate Binaural Loudness Balance Test (ABLB)

Procedure. The ABLB test is based on the phenomenon of "recruitment," which is defined as an abnormal rapid growth in loudness. The ear having a sensorineural loss with a cochlear site of lesion demonstrates recruitment. The ABLB consists of presenting pure tones at various suprathreshold levels, alternating the tone between the two ears, and asking the patient to indicate when the tones sound equally loud for both ears. Ideally, one of the ears should have normal hearing, and the other a sensorineural loss. In that way the loudness function can be compared; *i.e.*, the audiologist can determine whether the hearing-impaired ear demonstrates recruitment as compared to normal loudness growth in the normal hearing ear.

Interpretation

ABLB Results	Site of Lesion
Recruitment present	Cochlear
No recruitment	Retrocochlear*

* Normal and conductive hearing losses show no recruitment on the ABLB test.

Acoustic Reflex Decay Test

Procedure. Acoustic reflex thresholds are obtained at 500 and 1000 Hz (see following section, Impedance Audiometry, for procedure for obtaining acoustic reflex thresholds). A pure tone stimulus 10 dB above threshold is presented for 10 seconds. The audiologist observes the compliance change meter to determine if the reflex can be sustained for the full 10 seconds of stimulation. If the amplitude of the reflex decreases 50% in 10 seconds, reflex decay is present. The test is *not* performed at 2000 and 4000 Hz owing to the fact that many normal ears will display reflex decay at those frequencies.

Interpretation. Normal hearing ears will not demonstrate reflex decay. In ears with conductive losses, if reflexes are present, no decay will be observed. In retrocochlear lesions, abnormal reflex findings will be present.

Brainstem-Evoked Response (BSER) Audiometry

BSER is rapidly gaining clinical acceptance in the auditory evaluation of difficult to test populations and site of lesion testing. BSER consists of presenting pure tones of short duration through an earphone and picking up minute brainstem electrical responses which are computer analyzed, and displayed as a complex wave pattern. BSER does not yield a conventional audiogram, but rather specifies within a fairly close intensity range what the auditory thresholds are for particular frequencies. In retrocochlear lesions there is an asymmetry in the latency of responses between the two ears.

BSER is particularly useful with children, retardates, and other difficult to test populations. Responses are not affected by sedation and supply valuable information in terms of "quantity" of peripheral auditory function.

IMPEDANCE AUDIOMETRY

Impedance audiometry is an integral part of the auditory evaluation, particularly with infants, children, and other difficult to test populations. One of the most valuable applications of this test procedure is the identification of those patients in need of medical referral for middle ear disease. Impedance audiometry is an objective method of measuring the integrity of the middle ear system.

The impedance test battery consists of three separate evaluative procedures, tympanometry, static compliance, and acoustic reflex thresholds, the results of which should be viewed as a whole. The entire battery takes just a few minutes to administer and can be utilized easily and effectively with any age group. The following section presents a description of each portion of the impedance test battery, as well as how the tests are administered, and results interpreted.

Tympanometry

Tympanometry is an objective measure of the mobility (or compliance) of the tympanic membrane as air pressure is varied in the external canal. Tympanometry is useful in detecting various conductive mechanism abnormalities such as otitis media, tympanic membrane perforation, and ossicular chain disruption or fixation.

Procedure

An electroacoustic impedance meter with a headset attached is used to administer the impedance test battery. There are three openings in the probe tip portion of the headset, which are connected to the following: the first opening emits a constant pure tone, the second opening leads to an air pressure pump which allows changes in air pressure to be made within the external auditory canal, and the third opening leads to a pickup microphone which measures how much sound is reflected back into the external canal. Thus, the electroacoustic impedance meter, commonly referred to as an "impedance bridge," or simply "bridge," can be thought of as an instrument for measuring sound pressure level. The constant tone which is emitted from the probe tip is a low frequency 220-Hz tone with an intensity level of 80 dB SPL. The reason for the use of such a low frequency probe tone is that the middle ear is a "stiffness"-controlled system, and is therefore more sensitive to lower frequencies.

To perform tympanometry, the headset is placed on the patient's head, with the probe tip securely inserted into one ear to obtain an airtight seal. The air pressure meter is set to introduce +200 mm H_2O into the external auditory canal. The air pressure is gradually decreased in 50-mm steps from +200 mm H_2O to at least −200 mm H_2O (and when indicated, to −400 mm H_2O). As air pressure is varied the compliance change meter indicates the precise compliance changes of the tympanic membrane. The compliance changes are recorded for each 50-mm change in pressure.

The results from tympanometry are recorded on a graph called a tympanogram. Air pressure changes are recorded on the horizontal axis, and changes in compliance on the vertical axis. Thus, one can record the mobility of the eardrum as changes in air pressure are effected. The tympanic membrane reaches the point of maximum compliance when the air pressure in the external canal equals that in the middle ear. Thus, one can make an indirect measurement of existing middle ear pressure by observing where the highest point of compliance falls on the tympanogram.

Interpretation

Tympanograms are generally classified according to an "A-B-C" system.

Type A. The type A tympanogram represents a normal, intact, mobile eardrum. The maximum point of compliance is generally found at, or near, normal atmospheric pressure, ± 50 mm H_2O. Patients with normal hearing, as well as those with purely sensorineural impairments, will yield a normal type A tympanogram. Patients with conductive impairments *will usually not* demonstrate type A curves, *with one exception*—some patients with otosclerosis.

Type A_D. The type A_D tympanogram is found in ears with ossicular discontinuity, hence, the sub-D stands for "discontinuity." One may see this A_D curve in normal ears which have an unusually flaccid eardrum, such as those with a large monomeric membrane.

Type A_s. The type A_s tympanogram is found in ears which display a somewhat stiffened tympanic membrane. The sub-s in this instance stands for "stiffness." An otosclerotic ear may sometimes demonstrate an A_s curve. A thickened or heavily scarred drum, as well as tympanosclerosis, can also be the cause of an A_s curve.

Type B. A type B tympanogram represents a nonmobile tympanic membrane which does not have a point of maximum compliance. It is a fairly "flat" curve, and is frequently referred to as such. The reason for the flat appearance is that most of the sound pressure from the 220-Hz probe tone is reflected back into the external canal due to a very stiff middle ear system. Any one of the following conditions may produce a type B or "flat" curve:

1. Otitis media.
2. Perforation.
3. Pressure equalization tubes in the tympanic membrane.
4. Impacted cerumen.

Type C. The type C tympanogram is found in ears with intact, mobile eardrums; however, maximum compliance is reached at a negative point of pressure, i.e., ≥ -100 mm H_2O. Typically, a type C curve is caused by poor eustachian tube function, as shown by the negative middle ear pressure. A type C curve may or may not be associated with the presence of fluid in the middle ear.

Static Compliance

Static compliance determines the compliance of the middle ear system while at rest. In other words, a volume measurement is made in cubic centimeters.

Procedure

Two volume measurements are obtained. The first measurement is made by introducing +200 mm H_2O into the external canal (a condition creating poor compliance) and balancing the compliance needle straight up at zero. One then reads the cursor scale and notes the volume in cubic centimeters and records this as the C_1 value. The second measurement (C_2 value) is made with the tympanic membrane at its point of maximum compliance. The C_1 and C_2 measurements have no value when viewed independently. C_1 must be subtracted from C_2, resulting in a much smaller value, which reflects only the compliance of the ear at rest, and not the volume of the external canal.

Interpretation

The normal range for static compliance values is between 0.30 cc and 1.60 cc. A patient with stiffness of the middle ear system may demonstrate a value less than 0.30 cc. Likewise, if a middle ear system is extremely compliant, a static compliance value greater than 1.60 cc may be revealed. For example, patients with otosclerosis or otitis media will often have a static compliance value below the normal limit of 0.30 cc. Conversely, patients with ossicular discontinuity will demonstrate values above 1.60 cc.

Physical Volume Test

The physical volume test (PVT) is a unique application of impedance audiometry which can be performed during the evaluation of static compliance. The PVT is the C_1 value. The C_1 value usually does not exceed 1.0 cc. with an intact drum, because the impedance bridge is measuring only a tiny, hard-walled cavity between the probe tip and the drum membrane. However, if a perforation or a patent ventilating tube is present in the tympanic membrane, the bridge will make a volume measurement of a much larger cavity which now includes the middle ear space. Thus, a large volume of 4.0 cc, 5.0 cc, or greater will be recorded.

The PVT is very helpful in differentiating type B tympanograms. For example, a fluid-filled ear with an intact drum will yield a type B tympanogram, and an ear with a perforation will also yield a type B tympanogram. Hence, the only way to distinguish between the two would be to take a C_1 measurement. The ear with the perforation would show a considerably larger volume than the ear with the intact drum.

The PVT is also helpful in identifying whether or not a ventilating tube is open or blocked. Here again, the ear with a patent tube would show a large volume, and a small volume would be present if the tube were blocked.

Acoustic Reflex Threshold

Acoustic stimulation in one ear with a sufficiently loud sound (between 70 dB HTL and 100 dB HTL) will cause the stapedius muscle in the middle ear to contract bilaterally. This contraction of the stapedius muscle is referred to as the acoustic reflex and is innervated by the VIIth cranial nerve (facial nerve). The classical theory assigns a protective role to the acoustic reflex, stating that loud sounds cause the stapedius muscle to contract, which reduces the level of sound reaching the inner ear, thus protecting it from possible insult.

Procedure

The impedance headset is placed on the patient's head. Pure tones ranging in intensity from 65 dB HTL to 115 dB HTL, and covering the octave frequencies from 250 Hz to 4000 Hz are introduced into the earphone of the headset. Testing always begins at low intensity levels and ascends from there. Typically the test begins at 250 Hz up through 4000 Hz; however, frequently acoustic reflexes are obtained only at 500 Hz, 1000 Hz, and 2000 Hz. As the stimulus is presented to the earphone ear, the probe tip in the opposite ear records changes in the compliance of the tympanic membrane as the muscle contracts bilaterally. Thus, the examiner watches the compliance change meter as the stimulus is given. When there is a deflection of the needle, a reflex has occurred. It should be mentioned that the acoustic reflex test is always performed with the ear at maximum compliance so that changes in compliance of the drum may be most easily observed. Tympanometry administered prior to reflex testing establishes exactly where the point of maximum compliance lies.

Interpretation

Normal Acoustic Reflex Threshold. A normal acoustic reflex threshold will be obtained between 70 dB HTL and 100 dB HTL. The following conditions will present normal thresholds:

1. Normal hearing.
2. Mild to moderate sensorineural hearing impairment.

Elevated Acoustic Reflex Threshold. Acoustic reflex thresholds are considered elevated when the threshold level equals or exceeds 105 dB HTL. The following may present elevated thresholds:

1. Moderate to severe sensorineural impairment with accompanying recruitment.
2. Mild unilateral conductive hearing impairments (less than 30 dB). (This is quite variable as even a minimal amount of conductive involvement can obscure the measurement of compliance change of the drum.)

Absent Acoustic Reflex Threshold

When no acoustic reflex is present it may be due to one of the following:

1. Bilateral   profound   sensorineural

hearing loss (thus, the absence of acoustic reflexes in a child suspected of having a severe sensorineural hearing loss will confirm the suspicion).

2. Unilateral conductive hearing loss of 30 dB or greater.

3. Young children may not have acoustic reflexes (24% of these 5 years and younger).

4. Bilateral conductive hearing loss.

5. Acoustic tumor (reflex may be absent on the earphone ear).

6. Facial nerve paralysis (reflex may be absent on the "probe tip" ear).

7. Of the normal hearing population, 4% have no demonstrable acoustic reflex.

8. Fixation of the ossicular chain (otosclerosis, malleus ligament, etc.).

Ipsilateral Acoustic Reflex Threshold

In most clinical situations, the test for acoustic reflex thresholds is accomplished in a contralateral fashion, *i.e.*, the stimulus is presented to the earphone ear, and the reflex is recorded from the probe, or contralateral ear. However, there are instances in which one may wish to test only the ipsilateral pathways. In those cases, the stimulus is presented to the probe tip ear, and the reflex is recorded from the same ear. There are still many difficulties with ipsilateral reflex testing, and typically only the "presence" or "absence" of the ipsilateral reflex threshold is reported.

Acoustic Reflex Threshold Decay Test

A special application of the acoustic reflex is utilized in the auditory site of lesion test battery. Normally, the stapedius muscle should be able to sustain contraction for at least 10 seconds, without a significant decline in amplitude. However, in 10% of acoustic tumor cases, the stapedius reflex will decay to less than half of the original contraction amplitude in a 10-second time period. The acoustic reflex decay test is discussed in greater detail in this chapter, under Special Auditory Testing (Site of Lesion Testing).

Facial Nerve Function

Since the stapedius muscle receives its innervation from the facial nerve, it is possible to gain information on facial nerve function in patients with facial paralysis. The presence or absence of the reflex is useful in differentiating the site of lesion. Unlike the reflex decay test which tests the afferent nervous systems, the facial nerve function tests the efferent system. Therefore, the "probe" ear is the ear under test. If the reflex is absent on the side of the paralysis, the site of lesion is probably higher than the point where the nerve branches off to the stapedius tendon. If the reflex is "present," then one may assume that the damage is below the branching off point. This application of the acoustic reflex is particularly useful in monitoring facial nerve function in patients with deteriorating function, or those patients who have undergone a surgical procedure to restore facial nerve activity.

INTERPRETATION AND CORRELATION OF TEST RESULTS

This section is devoted to displaying examples of typical audiologic results correlated with various types of ear disease.

Normal Hearing

Normal hearing ranges from 0 to 15 dB.
Case 1 (Fig. 2.8.1):
Pure tone thresholds: air conduction (AC) and bone conduction (BC) thresholds within the range of normal, 0–15 dB.
Speech reception threshold (SRT): normal, agrees with pure tone average (PTA).
Speech discrimination: excellent, 100%.
Tympanograms: type A bilaterally.
Acoustic reflex thresholds: elicited at normal intensity levels (70–100 dB HL).
Weber test: midline.
Rinne test: positive, (AC > BC).

Conductive Hearing Losses

(A reminder that whenever there is a difference of 10 dB or more between the air and bone conduction thresholds, an air-

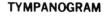
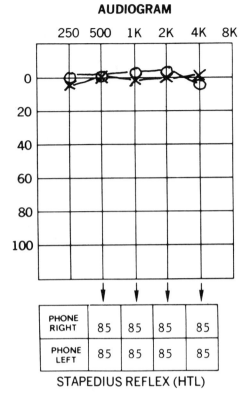
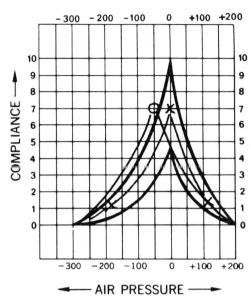
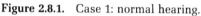

Figure 2.8.1. Case 1: normal hearing.

bone gap is present and the loss is a conductive loss.)

Mild Conductive Loss

A conductive loss is considered mild when it ranges from 15 to 30 dB.

Case 2 (bilateral loss) (Fig. 2.8.2):

Pure tone thresholds: BC thresholds normal; AC thresholds, 20 dB.

Speech reception threshold (SRT): 20 dB bilaterally, agrees with PTA.

Speech discrimination: excellent, 96% bilaterally (would expect this with mild conductive loss).

Tympanograms: type C bilaterally, showing significant negative middle ear pressure.

Acoustic reflexes: elevated reflexes bilaterally (110 dB) consistent with mild degree of conductive loss.

Weber test: midline.

Rinne test: positive (AC > BC), consist-

ent with degree of air-bone gap, *i.e.*, less than 25 dB.

Severe Conductive Loss

A severe conductive loss ranges from 45 to 65 dB. A purely conductive loss can never exceed 60 dB due to the fact that at approximately 60 dB one begins to hear sounds via bone conduction.

Case 3 (unilateral loss) (Fig. 2.8.3):

Pure tone thresholds: LE, AC, and BC thresholds normal; RE has maximum air-bone gap with BC at 0 dB and AC at 60 dB.

Speech reception threshold (SRT): LE normal; RE 60 dB.

Speech discrimination: LE excellent, 100%; RE good, 88%.

Tympanograms: LE, type A; RE, type A_D, suggesting either an unusually mobile TM, or ossicular discontinuity.

Acoustic reflexes: absent bilaterally,

consistent with degree of unilateral conductive loss.

Weber test: lateralized to RE, the ear with air-bone gap.

Rinne test: LE, positive (AC > BC); RE, negative (BC > AC).

Unilateral "Dead" Ear

A unilateral "dead" ear refers to an ear which has very little, or no measurable hearing. In many patients with one dead ear the hearing in the opposite ear is entirely normal.

Case 4 (right "dead" ear) (Fig. 2.8.4):

Pure tone thresholds: RE, NR to A/C or B/C; LE, AC and BC, 0 dB.

Speech reception threshold (SRT): RE, NR; LE, 0 dB.

Speech discrimination: RE, NR; LE, 100%.

Tympanograms: type A bilaterally.

Acoustic reflexes: stimulate RE, NR; stimulate LE, normal levels.

Weber test: lateralized to the only hearing ear, LE.

Rinne test: LE, positive (AC > BC); RE, heard in LE when fork placed on mastoid.

VESTIBULAR EVALUATION

The maintenance of equilibrium is dependent upon the interaction of three sensory systems: proprioceptive, visual, and vestibular. Although all of the pathways are not completely understood at this time, there are extensive, complex neural connections among these three systems which effectively contribute to man's orientation in space. It is no wonder, then, that the patient complaining of "dizziness" can often present a puzzling picture to the physician. Since the primary sensory receptors for equilibrium are located in the ves-

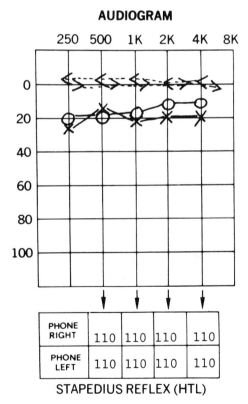

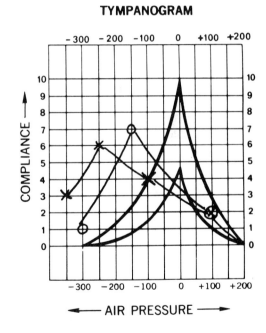

Figure 2.8.2. Case 2: mild conductive loss (bilateral).

tibular apparatus of the inner ear, the vestibular labyrinth is frequently the initial suspect area of dysfunction.

The peripheral vestibular system consists of three semicircular canals, the utricle, and the saccule. The receptors in the utricle and saccule are called *maculae*, and respond to linear acceleration, e.g., riding in a car, or going up or down in an elevator. Within the ampulla ending of each semicircular canal is located the *crista* which responds to angular acceleration (*i.e.*, rotation about a central axis).

Clinical Vestibular Tests

There are a number of evaluative techniques which can be quickly and easily utilized in any clinical setting to obtain some idea about the function of the vestibular apparatus. Of course one can always employ the Romberg, tandem walk, finger to nose, and pastpointing tests. These are generally considered to be tests of cerebellar function, and do not readily give information concerning the laterality of a vestibular lesion. The caloric test is perhaps the best method available for determining if a peripheral vestibular lesion exists, and localizing it to the right or left labyrinth. A screening caloric can be performed in a matter of minutes with little discomfort to the patient, and minimal equipment. In fact, a screening caloric procedure requires only cold tap water, a 20-ml syringe with a 15-gauge blunt needle, and that the patient be positioned with his head in the caloric test position, *i.e.*, the head tilted 60° backward from a sitting position, placing the horizontal semicircular canal in a vertical position which is necessary for maximal thermal stimulation, or the head elevated 30° from a supine position. The water can then be injected into the right external ear canal at a rate of approximately 1 ml per second, so that the cold water is

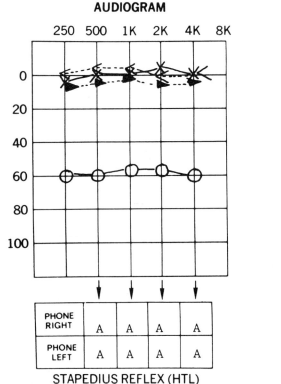

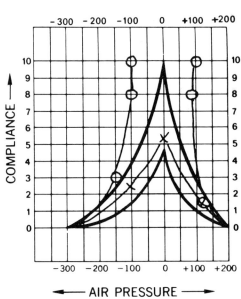

Figure 2.8.3. Case 3: severe conductive loss (unilateral).

AUDIOGRAM

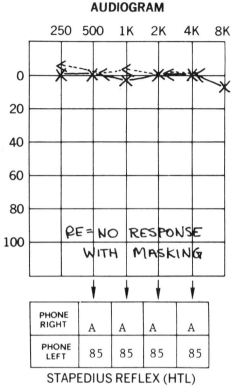

TYMPANOGRAM

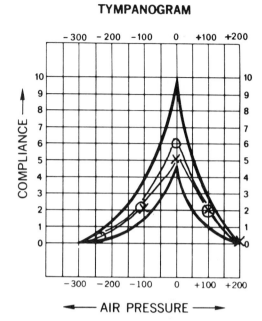

Figure 2.8.4. Case 4: right "dead" ear.

in contact with the tympanic membrane for 20 seconds. A rest period of at least 5 minutes follows the initial irrigation so that the temporal bone and endolymph fluid within the semicircular canals can return to normal temperature levels. The procedure is then repeated with the left ear. When cold water is used for the irrigations, a nystagmus beating away from the irrigated ear should result, *i.e.,* cold water in the right ear produces a left-beating nystagmus, cold water in the left ear produces a right-beating nystagmus. It should be noted that nystagmus is identified by the direction of the fast phase, as it is more readily observable than the slow phase. If this initial screening procedure does not yield an observable nystagmic response, the process can be repeated with ice water in an effort to effect maximal stimulation.

There are two important considerations when employing the caloric test as a screening device: (1) mental tasking for patient alertness, and (2) utilization of Frenzel's glasses. It is important to assign the patient mental tasks such as counting to 100 by 3's or 4's, so that he does not try to inhibit any eye movement or vertigo. The use of Frenzel glasses (+20 diopter lenses), in addition to providing easy visualization of the patient's eyes, also prevents the patient from visually fixing on an external object, thereby preventing diminution of the nystagmic response. Although results from this method of caloric testing are subjective and do not allow for quantitative measurements, it is a very useful procedure in determining whether the labyrinths appear to be functioning normally, or hypoactively. However, in those cases in which more definitive and precise information is required, a more complete vestibular evaluation can be obtained through the use of electronystagmography.

Electronystagmography (ENG)

Electronystagmography (ENG) is a clinical test of vestibular function and evaluates only the status of the semicircular canals. However, only indirect vestibular information is gained from ENG, as the measurements obtained result from semicircular canal effect on the ocular muscles. The use of ENG then, presupposes an intact oculomotor system.

ENG is an electrical recording of eye movements, and is based on the *corneoretinal potential*. The eye functions as an electrical dipole, with the cornea maintaining a positive charge and the retina a negative charge. If electrodes are placed around the eyes, the voltage change in the corneoretinal potential caused by eye deflection can be amplified and recorded. It should be noted that electrodes will record eye movements only in the plane of the electrode pair. Hence, if a pair of electrodes are placed at the outer canthus of each eye, only horizontal eye movements will be recorded. Similarly, for electrodes placed above and below the eye, only vertical eye movements will be recorded. A rotary type of nystagmus *cannot* be recorded through ENG because in pure rotary motion the eye rotates about its electrical axis, therefore, no voltage change occurs across the electrodes.

There are numerous *advantages* to employing the ENG procedure: (1) by measuring the slow phase velocity of nystagmus, quantitative measurements of vestibular function are obtained, (2) it can provide objective documentation of a patient's subjective complaints, (3) it can be used to monitor vestibular function in high risk patients such as those receiving gentamicin or streptomycin, (4) it evaluates the vestibular function of each ear independently, through bithermal caloric irrigations, (5) it permits recording of nystagmus with the patient's eyes closed, which may have been missed due to visual fixation if the patient's eyes were open.

However, ENG is not without its *limitations*. It is a lengthy, expensive test which causes discomfort to some patients. It is affected by most central nervous system active drugs (tranquilizers, antihista-mines, soporifics, analgesics, alcohol, etc.) and cannot be utilized with confidence on very young children. Although ENG's are rapidly becoming an integral part of the neurotologic evaluation, the various procedures included in the routine ENG evaluation still lack adequate standardization. Thus, one must always be sure to note the normative value which the clinician is using to interpret the ENG tracing.

ENG Test Procedure and Interpretation of Results

The ENG evaluation is carried out in a darkened room and takes approximately 1 hour to complete. An electrode is placed at the outer canthus of each eye to record horizontal eye movements; one is placed at the center of the forehead to act as a ground; and if vertical eye measurement is desired, two additional electrodes are placed above and below the one eye. If a patient has a nonfunctional eye, horizontal electrodes would be attached at the lateral and medial canthus of the functional eye.

The ENG testing procedure is essentially a series of ocular tests, positional tests, and caloric tests. The test procedures and interpretation of abnormal findings are described below. Certain abnormal findings will be suggestive of peripheral vestibular disease, while others suggest the CNS as the site of lesion. When speaking in terms of peripheral *versus* CNS site of lesion, the following differentiation is made: *Peripheral* refers to vestibular end organs, and/or the vestibular portion of the VIIIth nerve up to the point where it enters the brainstem, and *central* (or *CNS*) refers to any of the neural connections beyond that point. The ENG results *do not* diagnose anything. They only supply additional information to that obtained from the history, physical examination, x-rays, audiograms, and other laboratory studies.

Ocular Tests

Calibration

Accurate calibration is essential to ensure precise measurements of the slow phase velocity of the nystagmus.

Interpretation

Normal. The patient is able to shift his gaze between two points without difficulty, and without overshooting the calibration target.

Ocular Dysmetria (or Calibration Overshoots). Ocular dysmetria, commonly referred to as "calibration overshoots," can be detected through calibration. Ocular dysmetria relates to an over- or undershoot of the ocular rotation which occurs when visual fixation is transferred from one point to another. Due to the fact that most normal subjects display an occasional calibration overshoot, 50% of the calibrations must be overshot before ocular dysmetria is diagnosed. The presence of ocular dysmetria suggests CNS dysfunction, such as brainstem or cerebellar pathology.

Eyeblinks. In interpreting the calibration results, one must be cautious and rule out eyeblink artifacts as the potential cause for the overshoots. A vertical channel will differentiate the two because it records eyeblinks, but not the overshoots.

Gaze Test

Procedure

Gaze tests are carried out using 20° *alternating right and left* eye deflections.

Interpretation

Normal. A normal individual should not display any nystagmus on gaze testing. The ENG tracing should yield smooth lines.

Bilateral Horizontal Gaze Nystagmus. Bilateral horizontal gaze nystagmus is the most common form of nystagmus of CNS origin. The nystagmus beats to the right on rightward gaze, and to the left on leftward gaze. This type of nystagmus is usually indicative of brainstem involvement; however, if it is present as an isolated finding, one must rule out the effects of drugs, especially barbiturates.

Unilateral Horizontal Gaze Nystagmus. This type of nystagmus can be a peripheral or a CNS indication. The way in which a differentiation is made, is to have the patient close his eyes. If on eye closure a spontaneous nystagmus appears in the same direction as the gaze nystagmus, with a slow phase velocity greater than 7–8° per second, then the unilateral gaze nystagmus can be considered a manifestation of an intense spontaneous nystagmus, hence a *peripheral sign.*

Vertical Gaze Nystagmus. Vertical gaze nystagmus which is present on upward or downward gaze is abnormal, and also suggests CNS pathology, probably involving the brainstem. Upbeating vertical gaze nystagmus is more common than downbeating vertical gaze nystagmus.

(*Note:* One must rule out peripheral possibilities, as well as drug-induced abnormalities in interpreting gaze test abnormalities.)

Pendulum Tracking Test (or Sinusoidal Tracking Test)

Procedure

This test is accomplished by having a patient visually track a smoothly swinging pendulum (or any other suitable target) which does not exceed a 30° angle deviation from the center gaze. The patient must keep his head stationary and follow the pendulum back and forth with his eyes only. The value of this procedure is that it provides a quick screening measure of the integrity of the oculomotor system.

Interpretation

Normal. A normal person should be able to track the pendulum smoothly, yielding a smooth sine wave on the ENG tracing.

"Broken-up" Sine Wave Pattern. A tracing which displays a distorted sine wave pattern broken up by jerky eye movements can be indicative of a defective oculomotor system, or ocular dysmetria. However, here again, the effects of a strong vestibular spontaneous nystagmus or of drugs must be taken into consideration. Elderly patients also show poorly formed pendular tracking.

Optokinetic Testing

Procedure

The optokinetic (OPK) test is a sensitive test of oculomotor function. An optokinetic drum consisting of vertical black and white stripes is rotated from left to right, and right to left, at a slow and fast speed to elicit involuntary nystagmus. The left to right and right to left responses are compared, at both drum speeds, and symmetry is determined. The OPK test is an important part of the ENG procedure as it establishes the ability of a patient's oculomotor system to generate nystagmus.

Interpretation

Normal. The OPK nystagmus should be symmetrical at both slow and fast drum speeds, and should increase in intensity as the drum speed increases.

OPK Asymmetry. OPK asymmetry is clinically significant when the nystagmus in one direction exceeds the nystagmus in the opposite direction by 20° per second or more at a given drum speed. A significant OPK asymmetry suggests a CNS abnormality, or an intense spontaneous nystagmus of peripheral origin.

Reduced Response to Increased Stimulus. In this instance, the OPK response is symmetrical, but is abnormal due to the fact that the speed of the nystagmus never increases, or actually decreases with the increased speed of the drum rotations. This finding has been associated with brainstem disease and has been reported in patients with multiple sclerosis.

(*Note:* The effects of drugs, inattentiveness, intense spontaneous nystagmus, poor vision, and congenital nystagmus must be ruled out as a cause for the abnormal OPK response.)

Positional Tests

Procedure

The patient is placed, eyes closed, in a series of positions for at least 30 seconds per position. Typically the following positions are tested:
1. Sitting head center.
2. Sitting head right.
3. Sitting head left.
4. Supine head center.
5. Supine head right.
6. Supine head left.
7. Lateral right.
8. Lateral left.

Lateral body positions can be particularly useful in differentiating between nystagmus resulting from cervical involvement and/or vascular insufficiency, and positional nystagmus resulting from a vestibular lesion. The distinction rests on whether or not the nystagmus is present only when the neck is twisted, as in the supine positions, and disappears in the lateral positions in which the neck region is straightened out.

To overcome any central suppression of positional responses, the patient is given mental alerting tasks, such as counting backward from 100 by 1's, throughout the sequence of positional testing.

Nystagmus which is identified during positional testing is classified as either *positional* or *spontaneous* in nature.

Classification

Positional Nystagmus. This type of nystagmus is triggered when a patient assumes a particular head position. It may be present in some or all positions tested. The nystagmus can vary in intensity from position to position, it can disappear (fatigue) with repeated positioning, and it can also change direction (direction-changing positional nystagmus).

Spontaneous Nystagmus. This type of nystagmus is present all of the time, *regardless* of what position the patient is placed in. It does not change direction.

Interpretation

Normal. Most normal patients should not display a spontaneous or positional nystagmus. A small percentage of otologically normal patients do demonstrate a very low intensity spontaneous or positional nystagmus however, and drug- or alcohol-induced nystagmus must be ruled out.

Vestibular Spontaneous Nystagmus. This type of spontaneous nystagmus is usually associated with acute peripheral vestibular lesions and gradually disappears over an unspecified period of time.

Central Spontaneous Nystagmus. A central spontaneous nystagmus is most often associated with a brainstem or cerebellar lesion. A spontaneous nystagmus can only be considered a central finding after one has eliminated the possibilities of vestibular, or ocular (congenital nystagmus) origin.

Positional Nystagmus. Abnormal positional nystagmus is a nonlocalizing finding which may result from peripheral or central disturbances. Some examples of peripheral and central causes of positional nystagmus are listed below:

Peripheral

Chronic otitis media with cholesteatoma.
Labyrinthitis.
Meniere's syndrome.
Temporal bone fracture.

Central

Vascular disease of vertebral or basilar arteries (particularly involving the cervical vertebrae).
CNS degenerative diseases such as multiple sclerosis, syphilis.
Brain tumors.
Drug intoxication (particularly alcohol and barbiturates).

Positional Nystagmus of the Benign Paroxysmal Type. This type of nystagmus is a specific response to a specific maneuver and is usually indicative of a peripheral disturbance. The maneuver is referred to as the Hallpike head-hanging test. It involves having the patient sit on a table with his head turned to one side. He is then lowered very quickly to a supine position, with his head hanging over the table approximately 30° below the horizontal, for 10–15 seconds. This procedure is repeated with the head turned in the opposite direction. It is most useful to have the

patient's eyes open (with or without Frenzel's glasses) during this maneuver, as the nystagmic response is usually of a rotary type which, stated earlier, cannot be recorded through ENG. The classical abnormal or positive response to the Hallpike maneuver include the following:

1. Latency: the nystagmic response does not begin for a few seconds after the patient is moved into the test position.
2. Paroxysmal response: the nystagmus occurs in a sudden burst, builds for several seconds and then declines rapidly.
3. Vertigo: the burst of nystagmus is accompanied by a sudden onset of severe vertigo which may cause the person to try to get out of the position quickly.
4. Fatigability: when the positioning is repeated the nystagmus and vertigo will decrease or disappear.

The Hallpike test can be easily performed in any physician's office and does not require elaborate electrical recordings. When the test yields a classical positive response, the nystagmus usually beats toward the downward ear, which in most cases is also the affected ear. In addition, a positive response also supports a patient's subjective complaint of positional vertigo.

Bithermal Caloric Test

Procedure

The bithermal caloric test consists of obtaining a warm (44°C) and cold (30°C) caloric response from each ear. The patient is placed in the supine position with the head elevated 30°. Each ear is irrigated at 44°C, and 30°C, for 30–40 seconds, with a 5-minute rest period between each of the four irrigations. During each caloric irrigation the patient must have his eyes closed and must also perform some type of mental alerting task. The patient's ability to suppress his caloric nystagmic response through visual fixation is evaluated during at least two of the four responses (one from each ear). This is accomplished by having a patient open his eyes during the peak caloric response and fixate on an object for approximately 10 seconds, whereupon he again closes his eyes for the duration of the ENG recording. Caloric responses are usually recorded for 90 seconds following the termination of the irrigation.

The warm (44°C) irrigations produce nystagmus which beats toward the irrigated ear, i.e., right warm (RW) produces a right-beating nystagmus and left warm (LW) produces left-beating nystagmus. The reverse is true for the cold (30°C) irrigations, i.e., right cold (RC) produces a left-beating nystagmus, and left cold (LC) produces a right-beating nystagmus. A convenient method of remembering this is "COWS" (cold-opposite; warm-same).

Interpretation

For each caloric response the slow phase velocity is measured for the three strongest nystagmic beats occurring over a 10-second period, and then averaged. Slow phase velocity is reported in degrees per second. There are then four separate values (one from each of the four caloric responses), which are evaluated comparatively. Two comparative measurements are obtained: (1) comparison between the right and left ear responses (unilateral weakness or canal paresis), and (2) comparison between all right-beating and all left-beating responses (directional preponderance).

Normal Caloric Responses. The responses from each ear should be symmetrical. Normal persons may demonstrate peak caloric responses ranging from 15° per second to 50° per second.

Bilateral Weakness (BW). When warm caloric responses fall below 11° per second, and cold caloric peak responses below 6° per second, for both ears, or when the total peak response for all four irrigations is less than 40–50° per second, a bilaterally weak response is present.

A bilateral weakness may occur in CNS lesions, and also in certain peripheral vestibular lesions, such as: drug-induced ototoxicity, bilateral Meniere's syndrome, bi-lateral acoustic tumors, and bilateral temporal bone fracture. It should be noted that a small percentage of normal persons will reveal a bilaterally weak or absent response to caloric stimulation.

Unilateral Weakness (UW). A significant unilateral weakness (a difference of 20% or greater between the right ear responses and the left ear responses) is caused by a lesion in the vestibular end organ, or in the primary vestibular nerve fibers. A unilateral weakness is seen in patients with unilateral Meniere's syndrome, temporal bone fracture, vestibular neuronitis, or acoustic tumor.

A finding of a significant unilateral weakness is the most "concrete" finding which an ENG can yield. It localizes the site of lesion as peripheral in origin, and also identifies the diseased labyrinth.

Failure Fixation Suppression (FFS). All normal patients, as well as those with peripheral vestibular disorders, should be able to significantly reduce or abolish their caloric response nystagmus with visual fixation. Persons with CNS lesions may demonstrate no reduction, or sometimes an enhancement of nystagmus when visual fixation is performed. Thus, FFS is a good indication of CNS involvement.

Directional Preponderance (DP). A significant directional preponderance (a difference of 30% or more between the two right-beating responses and the two left-beating responses) is a nonlocalizing finding, as it can be associated with peripheral or CNS lesion. Hence, it has little clinical significance.

Bibliography

1. Barber, H. O., and Stockwell, C. W. *Manual of Electronystagmography.* The C. V. Mosby Co., St. Louis, 1976.
2. Northern, J. L. (Ed.). *Hearing Disorders.* Little, Brown, & Co., Boston, 1976.
3. Northern, J. L., and Downs, M. P. *Hearing in Children.* The Williams & Wilkins Co., Baltimore, 1974.

Chapter 3
Rhinology

Bruce W. Jafek
Arlen Meyers

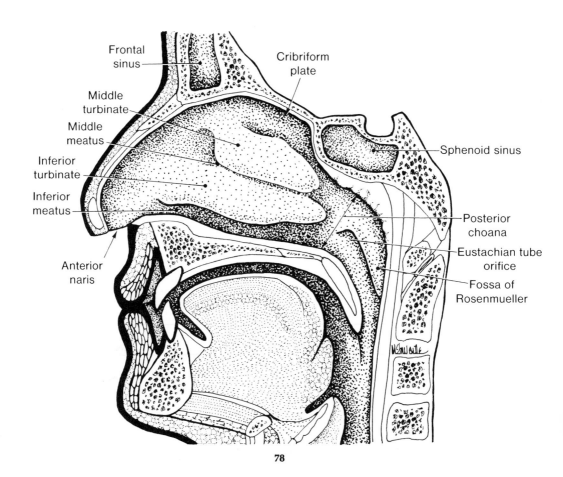

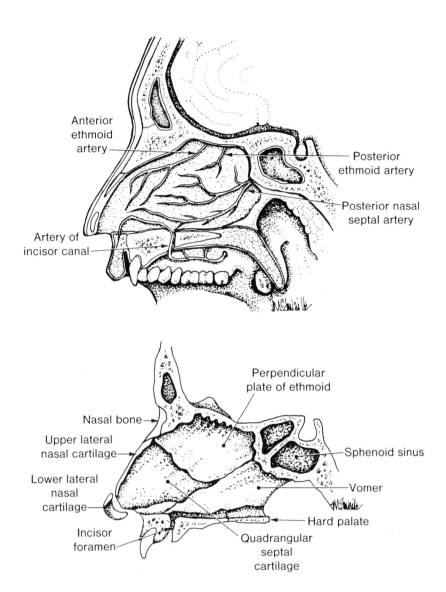

NASAL STUFFINESS

Functional abnormalities of the nose are common and can present as nasal stuffiness, rhinorrhea, postnasal drip, fullness, pressure and pain of the frontal-maxillary or intercanthal region. Although the physiology of the nose is poorly understood, it is clear that minor variations in nasal function result in bothersome, sometimes incapacitating symptoms.

Ciliary activity, production and flow of mucus, the humidifying capability of nasal mucous membrane, and the regulation of nasal airflow are all finely tuned nasal physiologic processes which are susceptible to pathologic alteration.

Diagnostic Approach

Subjective Complaints

Nasal stuffiness is most commonly caused by a structural abnormality of the nose or a physiologic dysfunction of the nasal turbinates (see Chapter Opening Figures). Several historical facts help elucidate those features responsible for nasal stuffiness.

Age. Nasal stuffiness beginning at age 20 to 65 is usually not attributable to a structural abnormality, unless there has been surgery or trauma. Nasal stuffiness in children should alert the physician to the possibility of a foreign body. This usually presents as unilateral nasal obstruction with purulent rhinorrhea. In adolescent males unilateral nasal obstruction which may be accompanied by epistaxis is suggestive of juvenile nasopharyngeal angiofibroma.

Sex. Females taking estrogen or who are pregnant may experience intermittent nasal stuffiness.

Seasonal variation. Allergic rhinitis is characterized by the presence of symptoms during predictable periods of the year. Seasonal variations may vary with geography. For the most part, however, symptoms of seasonal rhinitis are linked to the appearance of molds, spores, grasses, trees, pollens, and other irritants during predictable times of the year.

Irritating factors. Some patients with nasal stuffiness relate exacerbations of symptoms to particular events. For example, the symptoms seem worse on windy days, in damp places, and outside of the house, rather than inside. These historical clues can help differentiate various mold allergens.

Coexisting symptoms. Several organs respond to allergens simultaneously. Vertigo, dizziness, itchy eyes, sneezing, chronic cough, headaches, and laryngitis are sometimes manifestations which accompany nasal stuffiness secondary to allergies.

Drug history. Rhinitis medicamentosa is caused by chronic application of sympathomimetic drugs to the nasal mucosa. In addition, such substances as reserpine, estrogens, and phenothiazines may cause nasal stuffiness.

Nature of drainage. Whereas bacterial rhinosinusitis causes a purulent nasal exudate, allergic rhinitis usually produces a serous discharge. Atrophic rhinitis usually has little or no discharge, but significant crusting is present.

**Table 3.1
Evaluation**

Historical
  Generalized tendency, ecchymoses, etc.
  Family history
  Operative/trauma history
  Drop in hematocrit 2° to epistaxis
  "Easy bleeding or bruisability"
Physical examination
  Light, suction, anesthesia, *location*
Laboratory
  Screen: Prothrombin time, partial thromboplastin time, platelet count, hematocrit
  Detail: Specific factor assay, etc.
Other
  Angiography, hematology consultation

Other atopic diseases. Patients with seasonal allergic rhinitis frequently have a past history of other atopic manifestations. A family history of food intolerance, asthma, or bronchospasm should be sought.

Nonatopic disease. Association of nasal stuffiness with asthma, aspirin intolerance, and nasal polyps ("triad asthma").

Alternating nasal obstruction which may be related to position (when in the lateral decubitus position, the "down" side normally is obstructed) is suggestive of obstruction caused by mucosal swelling and not septal obstruction.

Objective Findings

Patients with nasal stuffiness should have a complete ear, nose, and throat examination. Examination of the nose should include anterior rhinoscopy and examination of the nasopharynx using a nasopharyngeal mirror or fiberoptic examining apparatus. This should be carried out before the topical application of 1% ephedrine or ¼% phenylephrine, which shrinks the mucous membranes and turbinates and allows a better view. Failure of the mucosa to shrink with the application of vasoconstrictors is important and should be noted. Be sure to note the presence, characteristics, and location of intranasal masses. The area of the middle meatus (below the middle turbinate) should be inspected carefully for the presence of polyps. When present, polypoid degeneration of the mucosa of the middle or inferior turbinate should be differentiated from true nasal polyps. The presence of what appears to be a unilateral polyp or polyps should be viewed with suspicion, as this more likely represents tumor. Whereas the nasal septum is rarely perfectly straight, significant deviation should be noted. The nasal valve, the junction between the nasal septum and the upper lateral cartilages, is a particularly important area which regulates nasal airflow. This location or deviation of the dorsal edge of the nasal septum may interfere with valve function, as can redundant or enlarged upper lateral cartilages.

The identification of intranasal pathology can, in addition, be aided by noting the presence, characteristics, and location of nasal secretions. The exudate in allergic rhinitis is usually clear. Bacterial or viral illness causes secretions which are more mucoid or purulent. Cerebrospinal fluid is clear and watery and gives a positive test for glucose.

The maxillary and ethmoid sinuses open into the middle meatus and the superior meatus. The sphenoid sinus ostium is located in the sphenoethmoid recess. Localization of drainage to the inferior, middle, or superior meatus helps to pinpoint the sinus involved. Palpation and transillumination of the paranasal sinuses sometimes reveals tenderness or opacification. Opacification of the sinus by transillumination might be indicative of a hypoplastic or absent sinus, however, and sinus x-rays 168are necessary to confirm the presence of are necessary to confirm the presence of sinusitis.

Assessment

Mechanical obstruction due to a deviated nasal septum is readily diagnosed by anterior rhinoscopy (posterior deviations of the vomer are very rare). Mechanical obstruction associated with functional obstruction due to mucous membrane swelling may be diagnosed by some relief of the obstruction by the application of vasoconstrictors. Normally, on the side opposite the deviation, there will be compensatory hypertrophy of the inferior turbinate.

Nasal obstruction due to mucosal swelling where the mucus is clear (uninfected) is usually related to allergic rhinitis, perennial (nonseasonal or nonallergic) rhinitis, hormonal imbalance, drug-induced mucosal swelling, or rhinitis medicamentosa. In addition to the history of nose drop use, the failure of the mucosa to shrink with the application of vasoconstrictors is suggestive of rhinitis medicamentosa. Allergic rhinitis may be diagnosed by the finding of eosinophils in the nasal smear, the presence of circulating eosinophilia and positive skin tests to inhalant allergens. Vasomotor rhinitis which represents an excessive response of the nasal mucosa to stimuli which normally produce some swelling (or sympathetic-parasympathetic mucosal imbalance) is usually accompanied by profuse clear rhinorrhea and sneezing with a nonseasonal pattern. The nasal smear is normal.

Mucosal swelling with purulent secretions (purulent rhinitis) is usually associated with purulent sinusitis. The nasal smear will reveal many polymorphonuclear leukocytes and bacteria. Sinus x-ray films will show either mucosal thickening or fluid levels in the sinuses. A culture of the nasal or preferably the sinus pus should be obtained. Aerobic and anaerobic cultures of sinus pus should be obtained. The usual organisms will be *Haemophilus influenzae, Pneumococcus, Streptococcus,* or *Staphylococcus.*

Unilateral polyp-like masses should be examined carefully as they are rarely simple polyps. When firm polypoid masses are seen in males, especially around adolescence, they should not be manipulated and *never* biopsied in the office. The nasopharynx should be inspected carefully and sinus x-rays films obtained as well as films of the nasopharynx. Where indicated, tomograms are obtained. The proper study of lesions suspected of being angiofibromas is by carotid arteriography. Friable lesions in other patients should be evaluated by biopsy and sinus x-rays and tomograms. These will usually be ethmoid or maxillary sinus carcinomas. They may be accompanied by purulent or serosanguineous nasal discharge.

Nasal polyps arising from the middle meatus, usually bilaterally, are most commonly either allergic polyps or polyps associated with non-reagin-mediated (triad) asthma. The history is helpful as is a family history, although reagin-mediated and non-reagin-mediated disease may occur in the same family and the same patient. Where asthma is present, the history of exacerbation with aspirin usage is diagnostic. Sinus x-rays usually reveal polypoid degeneration of the sinus mucosa. Skin tests to inhalant allergens should be performed. Pulmonary function studies are also obtained and any pus in the nose is cultured.

Plan

Septal deviation, where the symptoms are sufficiently bothersome to the patient, can be treated only surgically. Any mucosal disease should first be managed medically or the results will be disappointing.

Mucosal swelling due to allergy should first be managed by avoidance of the allergen (furnace filters, mattress and pillow pads, etc.). Secondly, medical management using antihistamines such as chlorpropheneramine, 4 mg q.i.d., and decongestants such as pseudoephedrine, 30–60 mg orally q.i.d., should be used. Rarely, hyposensitization by antigen injection may be necessary.

Drug-induced obstruction is treated by removing the offending drug where possible. This responds poorly to vasoconstrictors.

Rhinitis medicamentosa is difficult to treat. The patient is usually "hooked" on spray or drops. These must be stopped completely. Sympatomatic relief with vasoconstrictors by mouth is used. In stubborn cases, nasal dexamethasone spray is used three times a day for a few weeks (it is systemically absorbed). The patient must be warned that up to 3–6 months may be required for improvement.

Vasomotor rhinitis may respond to vasoconstrictors by mouth. If very severe, vidian nerve section may be beneficial.

Juvenile nasopharyngeal angiofibromas are treated surgically and may require intracranial resection as well as nasopharyn- geal approaches. Radiation may be necessary where there is significant intracranial extension of the tumor.

Squamous cell carcinoma of the ethmoid and maxillary sinuses is treated by irradiation and surgery where feasible.

Nasal polyps in reagin-mediated disease are treated by antihistamine vasoconstrictor (by mouth) followed by nasal dexamethasone spray. The polyps *frequently* recur. In non-reagin-mediated disease (triad asthma) the patients must be advised on aspirin avoidance. The asthma is the chief problem. The nasal polyps may be treated by nasal steroid spray or direct injection of the polyps with a long-acting steroid. If refractory, they should be removed. The steroid spray is then decreased to the minimum dose consistent with airway maintenance. Remember that adrenal suppression occurs with absorbable nasal steroids or polyp injection.

Where purulent rhinosinusitis is present, along with oral vasoconstrictors and antihistamines, antibiotics are used. The choices, depending upon culture results, are (in order of desirability): ampicillin, 250 mg q.i.d.; erythromycin, 250 mg q.i.d.; or tetracycline, 250 mg q.i.d.—all for 10 days.

Note that no mention is made of vasoconstrictor nose drops or sprays. They have no role in treatment of chronic rhinitis and should be restricted to use of less than 5 days for acute rhinitis or sinusitis.

Enlarged turbinates which don't respond to the above may require surgical treatment or electrocautery, but care must be used, as excessive removal of turbinates results in atrophic rhinitis with crusting, infection, and more obstruction, sometimes along with ozena, a foul-smelling purulent infection. Satisfactory treatment of this complication is almost impossible.

The complications of using long-term steroids must be borne in mind, as must the problems of vasoconstrictor use in hypertensive patients.

RHINORRHEA

Rhinorrhea (nasal discharge or "running nose"), probably the most common otolaryngologic complaint, is an inconvenient, but rarely serious, symptom and is often self-limited. Important historical considerations include unilateral or bilateral, intermittent or constant, associated pain or pruritus, drug use, or other systemic conditions (fever, etc.). The character of the discharge is important (bloody, purulent, clear) in the differential diagnosis along with its relation to recent or remote trauma.

Clear Rhinorrhea

Of great importance is the physiologic consideration that the nose and sinuses *normally* produce 1–1½ *pints* of mucus a day to humidify and filter the inspired air. This is normally carried to the nasopharynx by the *metachronal* beat of the respiratory cilia and then swallowed, or occasionally expectorated. Urban dwellers may produce more mucus. Medications given to "dry up" the nose, do so by decreasing the water content of the mucus, frequently making it thicker and more tenacious, and the patient *more symptomatic*. Additional considerations are given in the subsequent section on postnasal discharge.

Anterior rhinorrhea in symptomatic amounts implies either an excessive production of mucus, an abnormality in ciliary action, or nasal blockage. The latter are uncommon causes of clear rhinorrhea, as ciliary stasis (caused by smoking, infection, etc.) usually leads to local infection with resultant purulent rhinorrhea (see Purulent Rhinorrhea).

Subjective Complaints

Clear nasal discharge, unilateral or bilateral, intermittent or continuous, seasonal or perennial.

Objective Findings

Complete *nasal examination* with subsequent vasoconstriction (4% cocaine-moistened cotton packs or 1% ephedrine or ¼% phenylephrine for 5 minutes). The condition of the *nasal mucosa* is noted. High (ethmoidal) polypi are searched for. A *sinus series* is obtained in longstanding

cases. The patency of the posterior choanae (nasal openings) can be checked with a catheter in cases of total obstruction.

Assessment

Upper respiratory infection (URI), the "common cold" or coryza, is the most common etiology of clear rhinorrhea. The rhinorrhea is preceded by sneezing and nasal irritation and often by constitutional symptoms (fever, chills, etc.). The nasal mucosa is edematous and hyperemic. The profuse clear rhinorrhea becomes purulent as secondary infection, an outpouring of leukocytes and resolution occur. Various viruses are usually implicated in the early stages followed by secondary bacterial invasion (Staphylococcus, Streptococcus, Pneumococcus).

Allergic rhinitis is another frequent etiology. The *history* is usually positive for a family history of allergies; infantile eczema or "colic" or seasonal recurrence, especially at times of known elevated allergen levels, typically spring and fall, such as the"ragweed or hay fever season," etc. The symptoms may also be "perennial" (year-round), or have seasonal exacerbations of a continuous condition. The *nasal mucosa* is bluish and edematous. *Eosinophils* may be found in increased numbers (>2%) in the nasal secretions. *Skin tests* are usually positive, often showing multiple sensitivities.

Vasomotor rhinitis (VMR) presents with profuse watery rhinorrhea ("catarrh"). Heredity, infection, and psychologic or endocrine imbalances have been identified as predisposing factors. Atmospheric changes (humidity, temperature) or irritants (smoke, alcohol) may act as precipitating factors. The nasal mucosa may appear normal, but is more commonly hyperemic or hypertrophic. A frequent description is of a patient with nasal obstruction and rhinorrhea, "*carrying a box of Kleenex.*"

Hay fever is a nonspecific, lay term for recurrent (seasonal) rhinorrhea with other nasal symptoms (obstruction, sneezing, etc.) which can be included, on a general basis, with allergic rhinitis or possible

VMR, and usually includes conjunctival irritation and itching of the palate.

Nasal polypi may be accompanied by clear rhinorrhea, but are a manifestation of another condition (VMR,. allergies, etc.).

Cerebrospinal fluid (CSF) rhinorrhea is uncommon. A history of trauma (iatrogenic, surgical, or external) is nearly always present, although neoplastic and congenital etiologies have been described. It may occur intermittently, being classically described as "dripping with the head forward." The fluid contains glucose but no mucus or albumin. It "dries soft" on handkerchief.

Rhinitis medicamentosa results from prolonged use of vasoconstrictors (nasal sprays or drops) with resultant "rebound." The usual history is of a URI treated symptomatically followed by continued use of the drug beyond 3 weeks. The nose is sprayed "more frequently," as often as every half hour. The mucosa is bluish and edematous. The mucosal swelling usually fails to respond to spraying the nose with ephedrine (in long-standing cases).

Rare causes of rhinorrhea during the acute infective stages of rhinitis include rhinoscleroma, diphtheria, erysipelas, anthrax, etc. *Granulomas* (sarcoid, syphilis, etc.) may also produce clear rhinorrhea, but purulent rhinorrhea due to secondary bacterial infection is more common. *Tumors* should also be considered, but again purulence, epistaxis or a mass usually makes the diagnosis more obvious.

In the child, unilateral or bilateral rhinorrhea may be a manifestation of *choanal atresia*, especially if presence from birth can be documented. Bilateral atresia is usually accompanied by airway problems, as the infant is an obligate nasal breather for the first 2 or more weeks of life. The diagnosis is suspected if a catheter cannot be passed through the posterior choanae and can be confirmed on x-ray by putting a small mount of contrast material into the nose and noting an air-fluid level in the posterior nose on the lateral film of the child's head in the supine position.

A *foreign body* should also be suspected with unilateral rhinorrhea in the child, but this usually rapidly becomes purulent rhinorrhea.

Plan

Symptomatic relief can be obtained with decongestants in self-limited conditions (early coryza, etc.), with two cautions. The commonly used sympathomimetic drugs (pseudoephedrine) should be used with caution in hypertensives or older men with evidence of prostatic hypertrophy. Acute urinary retention or a hypertensive crisis may be precipitated. More important, these drugs often make patients *more symptomatic* as the mucus becomes thicker and more tenacious.

Combinations of decongestants with antihistamines are usually helpful in providing acute symptomatic relief in many cases of *allergic rhinorrhea*, seasonal or perennial, but the treatment should be directed toward eradication of the allergen. Avoidance is the most successful treatment, where the allergens are few and relatively infrequently encountered. When the allergens are more ubiquitous and the symptoms unresponsive to medical management, however, allergic consultation with hyposensitization, etc., may be required. Steroids may also be used to relieve the acute symptoms (hydrocortisone, 25–100 mg q.d.) and may even be required chronically in an extremely unusual case.

Vasomotor rhinitis may be extremely difficult to control. If an allergic component can be identified, it is handled as above. Submucosal resection of the inferior turbinates or vidian neurectomy have been recommended, while some recommend an intracranial (middle fossa) approach to the greater superficial petrosal nerve or transantral vidian neurectomy. Tranquilizers have often been used.

Rhinitis medicamentosa is handled by having the patient discontinue the use of the drug immediately. A "burst of steroids" is frequently required to control the extreme rebound congestion during this period (prednisone, 40 mg on the 1st day, decreasing by 5 mg per day until "finished," requires no. 36 5-mg tablets). Also useful is pseudoephedrine by mouth (30 mg q.i.d.) and topical dexamethasone spray (Decadron Turbinaire) t.i.d.

Of the less common causes, unilateral or bilateral *choanal atresia* is handled surgically. One side of bilateral atresia should be opened shortly after birth. Surgical correction of unilateral atresias can be postponed until age 5–10. Traumatic *CSF rhinorrhea* should be handled initially by elevating the head of the bed 45° and instituting daily spinal taps. In order to avoid masking meningitis, antibiotics are not given. If conservative measures are unsuccessful, or if a congenital basis is diagnosed, surgical repair with fascia may be required. Neoplastic origin is handled according to the treatment of the neoplasm. *Foreign bodies* should be removed with reversal of the changes and elimination of the symptom. Rhinorrhea due to *granulomas* or *infections* are handled by treating the systemic condition.

Purulent Rhinorrhea

Yellowish or greenish discoloration of the rhinorrhea implies infection in the upper respiratory tract (nose, sinuses, or nasopharynx). Brownish discoloration may be found in smokers with or without infection. The treatment is generally directed toward eradication of the infection and elimination of any predisposing factors.

Subjective Complaints

Purulent nasal discharge, often accompanied by posterior nasal discharge and constitutional symptoms (fever, malaise, etc.). May be unilateral or bilateral. *"Chronic"* implies rhinorrhea lasting over 6 months.

Objective Findings

Complete *nasal examination* with vasoconstriction. *Sinuses* (frontal and maxillary) are palpated bilaterally at the same time to compare tenderness. *Transillumination* of sinuses is rarely helpful. *Sinus x-rays* may show air-fluid levels in acute sinusitis, or mucosal thickening in chronic sinus disease. Bony erosion may be apparent in cases of neoplasia, or a radiopaque foreign body seen. *Systemic manifestations* should be sought (sarcoidosis, hypoimmune states, etc.).

Assessment

In general, unilateral symptoms imply mechanical obstruction, and bilateral symptoms imply systemic etiologies.

The history of unilateral purulent rhinorrhea in the child strongly suggests a *foreign body*. Examination under anesthesia may even be required to evaluate this possibility.

The possibility of *neoplasm* should always be considered, especially in unilateral purulent rhinorrhea in the adult. Biopsies should be obtained of suspicious areas.

Acute sinusitis is usually accompanied by constitutional symptoms (fever, malaise, etc.) with pain localized to the involved sinus. Fever and leukocytosis are unusual in early uncomplicated sinusitis. Malaise is common. X-rays are usually confirmatory. Purulent rhinorrhea may be minimal or absent if the sinus ostium is completely occluded. The usual organisms are gram-positive, Staphylococcus, Streptococcus, and Pneumococcus being most common. Culture with sensitivities is indicated when this diagnosis is suspected.

Atrophic rhinitis is usually found in the older patient, often a smoker. It is also an iatrogenic problem following excessive removal of nasal tissue, especially the inferior turbinates. Complaints of obstruction are frequent in spite of the fact that the airway is widely patent. Atrophy of the nasal mucosa with crusting is apparent on nasal examination.

Chronic rhinosinusitis is diagnosed when the condition has persisted for over 6 months. Varying states of mucosal change, including both atrophy and hypertrophy, are seen. X-rays usually show mucosal thickening of all of the involved sinuses. The organisms are usually mixed, including some anaerobes. Anosmia or objective parosmia may be noted.

Hypoimmune states may occasionally be found and an immune assay is indicated in chronic states.

Polypoid degeneration of the nasal mucosa is apparent on nasal examination and can be confirmed on x-ray.

Specific (uncommon) forms of *chronic rhinosinusitis* occasionally accompanied by purulent rhinorrhea includes syphilis, yaws, lupus vulgaris, tuberculosis, sarcoidosis, "chronic" diphtheria, scleroma, leprosy, rhinosporidiosis, and rhinoscleroma.

Fungal conditions are occasionally found, especially in the diabetic or patient with altered immune status, and include aspergillosis, actinomycosis, moniliasis, and even, amazingly, infections with Penicillium.

Granulomas include Wegener's and lethal midline granuloma.

Whenever one of the unusual infections is suspected, culture is indicated. Biopsy may also be required, especially where one of the specific or nonspecific granulomas is suspected.

Plan

Whenever a specific organism can be identified in *acute infections*, antibiotic therapy is indicated. This is usually *not* indicated, however, during the purulent resolution phase of coryza.

Management of the "*rare*" *forms of rhinosinusitis* (TBC, etc.) is that of the specific infection. Wegener's and lethal midline granuloma may respond to high doses of steroids, tapering these to determine the least effective dose, Imuran and Cytoxan. Radiotherapy may also be required. The prognosis is poor.

Atrophic rhinitis can be managed by irrigating the nose with physiologic saline followed by application of conjugated estrogen cream (Dienestrol vaginal cream) to the involved mucosa. Smoking must be discontinued.

Polyps should be removed when severe obstruction occurs. Subsequent treatment should be with irrigations and antibiotic management of acute infections. Local steroids (Decadron Turbinaire) may also be helpful in preventing recurrence, as well as intralesional injection with Kenalog.

Chronic rhinosinusitis is the most common cause of persistent purulent rhinorrhea. Antibiotics are rarely helpful except during the acute exacerbation. Decongestants may be somewhat helpful in relieving the congestion. Provision of drainage is the most effective form of therapy. This may be accomplished by having the pa-

tient "sniff up" physiologic saline (1 teaspoon of table salt in a pint of water) and blow it out forcefully. Surgical procedures include sinus irrigation (rarely helpful on a chronic basis), creation of a new ostium, or sinus obliteration. The choice of procedure depends on the individual case.

Hemorrhagic Rhinorrhea

This symptom, while ominous to the patient, rarely implies serious pathology. The nose should be carefully inspected and managed according to the principles presented in this chapter, under Epistaxis.

EPISTAXIS

Epistaxis (bleeding from the nose) is a common symptom. The successful management is dependent upon a sequential, practical approach that is logically and atraumatically applied. Site-of-bleeding classification (local, regional, or systemic) is helpful in stopping the acute bleed; etiologic classification is important in preventing its recurrence.

The initial assessment should always include *documentation* of the side of bleeding (right or left) and location (anterior versus posterior *and* high versus low). A *general plan* for evaluation is contained in Table 3.1 and for therapy in Table 3.2. Specific considerations are as follows:

Anterior Epistaxis with Associated Trauma

Subjective Complaints

History of trauma to nose usually with resultant deformity (swelling or displacement).

Objective Findings

Obvious displacement of nose or swelling; however, the nose may also have a nondisplaced fracture without deformity. *Nasal examination* utilizing *suction, light* (usually headlight) and *anesthesia* with vasoconstriction (4% cocaine-soaked gauze). Bleeding is often through traumatized mucosal edge. Check for septal hematoma.

Table 3.2
Management of Epistaxis

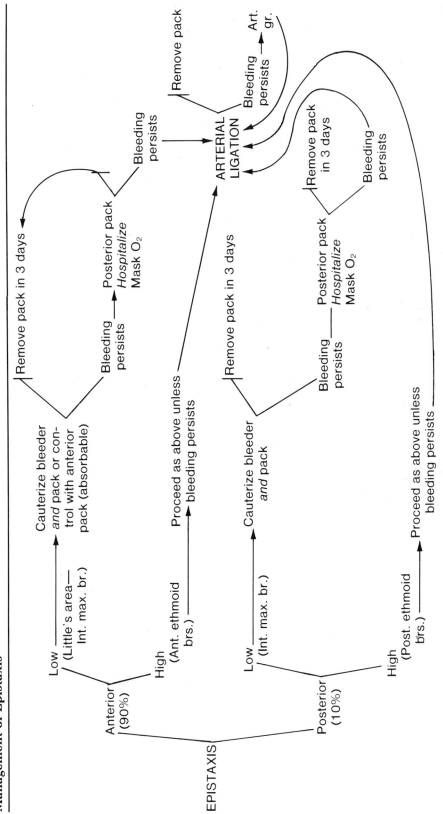

Assessment

Evaluate degree of deformity (external *and* internal). X-rays are usually obtained to try to confirm fracture, but may be difficult to interpret because blood vessel channels along the nasal bones simulate fractures and give minimal useful information. The diagnosis of fracture is therefore often a clinical diagnosis and x-rays may *or may not* be confirmatory. If displacement is identified, septal or external, relocation under local anesthesia will be necessary. Pretrauma pictures (as large as possible, anterior view) are helpful in confirming a previous "straight" nose.

Plan

Manage fracture as described for nasal trauma (see Chapter 11, Facial Trauma). Bleeding can usually be controlled with light absorbable anterior pack or cautery (see following). If posterior pack is required, arterial ligation is preferable to prolonged packing, which may lead to resultant deformity requiring secondary surgery. The fracture can be reduced and stabilized at the time of vascular ligation.

Low Anterior Epistaxis (90%) without Associated External Trauma

The most common site is Little's area (Kiesselbach's plexus). Bleeding may be initiated by minimal trauma. Usually a single bleeding point is seen in a vessel running up from the floor along the anterior (caudal) septal margin. The younger the patient, the greater the likelihood of this anterior bleeding source.

Subjective Complaints

Nosebleed; may be unilateral or bilateral, continuous or intermittent, minimal or profuse.

Objective Findings

Careful *nasal examination* with suction, light, and anesthesia to identify bleeding site and search for *possible neoplasm*. Suspicious areas should be biopsied. *General appraisal* for signs for systemic etiology (capillary hemangiomas, spider angiomas, ecchymoses, etc.).

Assessment

History: positive family history, easy bleeding or bruisability, or other history suggests bleeding diathesis (may require repetitive questioning before the patient or parents "remember"). *Physical examination* helps in ruling out other systemic problems or neoplasm. *Laboratory screen* should be obtained to include hematocrit, prothrombin time (protime), partial thromboplastin time (PTT), platelet count, and bleeding time. Detailed *specific factory assay* with *hematology consultation* is indicated when the screening tests are abnormal.

Plan

Pressure (pinching the nose for 5–10 minutes) and vasoconstriction/anesthesia (4% cocaine or 4% lidocaine + 1% ephedrine, if cocaine is unavailable, on cotton packed into the nose) are sufficient to control most anterior bleeds. The nose can then be examined carefully with *light and suction* and the bleeding point identified. It can then be touched with a silver nitrate stick or electrodesiccated to prevent rebleeding ("spot-welded"). Following application of the topical vasoconstrictor, the *specific site* of bleeding is cauterized. Electrocautery is better then chemical cautery ($AgNO_3$). *Do not cauterize the entire septum, paint-brush fashion.* The nose is then packed with absorbable packing (Surgicel) for 3 days. If the bleeding persists, hospitalize the patient and manage with a posterior pack as indicated under posterior epistaxis.

If a coagulopathy is identified, specific factor correction should be accomplished as rapidly as possible. Manipulative intervention in coagulopathies should be avoided whenever possible. If temporary packing is required, absorbable packing is preferred over nonabsorbable packing, as removal is not required. Gelfoam covered with powdered topical thrombin or Surgicel is useful in treating epistaxis when coagulopathies are the etiology. Epistaxis as the isolated manifestation of a coagulopathy is *very* uncommon.

High Anterior Epistaxis

Subjective Complaints

Vigorous epistaxis, which is primarily anterior, usually in the older hypertensive patient.

Objective Findings

Anterior bleeding from above the middle turbinate, often pulsatile and brisk. Usually unilateral.

Assessment

Evaluate patient for shock and other systemic disease. Immediate hematocrit and appropriate coagulation studies. Hourly repeat of the hematocrit until it equilibrates, as it has undoubtedly not yet stabilized. Complete nasal examination.

Plan

Type and cross 2 units of blood if initial hematocrit is depressed (<30%). Utilizing light, suction, vasoconstriction, pack nose with absorbable packing. If bleeding persists, place posterior pack and hospitalize (see below). If still persistent, otolarnygology consultation for consideration of arterial ligation. In face of acute bleed in elderly patient, signs of shock require monitoring of central venous pressure and appropriate transfusion. Also, Vaseline gauze packing may give superior hemostasis over any absorbable packing material in brisk bleeds.

Recurrent Anterior Epistaxis (Usually Pediatric)

Subjective Complaints

Daily or frequent nosebleeds, usually in the child. Patient may awaken in a.m. with significant blood on pillow.

Objective Findings

Nasal examination for foreign body (usually associated with purulence). General appraisal for systemic disease/signs of bleeding diathesis (telangiectasias, etc.). Identification of bleeding site, usually from bleeding point on large vein running from floor along anterior (causal) septal margin. Bleeder often on right with right-handed child.

Assessment

History helps to rule out bleeding diathesis. If bleeding point seen, additional evaluation rarely required except for hematocrit and screening blood coagulation studies (see above). Nose picking (trauma) may be etiology.

Plan

Bleeding point can be cauterized with chemical cautery (AgNO$_3$ stick) or electrodesiccated. Bipolar cautery helpful if active brisk bleeding encountered. *Use insulated nasal speculum if unipolar cautery used.* In younger child (<5 years old) general anesthesia may be required with elevation of the septal mucoperichondrium and cautery or division of feeding vessels following otolaryngologic consultation. Weber-Rendu-Osler syndrome (hereditary hemorrhagic telangiectasia) may require septal dermoplasty. If nose picking involved, cut child's fingernails short.

Posterior Epistaxis with Trauma

Subjective Complaints

Bleeding in *severely traumatized* patient (major maxillofacial injury).

Objective Findings

Usually brisk pumping arterial bleeding. Complete nasal/neurologic examination to identify *side* of bleeding. *Facial bone x-rays* usually required to define extent of maxillofacial injuries. Immediate blood studies should be obtained and vital signs monitored.

Assessment

Posterior epistaxis due to external facial trauma is extremely unusual. The patient usually has a major maxillofacial injury; the initial assessment, following control of the bleeding, should be of the neurologic status and facial bones. Concomitant neurologic injury (CSF rhinorrhea, concussion, etc.) is *usual*. Facial bone fractures should be handled as discussed under Facial Trauma. (Chapter 11). Arteriogram may be helpful.

Plan

A posterior pack is usually required (see below). Type and cross 2 units of blood and start iv. Plasma expanders or blood should be given as indicated by the initial hematocrit and state of vital signs. Broad spectrum antibiotics are started (posterior pack, possible CSF leak), e.g., penicillin, 1.2 M units every 6 hours. Central venous pressure (CVP) line may be required.

Posterior Epistaxis without Trauma (10%)

Subjective Complaints

Nosebleed, usually severe in older hypertensive smoker. Increased incidence during dry weather.

Objective Findings

Complete *nasal examination* with definition of *side* and site of bleeding. Evaluate for neoplasm (if unable to see due to active bleeding, recheck 3 weeks post-treatment). *Vital signs* to identify *hypertension* or *hypovolenic hypotension*. Systemic appraisal. Arteriography should be considered only if tumor is suspected or there is persistent bleeding in spite of packing. EKG should be obtained.

Assessment

Historical aspects include age, hypertension, coagulopathy, smoking history, medications, trauma, etc. The *physical examination* should determine the site of bleeding. *Laboratory studies* (hematocrit, hemoglobin, coagulation studies, blood chemistries, hepatorenal chemistries, etc.) should be obtained as a baseline immediately along with an EKG in patients over

40 or with sufficient cardiac history. The *vital signs* should be monitored frequently.

The presence of neoplasm should always be considered, although it is unlikely. The major exception is that juvenile nasopharyngeal angiofibroma should be suspected in the pubescent male with severe posterior epistaxis.

The patient's general status should be monitored closely as the pO_2 will decrease approximately 10 mm IIg *just by packing the nose* due to poorly understood nasopulmonary reflexes. This, on top of the hypovolemia hypotension, and preexisting chronic pulmonary disease (common in smokers) may precipitate a stroke or myocardial infarction. In *pregnant women, fetal monitoring* should be undertaken for signs of fetal distress.

Plan

Patient should be *admitted* and *typed* and *cross-matched* for 2 units of blood. An iv is placed and *plasma expanders* started if the patient is hypovolemic until the blood becomes available. CVP line in poor-risk patients. O_2 is given by mask. Bleeding is controlled with an absorbable *anterior pack*, if possible, or a *posterior pack*.

The posterior pack is placed as follows: The nose is first packed with 4% cocaine-moistened cotton or lidocaine-ephedrine mix (part of initial steps in identifying and controlling bleeding). A 30-ml 12–14 Fr Foley catheter is passed through the bleeding side and visualized in the pharynx. The tip has previously been cut off to decrease pharyngeal irritation. *Under vision*, the balloon is inflated with 10–12 ml of saline, and light tension is placed anteriorly. An additional 1–4 ml of saline are added until the soft palate bulges slightly (Fig. 3.1). At this point, the *nasopharynx* is occluded and bleeding comes anteriorly. The nose is then packed *bilaterally* with Vaseline gauze which is wrapped externally around the catheter approximately 2 cm to project from the nose. *Light tension* is maintained on the catheter and it is clamped with a C-clamp, which rests against the Vaseline, which rests, in turn, against the nose. Direct pressure of the clamp against the nose *must be avoided* to prevent pressure necrosis.

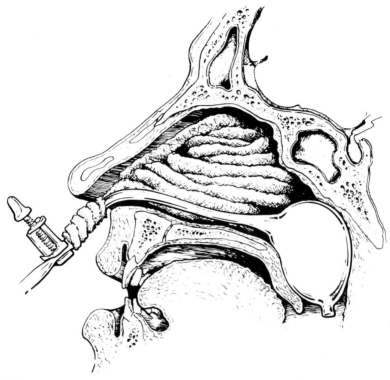

Figure 3.1

The pack remains in place for 3 days, during which *antibiotics* (penicillin VK, 250 mg *q.i.d.*, or erythromycin, 250 mg *q.i.d.*) and *sedation* (phenobarbital, 60 mg STAT, followed by 8–30 mg every 6 hours, depending on the level of consciousness, general physical condition, etc.) should be given.

The patient should be observed closely for complications of hypoxemia, hypoperfusion syndromes, nitrogen retention due to blood in the gastrointestinal (GI) tract, hypertension, disseminated intravascular coagulopathy (DIC), etc. The combination of nasal packing, sedation, immobilization and hemorrhage places severe stress on the cardiopulmonary and central nervous systems. Blood gas studies should be done on all patients with posterior packs.

The pack is removed on the 4th day and the patient is observed 24 hours before discharge. The post-hospitalization check at 3 weeks should include careful reexamination for neoplasm.

Medical consultation with initiation of antihypertensive therapy is indicated during the hospitalization if hypertension is found. *Smokers* should be advised to stop.

Arterial ligation may be required in cases of persistent or recurrent bleeding in spite of a *good posterior pack*. If this is required, otolaryngologic consultation is indicated. In an aged patient with poor general health or poor cardiopulmonary reserve, vascular ligation may be considered earlier.

The internal maxillary or external carotid artery is ligated if the bleeding is from the external carotid system, and the anterior ethmoid if from the ethmoid (internal carotid) system. Ligation procedures *don't* ligate the bleeder, they ligate *feeder*, decreasing the arterial pressure head; therefore, ligate as distally as possible. External carotid artery ligation is technically easier, and can be done under local anesthesia, but is slightly less successful and may cause CNS complications in the uncommon case of anomalies of the internal carotid system. In cases in which the bleeding point remains obscure, control *both* the internal carotid (ethmoid ligation) and the external carotid supplies (external carotid or internal maxillary artery ligation) in order to achieve maximal decrease in the arterial pressure to the bleeder.

Injection of the pterygomaxillary space to control posterior epistaxis is a *temporary measure*, offering control for 8–12 hours. It should *not* be used where internal maxillary artery ligation is being considered.

A successful ligation should allow unpacking of the nose *in the operating room* with discharge of the patient on the 1st postoperative day.

Increasing numbers of authors are recommending ligation as *the initial approach to posterior epistaxis* in order to avoid the morbidity and mortality associated with a posterior pack and to shorten the period of hospitalization.

In conclusion, the patient with posterior epistaxis is *sick*; 2% will die *during that hospitalization*, usually not of exsanguination, but rather owing to complications (gram-negative sepsis, stroke, myocardial infarction, etc.). These patients should be watched *closely*. It is essential that the physician not be lulled into a sense of complacency. It is *not* "just a nosebleed."

Several final points are important in the general management of the epistaxis patient:

1. Systemic etiologies should be managed *systemically*; local causes should be controlled *locally*.

2. Trauma, followed by infection, are the major causes of pediatric epistaxis. Epistaxis under the age of 2 is uncommon.

3. Cardiovascular causes (hypertension, etc.) are the most common causes of adult epistaxis.

4. The patient should have a careful ENT examination 3–4 weeks *after* pack removal, especially in cases in which the source of bleeding is obscure. This should include anterior and posterior rhinoscopy and sinus x-ray examination.

OLFACTORY DISORDERS

Disturbances in the ability to perceive odors, or smell, can be generally classified as *dysosmias* (*dys-*, impairment of; *-osmia*, sense of smell) or more specifically as decreased (*hyposmia*), lack of (*anosmia*), increased (*hyperosmia*), or perverted perceptions (*parosmia*). A more useful working classification is into conductive versus perceptive etiologies. Underlying disease states and site-of-lesion considerations are also important.

Hyposmia, Anosmia

Subjective Complaints

Decreased or absent ability to smell, often accompanied by impaired taste sensation (*dysgeusia*).

Objective Findings

Patency of airway (anterior, posterior, superior) must be assessed (conductive etiologies) along with the *condition of the mucosa* (erythema, edema, atrophic, etc.) which could either account for micro-obstruction (conductive) of the olfactory region or imply direct destruction (infection, granulomas, etc.). Any *discharge* (especially yellowish or greenish, implying an infection) is noted. The adjacent *sinuses* are palpated and percussed and any signs of systemic conditions (pregnancy, Addison's disease, etc.) evaluated. A complete *neurologic examination* is done.

Assessment

Conductive etiologies (Table 3.3) should be apparent on the physical examination. *Sinus x-rays* are helpful in reevaluating the extent of mucosal disease, infections, or obstructions (osseous). The cribriform plate region should be checked carefully for bony erosion (tumors or granulomas) or calcifications (olfactory groove meningioma) on these views. Additional *radiologic* (angiography, tomography, CAT scan), *neurologic* (lumbar puncture, EEG), or *allergic* (skin tests, etc.) evaluations may be necessary according to the findings on the initial screening examination and test battery. Appropriate consultations are obtained as indicated. Additional blood studies may be required if specific systemic disorders are suspected (e.g., Addison's, diabetes, etc.).

Olfactometry (testing of olfactory func-

Table 3.3
Classification of Dysosmias

A. By site of lesion
  1. Conductive
    a. Structural abnormality
    b. Physicochemical changes
  2. Perceptive
    a. End organ lesions
    b. Olfactory nerve lesions
    c. Central lesions
B. By etiology
  1. Non-disease states reported to affect olfactory acuity
    a. Hyperosmia
      (1) Hunger (?)
      (2) Nausea
      (3) Obesity
      (4) Occupational (perfumers, wine tasters)
      (5) Environmental
      (6) Nonobstructive nasal congestion
      (7) Hormonal (pregnancy state, etc.)
    b. Hyposmia
      (1) Presbyosmia
      (2) Hormonal (testosterone)
      (3) Satiety state (?)
      (4) Trace metal deficiency (zinc, copper, nickel)
  2. Disease states reported to affect olfactory acuity
    a. Hyperosmia
      (1) Adrenal cortical insufficiency (Addison's disease)
      (2) Virilizing nonhypertensive congenital adrenal hyperplasia ($\uparrow$ testosterone)
      (3) Mucoviscidosis (prior to nasal polyposis)
      (4) Epilepsy
    b. Parosmia (distasteful, distorted smell)
      (1) Objective
        (a) Sinusitis, atrophic rhinitis
        (b) Other infectious etiology
      (2) Subjective
        (a) Hysteria
        (b) Drug-induced (e.g., tetracyclines)
        (c) Epilepsy (especially temporal lobe)
        (d) Postinfectious perceptive
    c. Hyposmia and anosmia
      (1) Intranasal
        (a) Conductive
          Rhinitis: vasomotor, allergic, medicamentosa, bacterial
          Polyposis
          Septal deviation; nasal valvular collapse
          Endocrine vascular engorgement
          Neoplasm: adenoid cystic carcinoma, adenocarcinoma, nasopharyngeal carci-
            noma
          Chronic rhinitis (syphilis, sarcoidosis, TBC, rhinoscleroma)
        (b) Perceptive
          Postinfectious (viral)
          Pollutants: tobacco, SO_2, menthol, heavy metals
          Drug-induced: cocaine, formaldehyde, carbon monoxide, petrol derivatives,
            organic solvents, streptomycin
          Atrophic rhinitis, Sjögren's syndrome
          Radiation

Continued

Table 3.3 (Continued)

Trauma
Neoplasm: esthesioneuroepithelioma, Schwannoma, neurofibroma
Diabetes
Diphtheria
(2) Extranasal-intracranial
    (a) Selected congenital anosmia
    (b) Familial dysautonomia (usually hyposmic)
    (c) Trauma: concussion (50%)
    (d) Diffuse senile atrophy
    (e) Infection: meningitis, frontal/ethmoid sinusitis with secondary osteomyelitis, viral (influenza)
    (f) Cerebrovascular accident
    (g) Tumors: vascular, meningioma, intracerebral (frontal lobe), osteoma, paraoptic chiasmal (craniopharyngioma, pituitary, aneurysm)
    (h) Drug-induced: amphetamines
    (i) Epilepsy
    (j) Hydrocephalus
    (k) "Little strokes"; transient ischemic attacks (TIA's)
(3) Extranasal-extracranial
    (a) Familial dysautonomia
    (b) Turner's syndrome
    (c) Congenital hypogonadotrophic eunuchoidism
    (d) Diabetes mellitus
    (e) Pseudohypoparathyroidism
    (f) Hypogonadal females
    (g) Vitamin A deficiency: postgastrectomy, Whipple's disease, abetalipoproteinemia
    (h) Iatrogenic: postlaryngectomy
    (i) Psychogenic: hysteria, schizophrenia

tion) can be extremely complex. On a research basis, temperature, humidity, purity of the odorant, flow rate, stimulus duration, and concentration all must be controlled. As a matter of fact, most researchers in this area begin by devising their own tests, making meaningful comparison of results or treatment regimens virtually impossible. Examples are included in the bibliography.

In a more practical way, the following test battery (with considerations of each) is useful in the office setting:

1. Coffee (complex odorant; excellent recognition index); patient should close eyes to avoid visual clues; fresh "instant" coffee may be used.

2. Oil of cloves (a complex odorant with good recognition index): olfactory (cranial nerve I) stimulant.

3. Phenylethyl alcohol: cranial nerve I stimulant; pleasant odor—like roses; widely used in research.

4. Amyl acetate: cranial nerve I stimulant; more subtle (like bananas).

5. Distilled water: use as a control.

6. Menthol: trigeminal (cranial nerve V) stimulant (control).

7. Acetone: cranial nerve V stimulant (control).

All odorants are kept in similar glass-stoppered bottles and the patient is allowed to "sniff" each. It is recognized that there is no "standard sniff," but this technique is useful within the context of a screening battery with the interpretations as given below.

Anosmic patients should *perceive*, but not necessarily *identify*, the two trigeminal controls, but not the cranial nerve I stimulants, nor the distilled water. Hyposmic patients should perceive most and recognize some odorants. Hysterical patients will be inconsistent in their replies, often reacting to such stimulants as acetone, but denying perception. Ammonia, which strongly stimulates cranial nerves V, is helpful in additional evaluation of the hysterical patient.

Quantitative testing is more time-con-

suming and is generally used only in research setting; protocols can be found in
the references.

Plan

When a *conductive defect* is correctly
identified, surgical correction or medical
treatment should allow return of smell.

Correction of an *underlying disease
state* may also eliminate the symptom.

Where no definite etiology can be found
("idiopathic anosmia or hyposmia"), various empirical regimens have been found
to be helpful in some cases. Each can be
tried in sequence for 1 month:

1. Zinc sulfate, 220 mg *t.i.d.*
2. Vitamin A, 100,000 units *q.d.* × 2
weeks, then decrease to 50,000 units *q.d.*
3. Repetitive cocainization (10% cocaine—2 drops to olfactory region to eliminate "efferent feedback inhibition").

If the condition persists for longer than
1 year it is usually permanent.

Hyperosmia

Subjective Complaints

Complaints that odors are "too sharp"
or the sense of smell "too sensitive." Differentiate from parosmia (*distorted*, perverted or foul odors).

Objective Findings

Inspection of patency of airway, condition of mucosa, discharge, neurologic examination, *signs of systemic condition.*

Assessment

Almost exclusively perceptive etiology.
Physical examination rarely contributory
except for determining associated systemic condition (Table 3.3). May be psychogenic or hysterical.

Plan

Correction of associated disease state
should correct hyperosmia if identified.
Otherwise no specific therapy.

Parosmia

Subjective Complaints

Perverted or distasteful smell. May be
intermittent or continous.

Objective Findings

Complete nasal and neurologic examination. If smell is also perceived by examiner, local nasal etiology is strongly suggested (infectious, etc.) (Table 3.3).

Assessment

Sinus series and complete *neurologic
workup* to include skull x-rays and EEG is
indicated to evaluate temporal lobe. May
represent postinfectious perceptive etiology. Psychogenic dysosmias often take
this form. Symptom more likely to have
central etiology, although this may remain
obscure.

Plan

Vitamin A, 100,000 units *q.d.* for 2 weeks
followed by 50,000 units for an additional
2 weeks is helpful in some postinfectious
parosmias. Correction of the underlying
condition (polyposis, infection, sinusitis,
etc.) is usually curative in objective parosmias. Psychogenic parosmia may be extremely difficult to diagnose, but once
found, psychiatric referral is indicated.

In conclusion, olfactory disorders are
hard to evaluate and harder to treat successfully except where a reversible conductive or systemic etiology can be definitely identified. In these cases, however,
the symptoms are often recurrent because
of recurrence of the underlying condition.

Bibliography

Nasal Stuffiness

1. Baker, D. C., Jr. Steroid therapy in otolaryngology. *Trans. Am. Acad. Ophthalmol. Otolaryngol*
76: 297–300, 1972.
2. Fabricant, N. D. The physiological approach to
nasal medication. *Am. J. Med. Sci. 230:* 436–440,
1955.
3. Goode, R. L. Diagnosis and treatment of turbinate dysfunction. *American Academy of Ophthal-*

mology and Otolaryngology (AAOO) Self-instruction Package, 1977.
4. House, H. P. Submucous resection of the inferior turbinal bone. Laryngoscope 61: 637–648, 1951.
5. Ozenberger, J. M. Cryosurgery for the treatment of chronic rhinitis. Larynoscope 83: 508–516, 1973.

Rhinorrhea

1. Ballenger, J. J. (Ed.). Diseases of the Nose, Throat and Ear, ed. 12, pp. 105–237. Lea & Febiger, Philadelphia, 1977.
2. English, E. M. Otolaryngology, pp. 275–312. Harper & Row, Hagerstown, Md., 1977.
3. Scott-Brown, W. G., Ballantyne, J., and Groves, J. Diseases of the Ear, Nose and Throat, ed. 2, pp. 173–314. Butterworth, London, 1972.
4. Simpson, J. F., Robin, I. G., Ballantyne, J. C., and Groves, J. A Synopsis of Otolaryngology, ed. 2, pp. 135–233. John Wright & Sons, Bristol, 1967.

Epistaxis

1. Cassisi, N. J., Biller, H. F., and Ogura, J. H. Changes in arterial oxygen tension and pulmonary mechanisms with the use of posterior nasal pack-ing. Laryngoscope 81: 1261, 1971.
2. El Bitar, H. The etiology and management of epistaxis; a review of 300 cases. Practitioner 207: 800, 1971.
3. Juselius, H. Epistaxis, a clinical study of 1724 cases. J. Laryngol. Otol. 88: 317, 1974.
4. Pinsker, O. T., and Holdcraft, J. Surgical management of anterior epistaxis. Trans. AAOO 75: 492, 1971.
5. Rosnagle, R. S., Yanagisawa, E., and Smith, H. W. Specific vessel ligation for epistaxis; survey of 60 cases. Laryngoscope 83: 517, 1973.

Olfactory Disorders

1. Doty, R. L. Intranasal trigeminal detection of chemical vapors by humans. Physiol. Behav. 14: 855, 1975.
2. Doty, R. L. Mammalian Olfaction, Reproductive Processes and Behavior. Academic Press, New York, 1976.
3. Douek, E. The Sense of Smell and Its Abnormalities. Churchill-livingstone, Edinburgh, 1974.
4. Henkin, R. I., Schechter, P. J., Hoye, R., and Mattern, C. F. T. Idiopathic hypogeusia with dysgeusia, hyposmia and dysosmia. JAMA 217: 434, 1971.

Chapter 4
Facial Paralysis

Robert E. Mischke

IDIOPATHIC (BELL'S) PARALYSIS

Subjective Complaints

Facial weakness of spontaneous onset by history involving one side of face. May be complete or incomplete. No history of draining ear, associated trauma. Possible history of prior episode, or association of diabetes, pregnancy, hypertension, or family history.

Objective Findings

Facial paralysis—complete or incomplete. Note facial tone and tearing on involved side. Examine ear canal and tympanic membrane to rule out disease. Rule out other neuropathy by cranial nerve examination and complete neurologic examination. Differentiate between central paralysis (lower face involved ipsilaterally) and peripheral etiology (forehead not spared as in central).

Assessment

Audiogram to evaluate cochlear division of VIIIth nerve. X-rays—preferably polytomography of temporal bone—to rule out lesion of internal auditory canal and fallopian (facial) canal. If complete paralysis, topographical analysis of facial lesion important: Shirmer test to evaluate lacrimation (greater petrosal branch); stapedial reflex to evaluate stapedial branch; taste test or salivary flow to evaluate third branch (chorda tympani). Nerve excitability testing critical to differentiate between neuropraxia (physiologic block) and neurotmesis (nerve death). If partial paralysis, determine which branches are involved so that progression or resolution may be noted. Nerve excitability testing appropriate. Electromyogram (EMG) is helpful after 14–21 days in identifying fibrillation potentials (nerve death). Electronystagmography (ENG) may be done to check vestibular division of VIIIth nerve.

Plan

If incomplete paralysis or complete paralysis with normal or near normal nerve excitability, may institute steroid therapy (controversial, although most use): prednisone, 60 mg per day, phasing out in decrements in 10–14 days. Follow very closely (at least every other day) during first 2 weeks to rule out progression to nerve death.

If complete and nerve excitability definitely abnormal or absent (or if EMG shows fibrillation potentials 2 and 3 weeks after onset) refer immediately to otologist or otolaryngologist for consideration of surgical decompression.

TRAUMATIC FACIAL PARALYSIS

Subjective Complaints

Facial paralysis associated with head trauma. Check for history of loss of consciousness, drainage from ear. Note whether immediate or delayed onset. (If delayed, handle like Bell's). Head trauma may be due to birth, gunshot wound, skull fracture, or surgery.

Objective Findings

Determine if complete or incomplete. Examine ear canal and (TM) for lacerations, hemotympanum, and CSF otorrhea. Check for other cranial nerve or neurologic deficits. Note as soon as examination is possible condition of facial movement to differentiate immediate and delayed paralysis.

Assessment

Topographical analysis of paralysis (see Idiopathic (Bell's) Paralysis). X-rays for temporal bone—base of skull fracture. Polytomography best. Audiogram for hearing level. ENG, if condition permits, to evaluate labyrinth.

Plan

If CSF otorrhea: broad spectrum antibiotic coverage and sterile dressing immediately. Delayed onset: management like idiopathic (Bell's) paralysis. Immediate onset: requires referral to otologist or otolaryngologist for surgical exploration as soon as condition allows.

HERPES ZOSTER OTICUS (RAMSAY HUNT SYNDROME)

Subjective Complaints

Facial paralysis associated with painful herpetic lesions in ipsilateral concha and external meatus. May have other sensory nerve distribution.

Objective Findings

Herpetic lesions of concha and external meatus of involved side. Determine complete or incomplete paralysis.

Assessment

Determine involvement of VIIth nerve topographically. Check hearing and ear canal and TM to rule out otitis media, etc.

Plan

Manage same as Bell's

FACIAL PARALYSIS DUE TO CHRONIC OTITIS MEDIA

Subjective Complaints

History of draining ear or chronic ear infections usually preceding onset of facial weakness.

Objective Findings

Evidence of otitis media by actively draining, infected middle ear with perforation or by cholesteatoma. (May be dry.) Evaluate complete or partial paralysis.

Assessment

Hearing test. X-rays of mastoid and middle ear and facial canal.

Plan

Antibiotics. Refer for *immediate* surgical exploration.

FACIAL PARALYSIS ASSOCIATED WITH NEOPLASM

Subjective Complaints

History of facial paralysis, possible recurrent and may be associated with hearing loss, progressive, dizziness, facial twitching. May have draining ear (facial neuroma or glomus eroding into canal).

Objective Findings

Check completeness of paralysis, other cranial nerves including corneal reflex and complete neurologic. Examine ear canal and drum carefully.

Assessment

Audiogram for unilateral hearing loss or poor discrimination. Acoustic reflex decay test for positive decay. Polytomography of internal auditory canal for cerebelopontine angle lesion (acoustic neuroma), fallopian canal for facial neuroma, and jugular foramen for glomus tumor.

Plan

If suspect acoustic neuroma, refer for posterior fossa myelogram and surgery. If suspect glomus tumor, facial neuroma, refer for evaluation and possible surgery.

FACIAL LACERATION CAUSING PARALYSIS

Subjective Complaints

History of facial laceration (or surgery in area) associated with complete or partial facial weakness.

Objective Findings

Evaluate completeness of facial paralysis and determine where nerve most likely injured.

Assessment

Topographical analysis (see first section, Bell's Paralysis) to be sure nerve not injured proximal to suspected area.

Plan

Refer for immediate microsurgical anastomosis of lacerated nerve.

CONGENITAL FACIAL PARALYSIS

Subjective Complaints

History of facial abnormality at birth. Paralysis of face may be associated with paralysis of lateral gaze (Möbius syndrome), hypoplastic mandible, or microtia (Treacher Collins syndrome).

Objective Findings

Evaluate development of ears and ear canal for microtia and atresia or stenosis. Evaluate development of other cranial nerves and mandible-maxilla complex. Observe for other congenital abnormalities.

Assessment

X-rays usually not indicated until later when surgical correction contemplated.

Plan

Refer for evaluation of hearing and follow-up management.

CENTRAL ETIOLOGY OF FACIAL PARALYSIS

Subjective Complaints

History of stroke with facial weakness. History of simultaneous double vision, hemiparesis, etc.

Objective Findings

Central facial paralysis with sparing of ipsilateral forehead. May have other neurologic deficits such as VIth nerve paralysis or hemiparesis.

Assessment

X-ray of skull and temporal bone, audiogram, stimulate nerve if complete, spinal fluid analysis, CAT scan.

Plan

Refer for otologic and neurologic evaluation if does not fit pattern of simple stroke to rule out tumor, demyelinating disease, etc.

MELKERSSON'S SYNDROME

Subjective Complaints

History of recurrent facial weakness associated with swelling of face and fissured tongue.

Objective Findings

Facial paralysis, fissured tongue, and facial edema.

Assessment

X-rays and hearing test to rule out tumor.

Plan

Steroids (as for Bell's); return of function usually excellent in this syndrome.

MALIGNANT EXTERNAL OTITIS CAUSING FACIAL PARALYSIS

Subjective Complaints

History of ear infection associated with progression to toxic state, facial weakness; often patient is elderly diabetic.

Objective Findings

Facial paralysis with draining necrotic area, posterior ear canal.

Assessment

Culture usually reveals Pseudomonas. X-rays for evaluation of erosion. Evaluate for diabetes if not known.

Plan

Treatment must be aggressive to avoid mortality-gentamycin, 3–5 mg per kg per day and carbenicillin, 4–6 g every 4 hours, and possible surgical debridement. Immediate consultation or referral advisable.

GUILLAIN-BARRÉ SYNDROME

Subjective Complaints

History of bifacial palsy associated with ascending paralysis.

Objective Findings

Ascending paralysis, and bifacial paralysis.

Assessment

Spinal fluid; neurologic examination.

Plan

Steroids; observe for respiratory distress.

MULTIPLE SCLEROSIS

Subjective Complaints

History of facial weakness—may be associated with other symptoms or weakness or pain in upper or lower extremity. May have history of dizziness.

Objective Findings

Facial paralysis, tone usually good. Check for other neuropathy. Multiple neuropathies important for diagnosis. Complete neurologic examination.

Assessment

Audiogram, ENG, x-rays, visual evoked response.

Plan

Steroids and observation.

Chapter 5
Facial Pain and Headache

Gerald M. English

Headache and facial pains are common complaints in clinical practice. There are few symptoms that bring patients more readily to a physician than a headache or facial pain.

There are several reasons why these problems may be confusing and difficult to diagnose. The innervation of the head and neck is complex. There are many pain-sensitive structures in this region that have widely interrelated neural pathways. Referred (heterotopic) pains are very common and the various pain syndromes may be quite similar. There are a number of associated symptoms that cloud the clinical presentation, including tachycardia, chest pain, nausea, vomiting, abdominal pains, sweating, weakness, fatigue, anxiety, and depression. The patient may not relate these symptoms to the head pain, and may present these problems as the primary symptom.

A systematic, thorough investigation is the best means of making a proper diagnosis; and the history is probably the most important element of that examination. The problem-oriented method is particularly helpful in assessing these problems. This method will ensure that the pain is not overlooked or ignored. As the investigation proceeds each item on the problem list is appraised and a plan should be formulated for that particular symptom.

NASAL PAIN

Subjective Complaints

This pain is described as tight, burning sensation of the upper nose and forehead. It is often associated with nasal airway congestion and rhinorrhea. All symptoms are worse at night. Sneezing and blowing the nose may increase the pain. An application of topical decongestant or exercise sometimes relieves the discomfort. Spontaneous nasal bleeding, or bleeding with blowing the nose, is common. A decreased sense of smell (anosmia) is also common. Other abnormalities (parosmia and dysosmia) of the sense of smell are less common but do occur.

Objective Findings

Examination may reveal several abnormalities. The most common are edema and erythema of the nasal mucous membrane, and a deviated or perforated nasal septum. The secretions within the nasal chambers and nasopharynx vary from clear and watery to cloudy and discolored. There may be crusting of the nasal mucous membrane. When the secretions are purulent and present in the area of sinus drainage (superior and middle meatus), a diagnosis of sinusitis should be considered. Occasionally, there is tenderness of the nose when an acute rhinitis is present. If the mucosal edema or engorgement subsides with topical decongestants, a noninfectious etiology is more likely. Polyps may be present, and they do cause some vague discomfort. Nasal polyps are not pain-sensitive to palpation, and they do not bleed readily.

Assessment

The history will usually suggest whether the nasal disease is from an infectious, allergic, or traumatic etiology. A nasal and nasopharyngeal culture should be obtained when infection is suspected. These studies will reveal both normal and pathogenic organisms. Nasal smears may reveal an elevated eosinophil count or large numbers of inflammatory cells. X-ray examinations, including xeroradiograms, will often demonstrate a deviated nasal septum, hypertrophied turbinates, and sinusitis, as well as other abnormalities. The sinuses should be clear unless sinus diseases are present.

Plan

The treatment should be as specific as possible. Analgesics (aspirin, Acetaminophen, Darvon, codeine) are helpful and narcotics are rarely required. If an allergic etiology is diagnosed, antihistamines (Chlor-Trimeton, Pyribenzamine, Benadryl, etc.) are essential for the initial management. Allergy testing and desensitization should be considered for those patients who do not respond to medical treatment or have advanced disease. Topical decongestants (Neo-Synephrine, Otrivin, Afrin) and systemic decongestants, pseudoephedrine hydrochloride (Sudafed) and phenylephrine hydrochloride (Neo-Synephrine) will often reduce the engorgement and improve the nasal airways. Steroids, either topically (Decadron Turbinaire, Vanceril) or systemic (prednisone, Medrol) on a short-term declining schedule should be reserved for those patients who do not respond to simpler methods of treatment. When the patients fail to respond, and there are few or no nasal abnormalities, a psychogenic etiology should be suspected. Nasal septal surgery or turbinectomy is reserved for patients with specific abnormalities or advanced disease. Nasal septal perforations can sometimes be repaired surgically or treated with a Silastic stent.

SINUS PAIN

Subjective Complaints

Headaches from sinus disease are rare but local facial pain is common. The location of the pain is related to the sinus involved and referred pain is more or less specific for the various sinuses (Fig. 5.1 and Table 5.1). The other symptoms of sinus disease include rhinorrhea, postnasal drainage, epistaxis, facial swelling, or redness and fullness of areas of the face or ear. Sinus pain characteristically begins in the morning or early afternoon. It subsides later in the early or late evening. The pain is often increased by shaking the head, bending over, or straining and coughing. A tight collar that increases venous pressure in the head and neck may also increase sinus pain. Menstruation, cold air, sexual excitement, and alcohol all produce engorgement of the nasal mucosa and, thereby, increase the intensity of the pain. The barometric changes encountered during flying or scuba diving will often cause patients with thickened sinus mucosa to have extreme pain. This pain is a diffuse, sustained, deep-aching, and non-pulsatile sensation. Lacrimation, photophobia, and hyperalgesia are common.

Objective Findings

The clinical findings vary depending upon the sinus involved and whether the affected sinus ostium is open or closed. These clinical findings are also related to whether or not the disease is acute or chronic. Ocular, visual, nasal, neurologic, dental, and local signs are seen in various combinations (Table 5.2).

Assessment

An x-ray examination of the paranasal sinuses is essential for diagnosis. Specimens from the sinuses should be cultured to identify the causative agents. When a neoplasm is suspected, tissue biopsies from the sinus should have a histopathologic examination.

Plan

Simple analgesics (aspirin, Acetaminophen, codeine) will usually relieve the discomfort. Antibiotics are useful for those patients with an active infection. Decongestants, either topically or systemically, will help relieve nasal engorgement and improve drainage of the sinuses through the natural ostia. Increased humidity will made the nasal and paranasal sinus secretions less tenacious, and this facilitates removal of the materials from the nose and sinuses. Drainage and irrigation of the sinuses are often necessary, both for treatment and for diagnosis of the specific etiology. These techniques should be performed by an otolaryngologist, or a physician with specialized training and experience.

ORAL DENTAL PAIN

Subjective Complaints

The pain from oral or dental diseases is usually more severe at night. These pains occur at the site of the disease (teeth, man-

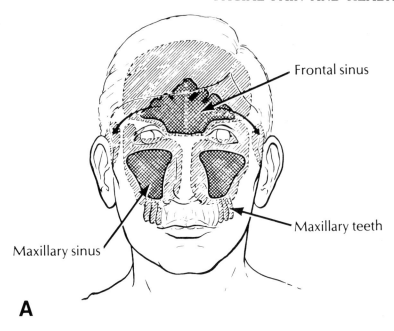

A

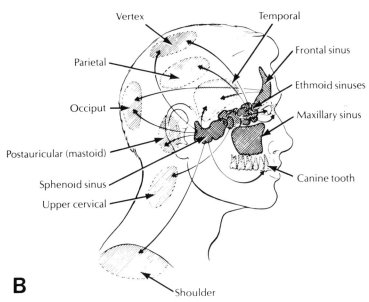

B

Figure 5.1.   *A and B*, areas to which sinus pains are referred. (From English, G. M.: Pain of the head and neck In *Otolaryngology, A Textbook*. Harper & Row, Hagerstown, Md., 1976. Reproduced with permission.)

dible, maxilla, tongue, palate, or mucosa), but may be referred to distant areas (Fig. 5.2). Thermal or mechanical stimulation (chewing and swallowing) often aggravates or intensifies the pain. Hot and cold foods and drink are the most notorious offenders. A history of dental disease, trismus, difficulties with chewing (mastication), dry mouth (xerostomia), or increased salivation (ptyalism) are fairly common.

Table 5.1
Homotopic and Heterotopic Pains Associated with the Paranasal Sinuses

Sinus Involved	Local Pain	Referred Pain
Maxillary	Cheek, nose, upper lip and upper teeth	Retro-orbital and mandibular teeth
Ethmoid	Retronasal and retro-orbital	Occipital and upper cervical
Sphenoid	Retro-orbital and retronasal	Bitemporal, frontal, vertex, occipital, shoulder, mastoid, and canine toothache
Frontal	Frontal and supraorbital	Bitemporal and occipital headache

(From English, G. M.: Pain of the head and neck. In *Otolaryngology, A Textbook*. Harper & Row, Hagerstown, Md., 1976. Reproduced with permission.)

Table 5.2
Clinical Findings in Sinus Diseases

Sinus Involved	Clinical Signs
Maxillary	Ocular abnormalities, including diplopia, proptosis, and epiphora Nasal obstruction and rhinorrhea Epistaxis Loose teeth and ill-fitting dentures Palatal, facial, and gingivobuccal swelling Hypesthesia of the upper teeth, the cheek, and the upper lip Trismus
Ethmoid	Evidence of pansinusitis, except in children Orbital swelling and orbital tenderness Proptosis and diplopia Nasal obstruction and purulent rhinorrhea Tenderness over inner canthus of eye
Sphenoid	Stiffness of the neck Postnasal drainage Forgetfulness Perversions of the sense of smell Cough Anorexia and vertigo Visual disturbances
Frontal	Nasal obstruction and rhinorrhea Pus in the nasofrontal duct and anterior part of the middle meatus Tenderness over the frontal sinus along its floor Pitting edema over the frontal sinus Redness and local tenderness Signs of meningitis or intracranial infection

(From English, G. M.: Pain of the head and neck. In *Otolaryngology, A Textbook*. Harper & Row, Hagerstown, Md., 1976. Reproduced with permission.)

Objective Findings

Dental caries, ulcerations of oral mucosa, and mass lesions are the most common clinical findings. Palpation and percussion of the teeth or other oral structures will often elicit the symptom of pain. Edentulous patients may have retained tooth fragments that are inciting the pain.

Assessment

An x-ray examination of suspicious areas will usually reveal any underlying

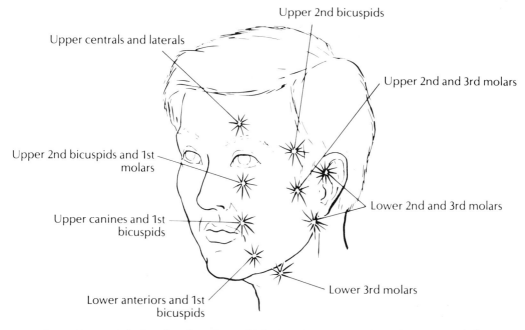

Upper 2nd bicuspids

Upper centrals and laterals

Upper 2nd and 3rd molars

Upper 2nd bicuspids and 1st
molars

Lower 2nd and 3rd molars

Upper canines and 1st
bicuspids

Lower 3rd molars

Lower anteriors and 1st
bicuspids

Figure 5.2. Areas of the head and neck to which dental pains are referred. (From English, G. M.: Pain of the head and neck. In *Otolaryngology, A Textbook*. Harper & Row, Hagerstown, Md., 1976. Reproduced with permission.)

dental or bone disease. Many patients should be referred to a dentist for more extensive studies and treatment. Laboratory tests, including complete blood count, serologic test for syphilis, and biopsy of suspicious lesions will help determine the proper diagnosis.

Plan

Those patients who have pain from dental disease will require appropriate dental care, but analgesics will make the patient more comfortable until the dentist can begin treatment. Antibiotics should be used in those patients who have infection. A biopsy of suspicious lesions and histopathologic study of the tissue is essential. Neoplasms must be differentiated from the oral lesions of pernicious anemia, polycythemia, agranulocytosis, leukemia, avitaminosis (vitamin B_2 complex-pellagra and vitamin C-scurvy). Specific therapies for those problems are beyond the scope of this book.

TEMPOROMANDIBULAR JOINT PAIN

Subjective Complaints

The pain varies from a dull, recurring ache over the temporomandibular joint to an intense, agonizing, short spasm of pain that radiates into the cheek, temple, lower jaw, ear, mastoid area, or upper neck. The pain is often associated with chewing, talking, or yawning. There may be an associated trismus or stiffness of the jaw. Malocclusion, subluxation, and "clicking" of the joint also occur. Anxiety, grinding the teeth (bruxism), dental repair, or extractions and trauma to the mandible are the most common causes of this disease.

Objective Findings

Clicking, crepitus, tenderness on palpation, malocclusion, poorly fitting dentures, and loss of teeth are the most common clinical findings. A normal external auditory canal and tympanic membrane in patients with an earache should alert the physician to consider this disease as the cause of the otalgia. Tenderness and spasm of the muscles of mastication and a diminished range of motion of the mandible are common clinical findings in this disease.

Assessment

An x-ray examination of the temporomandibular joint will reveal any structural or degenerative changes in the joint. Both an open and closed mouth view are essential for a complete examination. Dramatic but temporary relief of the pain can be obtained with an injection of a small amount of local anesthetic (Xylocaine 2%) into the joint area or the petrotympanic fissure. This technique may be necessary to establish the correct diagnosis.

Plan

Analgesics are helpful but narcotics are rarely necessary. Temporomandibular joint exercises (Table 5.3) will help the patient relax the muscles of mastication and increase the range of motion of the lower jaw. These exercises should include chewing on both sides of the jaw. Muscle relaxants will reduce muscle spasm and fatigue. A bite plate or block can be used to reduce bruxism during sleep. Correction of occlusion discrepancies or problems by replacing missing teeth and restoration of the dentures is required for relief in appropriate patients.

Steroid injection into the affected joint is helpful but it should be followed by appropriate treatment of the causes of the disorder. Surgical treatment consists of condylectomy or condylotomy, and this form of therapy should be reserved for those patients who do not respond to other methods of treatment (Fig. 5.3).

CAROTIDYNIA

Subjective Complaints

The attacks of pain are periodic, unilateral and not ordinarily associated with visual disturbances. A dull, aching sensation is usually described. The pain is referred to the eye, deep malar region, and spreads to the back of the ear and down the neck. Gastrointestinal symptoms such as abdominal pain, nausea, vomiting, and diarrhea are common. There is often a history of confusion, lethargy, depression, and insomnia. The patient is usually asymptomatic between the attacks of pain.

Objective Findings

There are swelling and tenderness of the carotid artery on the affected side. The pain is accentuated by palpation of the carotid artery and can be produced by pressing the carotid artery backward against the cervical transverse process. A conspicuous pulsation of the carotid artery is present in some individuals.

Assessment

These patients have many of the general features of migraine headache. This pain,

Table 5.3
Exercise Program for Temporomandibular Joint Disorders

1. Open and close the mouth as widely and as rapidly as possible.
2. Open the mouth against slight pressure applied by placing the open palm beneath the chin.
3. Close the mouth against slight pressure applied by placing the open palm above the chin.
4. Move the mandible from side to side without resistance; then move it from side to side with pressure from the palm of the hand against the side of the chin.
5. Protrude the jaw with and without resistance.
6. Chew a small piece of wax on each side, and then in the center for 3–5 minutes.

Repeat each exercise five times, twice a day. Increase at a rate of five times each week to a maximum of 25 exercises twice a day.

(From English, G. M.: Pain of the head and neck. In *Otolaryngology, A Textbook.* Harper & Row, Hagerstown, Md., 1976. Reproduced with permission.)

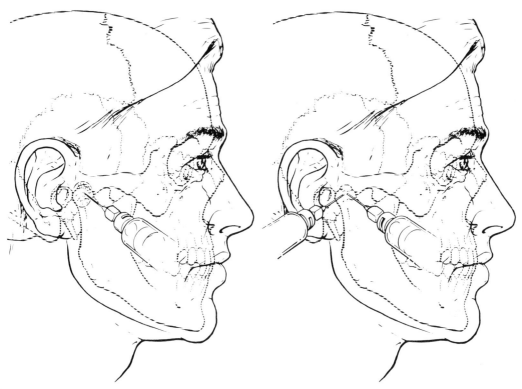

Figure 5.3.   Injection of the temporomandibular joint. *A (left)*, a wheal is raised one fingerbreadth in front of the tragus and just below the zygomatic arch. *B (right)*, the needle is inserted behind and in front of the condyle. (From English, G. M.: Pain of the head and neck. In *Otolaryngology, A Textbook*. Harper & Row, Hagerstown, Md., 1976. Reproduced with permission.)

however, does not subside with ergotamine tartrate. The patients appear to be quite ill. The face is pale, sallow, and often covered with a light oiliness or sweat. There may be a slight edema of the affected side of the neck and face. The patient complains of a lack of vigor and exhibits overall lassitude. Laboratory and x-ray examinations are usually normal.

Plan

Analgesics are necessary for symptomatic relief. When the pain is of low intensity, 0.3–0.6 g of aspirin or 60 mg of codeine are sufficient for control of the symptom. These patients do not obtain relief from ergotamine tartrate. Ergotamine tartrate may be used to help differentiate carotidynia from other vascular headaches (migraine, cluster headache). They may have an exacerbation of their symptoms with various vasodilators. Reassurance regard-

ing the nature of the disorder will help relieve the patient's anxiety. A change in life style may be beneficial when stress is a factor precipitating the pain. Avoiding tight, constricting collars or other garments may be helpful. There is no specific therapy but steroids and other anti-inflammatory agents are sometimes helpful.

NEURALGIAS

Trigeminal Neuralgia (Tic Douloureux)

Subjective Complaints

This is an episodic, unilateral recurrent facial pain that occurs most commonly in patients between the ages of 30 and 60 years. The pain is experienced chiefly over the area of the face supplied by the second division of the trigeminal nerve and less often in those areas supplied by the first and third divisions of the Vth cranial nerve (Fig. 5.4). The pain is a high intensity "jab" of 20–30 seconds' duration. It is also described as an aching, burning sensation that may occur spontaneously. Cold air, a light touch, chewing, swallowing, laughing, talking, yawning, sneezing, and blowing the nose or drinking cold water will often precipitate an attack of pain. The most common "trigger" site is the lateral border of the nose. The attacks may occur at any time during the day or night but seldom begin during sleep unless the face is inadvertently rubbed. Anxiety, tension, fatigue, and stress may cause the attacks of pain. The pain may disappear for weeks or months but spontaneous recovery is rare.

Objective Findings

There is no demonstrable neurologic defect of motor or sensory function. Occasionally, a mild hyperalgesia during the attack and a minimal hypalgesia of the face between attacks is noted. During the attack, the cheek is reddened, the tongue

is furred, and the eyes are watery. There is a cramped facial expression. Between attacks, the patient holds his face immobile and talks cautiously through closed lips and jaws. The affected side of the face is often soiled and unshaven. These patients report that the face washing or shaving precipitates the pain.

Assessment

Laboratory and x-ray examinations are normal.

Plan

Because the pain has such a short duration, analgesics are of limited value. Trichloroethylene inhalations often give prompt but temporary relief. Dilantin (100 mg three times daily) may be beneficial. Benadryl has also been used with some success. Carbamazepine (Tegretol), 400 mg per day up to 800 mg per day, may give complete or partial relief of the pain. Those patients who do not respond to medical therapy should have injection or surgical ablation of the affected nerve. These pro-

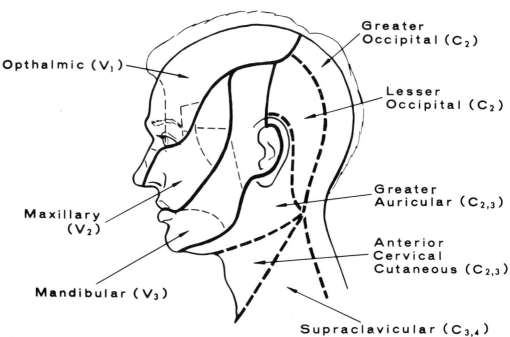

Figure 5.4. The approximate cutaneous distribution of the three divisions of the Vth cranial nerve and the cervical nerves to the face and scalp.

cedures require the special skills of a neurosurgeon (Fig. 5.5).

Glossopharyngeal Neuralgia

Subjective Complaints

This is a severe, episodic pain in the region of the tonsil and ear. The pain is usually initiated by yawning, swallowing, or food and water that come in contact with the tonsillar area. The quality, onset, duration, and frequency of the pain are quite similar to those of trigeminal neuralgia. Syncope may occur during the attack from cardiac slowing or cardiac arrest.

Objective Findings

There are no neurologic abnormalities. Palatal and pharyngeal mobility are unimpaired and the "gag" reflex is intact.

Assessment

Laboratory studies and x-ray examinations are usually normal.

Plan

Analgesics are of limited value. A topical anesthetic spray (Cetacaine) applied to the trigger zone may give temporary relief. The other forms of treatment for this neuralgia are similar to those used for trigeminal neuralgia.

Sphenopalatine Neuralgia (Lower-Half Headache, Sluder's Headache)

Subjective Complaints

This pain involves the lower one-half of the face below the ear. It is episodic, recurrent and lasts from a few minutes to several days. There are two sites of maximum pain: (1) the orbit and base of the nose, and (2) the mastoid process. The most common site is the orbit and nose. In addition to an earache, fullness in the ear, tinnitus, and vertigo are sometimes reported. Unilateral nasal airway congestion and rhinorrhea are also present during the attack. The pain may spread down the neck to the shoulder. Itching of the skin, taste disturbances, and stiffness and weakness of the shoulder muscles are not rare. The pain may emanate from the teeth of the upper and lower jaws with an associated tingling of the skin of the lower jaw.

Objective Findings

Examination will not reveal any specific abnormalities. There are occasional patients who have a deviated nasal septum or nasal septal spur. This is important to detect because these patients often respond to appropriate surgical treatment of the nasal abnormality.

Assessment

The pain is usually relieved by an application of cocaine to the sphenopalatine ganglion region in the posterior nasal chamber. Injections of the sphenopalatine ganglion with a local anesthetic (Xylocaine) through the greater palatine canal will produce prompt relief of the pain. (Fig. 5.6).

X-ray examinations of the nose, paranasal sinuses, teeth and ear are usually normal.

Plan

Analgesics are of limited value. Cocainization or injections of the sphenopalatine ganglion will give relief. Nasal septal operations have been reported as an effective treatment for the pain in some patients. Resection of the sphenopalatine ganglion may be of value but should be reserved for patients with pain that does not respond to other forms of treatment. A neurosurgeon or otolaryngologist should be consulted regarding this procedure.

Vidian Neuralgia

Subjective Complaints

This pain is located in the nose, face, eye, ear, head, neck, and shoulder. The attacks are episodic, unilateral, and often nocturnal. The pain is not precipitated by external stimulation. A unilateral nasal

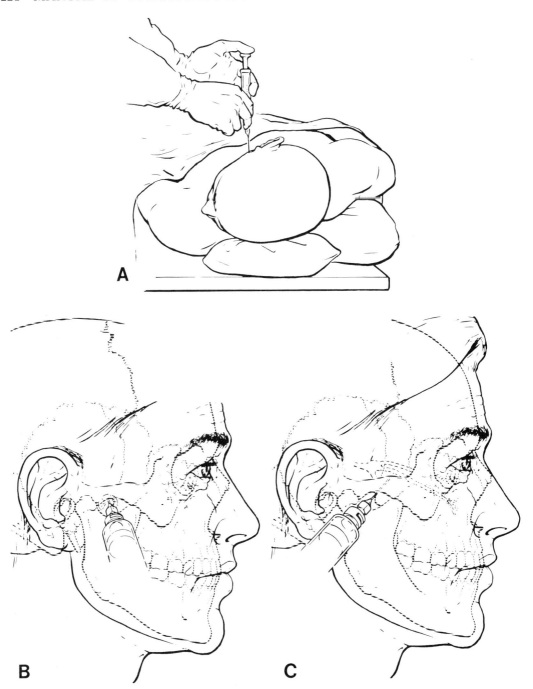

Figure 5.5. *A*, the proper position of a patient for a maxillary nerve block in the pterygopalatine fossa. *B*, a wheal is raised 3 cm in front of the tragus and 1 cm below the arch of the zygoma. *C*, a needle is passed through the anesthetized area below the arch of the zygoma into the pterygopalatine fossa. If bone is encountered at 5 or 5.5 cm, the needle is impinging upon the pterygoid plate of the sphenoid bone and it can be moved forward until it "falls" into the fossa. A sudden pain in the upper lip will indicate proper placement of the needle. (From English, G. M.: Pain of the head and neck. In *Otolaryngology, A Textbook.* Harper & Row, Hagerstown, Md.: 1976. Reproduced with permission.)

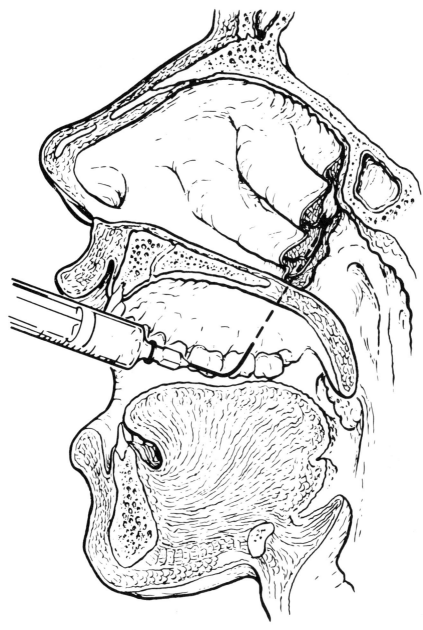

Figure 5.6.   A sphenopalatine ganglion block. The needle is inserted through the greater palatine foramen. This foramen lies medial to the last molar tooth and can occasionally be identified as a slight dimple in the mucosa. The needle is inserted to a depth of 1.25 inches, and 1 cc of solution is injected slowly. Paresthesia may be produced along the distrubution of the maxillary nerve when the needle touches the ganglion. (From English, G. M.: Pain of the head and neck. In *Otolaryngology, A Textbook.* Harper & Row, Hagerstown, Md., 1976. Reproduced with permission.)

airway congestion and rhinorrhea are often associated with this pain. This pain syndrome is similar to the pain of sphenopalatine neuralgia and may be indistinguishable from that entity.

Objective Findings

There is no associated loss of sensory or motor function. Engorgement of the nasal mucosa and increased secretions are seen on one side of the nose in some patients.

Assessment

An x-ray examination of the paranasal sinuses may reveal sphenoid sinus disease. This has been specifically related to Vidian neuralgia, but the incidence of the sinusitis and pain syndrome has not been established.

Plan

The treatment is similar to that for sphenopalatine ganglion neuralgia. Medical and surgical treatment of sphenoid sinus disease seems to be an effective method of controlling the pain in some patients.

VASCULAR HEADACHES

Classic Migraine

Subjective Complaints

There is often a family history of migraine. The migraine attack is always preceded by an aura or prodromal symptom of a visual or an auditory nature. Childhood complaints of carsickness and "bilious" spells are often harbingers of migraine attacks later in life. The attacks may begin with the first important life change. Stress situations, such as leaving home to enter the Armed Services or beginning the first job, are often associated with the onset of attacks. There may be an increased number of attacks during the first few months of pregnancy, and they generally tend to increase during stressful periods. The headaches decrease during periods of calm and with advancing age.

Objective Findings

The patients usually look very ill, with a face that is pale and covered with sweat. They support the head with the hands to reduce movements that accentuate the pain. Flushing of the face, distention of the superficial temple artery, and congestion of the conjunctivae or the nasal mucous membrane are common.

Assessment

Physical examination, laboratory studies, x-rays, and electroencephalograms are usually normal.

Plan

The treatment of both classic and common migraine headache is designed to reduce the frequency and severity of the attacks and to relieve the pain of the acute attack. Interval treatment or prophylaxis can be accomplished with methysergide maleate. This is a serotonin antagonist and a useful agent for the interval treatment of migraine. This substance does not produce overt vasoconstriction. Because of its possible adverse effects, including retroperitoneal fibrosis, this drug should be considered only for those patients who have one or more severe attacks per week and those individuals who have uncontrollably severe attacks. Cyproheptadine hydrochloride has been used as a prophylactic agent against migraine. This potent serotonin and histamine antagonist has not proved significantly superior to other agents. Pizotyline, a tricyclide derivative, has an action similar to that of cyproheptadine hydrochloride. It has not proved to be more effective than methysergide maleate.

Common Migraine

Subjective Complaints

The prodomes are vague and vary. These symptoms may precede the attack by several hours or even days. The headache usually starts when the patient awakens in the morning. The intensity increases over a span of several hours. Occasionally, a patient may be awakened from a sound sleep with a full-blown headache. There are various associated symptoms, such as vomiting, polyuria, chills, and prostration. The headache usually lasts most of the day or until the patient goes to sleep. The pain may continue for several days. The headache is usually unilateral and covers areas supplied by several sensory nerves. The headache is often associated with nasal congestion and rhinorrhea on the affected side. There is occasionally unilateral lacrimation and conjunctival congestion. These phenomena might suggest a diagnosis of sinus headache unless they are recognized as an integral part of the migraine attack. The patient may complain of photophobia, phonophobia, or both. Eighty percent of the patients have a family history of migraine. There may be a youthful history of carsickness and "bilious" attacks. Life stresses, such as puberty, school work, job responsibilities, marriage, and child-rearing, often bring on migraine episodes. During pregnancy, there is relief in about 80% of patients. There may be temporary remissions during a *bona fide* illness, such as coronary thrombosis, pneumonia, jaundice, cholecystectomy, hysterectomy, prolonged orthopedic operations, or other debilitating ailments which serve to convince the patient that he is "a legal invalid" for a short period of time. A long vacation or leisurely travel often provides relief from the attacks. Menopause may be a time of accentuation of the attacks, and the postmenopausal phase may be one of either relief or continuation of the attacks. Arterial hypertension may increase both the frequency and severity of the migraine headache.

Objective Findings

There are no specific clinical findings associated with this disease.

Assessment

Laboratory x-rays and other diagnostic studies are usually normal.

Plan

The treatment for this form of migraine is essentially the same as that described for classic migraine.

Cluster Headaches

Subjective Complaints

A short period (5 minutes) of burning pain in the temple or eyes followed by a rapidly increasing and excruciating steady or throbbing pain is described by most patients. The pain may radiate into the neck. The attacks often arise with clock-like regularity during sleep or after relaxation or naps. The pain lasts from a few minutes to a few hours (30–90 minutes) and rarely more than 2 hours. The attacks are precipitated by alcohol, nitrates, or histamine. Increased salivation, nasal airway congestion, and rhinorrhea are common. The headaches often follow periods of prolonged strain, overwork, and emotional stress.

Objective Findings

An ipsilateral prominence of the temporal blood vessels, conjuctival injection, lacrimation, miosis, edema, unilateral sweating, and engorgement of the turbinates are present. There are no neurologic abnormalities. Peptic ulcers and ulcer symptoms are common in patients with cluster headache.

Assessment

Laboratory, x-rays, and other studies are normal.

Plan

Antihistamines, analgesics, narcotics, sedatives, and tranquilizers are ineffective in relieving cluster headaches. Ergotamine preparations are quite effective in aborting or alleviating the attack. The oral administration of 1–2 mg of ergotamine tartrate an hour or so before the anticipated attack is useful when the attacks recur at consistent times of the day. Ergotamine tartrate, 1–2 mg, before retiring will prevent attacks that awaken the patient during sleep. The usual range of dosage of ergotamine tartrate is 1–4 or 1–5 mg per day. The patient should be carefully observed and cautioned about the early signs and symptoms of ergotism. These include pallor, numbness, tingling, or cyanosis of the digits.

Methysergide has been used with some success as a prophylactic for cluster headache. The usual dose is 2 mg, three times daily. It can be used for 6–8 weeks and then gradually tapered, reduced, and discontinued.

Those patients who become refractory to ergotamine tartrate and methysergide may respond to diazepam (Valium), corticosteroids, diphenylhydantoin (Dilantin) or cyanocobalamin (vitamin B_{12}).

Psychotherapy should always be considered in patients with cluster headache.

MUSCLE CONTRACTION HEADACHE (TENSION)

Subjective Complaints

The pain is located in the frontal, parietal, occipital, or temporal areas. This is a steady, nonpulsatile pain that may be either unilateral or bilateral. A tight "bandlike" or "viselike" sensation is usually described. The headache is precipitated by brushing or combing the hair and wearing a hat. Support of the head with the hands may relieve the pain. The patients usually purposely limit the range of head movement. Dizziness, tinnitus, and increased lacrimation may accompany the pain. Tension, anxiety, or specific stressful situations may precipitate the pain. Irritability, restlessness, and sleep disturbances are common in these patients.

Objective Findings

There may be signs of muscle contraction. Tenderness of the neck and scalp may be demonstrated by gentle palpation. No other specific abnormalities are present.

Assessment

X-ray examinations of the skull and neck are usually normal. Some patients may demonstrate degenerative changes in the cervical spine.

Plan

Muscle relaxants, mild sedatives, analgesics, and physical therapy are useful. Psychotherapy should be considered if the individual patient warrants it.

Bibliography

1. Beeson, P. B., and McDermott, W. (Eds.). *Cecil and Loeb Textbook of Medicine*, ed. 13, pp. 155–160. W. B. Saunders Co., Philadelphia, 1971.
2. Brain, R. *Diseases of the Nervous System*, pp. 286–290. Oxford University Press, London, 1956.
3. Diamond, S., and Baltes, B. J. Headache an emergency? *Emergency Med.* 4: 87, 1972.
4. English, G. M.: Pain of the head and neck. In *Otolaryngology, A Textbook*, pp. 756–775. Harper & Row, Hagerstown, Md., 1976.
5. Finneson, B. E. *Diagnosis and Management of Pain Syndrome*, pp. 1–72. W. B. Saunders, Philadelphia, 1962.
6. Muelig, W. A. Why is the head aching? *Emergency Med.* 4: 170, 1972.
7. Vanden Noorst, S.: A face in pain. *Emergency Med.* 4: 170, 1972.
8. Wolff, H. G. *Headache and Other Pain*, ed. 2, pp. 227–466. Oxford University Press, New York, 1963.

Chapter 6
Trismus

Richard Cundy

Trismus is a symptom which is the inability to open the mouth. It is often a manifestation of a true ankylosis which is the pathologic involvement of articular structures of the temporomandibular joint. False ankylosis or pseudoankylosis can cause trismus as a result of extraarticular abnormalities which prevent adequate jaw motion. Although there are many causes of trismus, the most common are listed below.

1. Trauma.
2. Dental problems.
3. Infection.
4. Temporomandibular joint syndrome.
5. Arthritis.
6. Tumors.
7. Radiotherapy.
8. Central nervous system lesions.
9. Systemic diseases.
10. Congenital causes.
11. Psychologic causes.

Subjective Complaints

The etiology of trismus can be so varied that a complete history relating to all of the above conditions must be elicited from the patient. Since trismus does limit jaw motion, it can limit the ability to speak, and many questions can be answered only by shaking of the head to indicate yes or no.

Trauma. Traumatic injuries to the jaw and the temporomandibular joint are the most common causes of trismus in patients who present to a physician. A history of injury to the jaw, ear, cheek, or other parts of the head or neck is offered voluntarily, but in marital disputes the injury may be denied. The patient is usually aware if he has been struck by a fist or foreign body, but many times in auto accidents the patient will remember only striking his head against the windshield or dashboard, completely forgetting that his chin was the foremost part of the head in the accident. The patient may have been unconscious, and questions to witnesses or ambulance attendants may be necessary to determine where the patient was riding in the vehicle in order to reconstruct the manner of injury. History of an ecchymosis or tender spot which now has improved may lead to the diagnosis, and the patient may say that swelling was marked at one point of the jaw but has since resolved. He may state that difficulty in swallowing or shortness of breath accompany his injury but if these are severe, the patient may be very incapacitated from speaking. He may be spitting blood, gurgling, or have severe pain when trying to open his jaw to speak.

Dental Problems. The patient may complain of a lopsided or asymmetrical appearance to the jaw occurring after sleep or yawning. Many patients will state that their teeth do not fit together properly. Some seem to grind their teeth (bruxation), especially when nervous, or during sleep. The spouse may complain that he/she spends the night listening to this annoying sound. The initial symptom may be pain in the ear due to the proximity of the temporomandibular joint to the adjacent external canal wall. Spasm and pain in the musculature may cause the patient to state that the soreness extends either into the temple or down into the cervical area. One must ascertain whether a new set of dentures has just been fitted or whether major dental work in which the teeth were remodeled, capped, or ground down has taken place. Occasionally, a patient will state that prior to the remodeling of his present dentures the jaw felt normal; but since that time he has had marked difficulty in fully opening his mouth.

A tooth extraction often leads the patient to seek medical help when pain or swelling persists. The most common site is the third molar although any tooth nerve can stimulate a reaction which can lead to trismus. Usually the tooth socket starts hurting on the 2nd or 3rd day and may be accompanied by fever or chills as well as swelling near the site of the tooth removal. Dysphagia may occur with a fairly rapid onset. Chewing may be restricted, especially by any feeling of swelling near the occlusal surface in the posterior part of the mouth. A history of an injection placed in the posterior alveolar surface or near the condyle may cause a pain as well as swelling from either nerve or muscle damage. If a hematoma is developing, the patient will complain of a swelling in the posterior alveolar ridge and trismus will be accompanied by deviation of the jaw to the ipsilateral side due to spasm in the muscle.

Infection. Since infections may play a great role in the cause of trismus, a careful history with special attention to contacts with communicable diseases should be elicited. Peritonsillar abscesses may cause trismus in a great number of cases and any history of treatment for a sore throat should be elicited. When this is the case, symptoms of fever, dysphagia and pharyngeal soreness are usually offered spontaneously, but one must determine whether the patient was inadequately treated with antibiotics for any infections of the throat. A sour or bitter taste in the mouth indicating pus is occasionally offered, and again dental abscesses from tooth removal or filling can often be the anticipated cause. History of trauma must be brought out in infected cases since osteomyelitis may be developing and this would manifest itself in marked pain, tenderness, and swelling.

Tetanus. Tetanus is a disease which is usually caused by foreign body penetration. Metallic objects are the most common penetrating substances which can cause this fatal disease. Even though tetanus is an uncommon disease in the United States (200 cases per year), it is very common in other parts of the world and over 300,000 cases per year are reported. Careful questioning as to immunization, both recent and in the past, must be done to determine whether the patient would be susceptible to this disease. Although the exotoxin (tetanospasmin) incubates in from 2 up to 56 days, most symptoms occur within the initial 3 weeks of exposure. The patient may complain of trismus associated with neck stiffness, dysphagia, or increasing inability to move the face, as well as respiratory difficulties. As symptoms are progressive, opisthotonos can occur and spasms of the musculature become extremely painful. If cephalic tetanus occurs (trismus and unilateral facial palsy) within 7 days after contamination, then a grave prognosis is present.

Arthritis. Rheumatoid arthritis can eventually involve the temporomandibular joint and the patient should be questioned as to whether any other rheumatoid joints have been present. On the other hand, osteoarthritis of the temporomandibular joint is due to chronic irregular movement or trauma and this can be determined with many of the preceding questions. Pain in the ear is often the main complaint, since the anterior wall of the ear is the posterior joint surface. The patient may state that his pain becomes markedly better with aspirin but not with phenacetin, indicating a joint inflammation problem.

Tumors. Tumors of the parotid or the mandibular condyle may impinge into the joint space or the surrounding musculature and cause trismus. One should elicit a history of masses or previous surgery for a tumor. If a patient had a malignancy requiring *radiotherapy*, significant fibrosis may have occurred in the masticator muscles to create a severe disability opening the jaw.

Central Nervous System Lesions and Systemic Diseases. Since these can result in trismus, a general history should be included. Any symptoms of multiple sclerosis, epilepsy, or polio should be attained—since all may create trismus. Headache is often associated with central nervous system lesions which cause trismus, and pain along the distribution of the maxillary or mandibular nerve is sometimes present. Generalized bone disease or muscle tetany can occur, since hypocalcemia and hypomagnesemia both can have associated trismus. Syphilis as well as temporal arteritis may create difficulty in opening the jaw.

Congenital Causes. Congenital causes of trismus are quite rare. Usually they are detected very early in life and are associated with syndromes which are very easily diagnosed. The first branchial arch syndrome with maldevelopment of the ear and mandible limits mandible excursion. The Pierre Robin syndrome with an underdeveloped mandible may lead to difficulty in opening the mouth, giving the impression of glossomegaly. A very rare syndrome called pseudocamptodactyly may have marked mouth opening limitations and has been reported only in certain Kentucky-Dutch children. As the jaw develops in some children, the coronoid process may become so long that it impinges upon the zygomatic arch and its musculature, thus creating marked difficulty in jaw movement.

Psychologic Causes. If all these questions have failed to stimulate any thoughts toward a specific diagnosis, one must always be aware that conversion reactions and other types of hysterical problems can cause trismus. The patient usually is very inconsistent in giving the history and does not seem appropriate in the description of symptoms. Patients may be showing a lack of reasoning or they may be emotionally distraught while discussing their complaints. One must subsequently go deeper into the cause of anxiety or extreme stress which is causing their particular symptom.

Objective Findings

As in any patient with a significant symptom, a physical examination should not be solely confined to the area of complaint. As mentioned before, many systemic and central nervous system diseases can be manifested as trismus and this should be anticipated when examining the patient.

Often, just general observation of the patient will start the physician on the proper road to diagnosis. There may be a history of trauma with ecchymoses, swelling, or lacerations around the jaw or face. When he is speaking, the patient's occlusion may be quite asymmetrical or the jaw may deviate to one side when trying to open the mouth. In severe injuries or in infections, the patient may be leaning forward with a posture of air hunger. One may observe a hypertrophy of the masseter muscles, although often this cannot be determined until palpation is done.

The palpation of the mandible must be done very gingerly since oftentimes fractures have torn the periosteum and extreme pain can be elicited by touching the tender site. Stepoff deformities of the mandible will tip off the physician to a fracture. Tenderness is usually elicited over a fracture site, even though it may not be displaced. Palpation of the temporomandibular joint in both opened and closed positions will determine whether any joint pathology seems to be present. Examina-

tion of the ear canal may reveal a laceration indicating a posterior joint space fracture into the ear canal. Palpation of the muscles around the jaw and the neck may reveal hematomas, fibrotic tissue, or marked spasm. The parotid gland should be carefully palpated for any tumors, swellings, or bony deformities. Fluctuation is often a sign of an abscess.

Intraoral examination can be an extremely difficult procedure in patients with severe trismus. Initially, the dental occlusion should be evaluated in both the open and the closed positions. Two tongue blades can be placed laterally in the buccal space to reveal both sides of the occlusal surfaces. Any premature contact of the cusps may cause blocking or bumping of the joint surfaces and these should be noted. Occasionally, overclosure can occur, especially in patients who have lost posterior teeth. The alveolar ridge and gingiva should be carefully examined for any dry sockets or swelling which may indicate early abscess or infection. Lacerations of the gingiva may be from a mandibular fracture.

Peritonsillar cellulitis, swelling, or edema of the uvula may indicate an impending abscess and may be creating spasm in the occlusal musculature. Retromolar trigone abscesses present in the space between the lower and upper jaw and will more infrequently cause uvular edema.

There are patients in whom trismus may be so severe that adequate examination of the intraoral and posterior pharyngeal areas cannot be accomplished, and various other measures must then be undertaken. Bite blocks can be inserted between the molars to try to wedge them apart, but overactive use of these can cause severe pain and create a severely distressful situation. An oropharyngoscope can be inserted between the slightly opened teeth to visualize the posterior part of the pharynx. This will usually give enough visualization to determine if there is a peritonsillar or retromolar abscess. A fiberoptic pharyngoscope or laryngoscope can also be used in the same manner and these give the advantage of having a flexible light source. The nasopharyngoscope, which is thinner but can be inserted through the nostril along the floor of the nose into the nasopharyngeal space, has its limitations in that the palate often causes an obstructed view of the posterior pharynx. The fiberoptic scope again can be of some value in this situation if it can be manipulated to visualize the lateral pharyngeal spaces.

Assessment

After the history and physical have been completed, the diagnosis is usually apparent. Laboratory studies may be useful and should include a complete blood count (CBC) and urinalysis. In cases of tetany, calcium and magnesium levels should be determined. If rheumatoid arthritis (RA) is suspected, sedimentation rates, RA factors, and antinuclear antibody (ANA) levels should be run. Syphilis tests will probably be run as a routine on most hospital admissions. If infection is entertained as a diagnosis, a culture of the intraoral surface may be of some help, but more information can be gained if pus is present. Aspiration may be required to obtain a true culture of an abscess or cellulitis. Clostridium tetany is a gram-positive anaerobe and can be cultured from the penetrating wound in cases of tetanus.

The most helpful diagnostic tool in trauma cases is the x-ray. Temporomandibular joint x-rays may demonstrate a dislocated mandible or arthritis of the joint surfaces. Mandibular x-rays are essential in demonstrating fractures of the bone or joint space. Two mandibular fractures are commonly found, one being near the joint on the opposite side of a main fracture of the body or angle of the mandible. The coronoid process should be observed for its relationship to the zygomatic arch in both the open and closed positions. In dental problems or in situations in which a mandibular fracture is suspected but not confirmed, a Panorex should be done. Most oral surgeons and some hospitals have this type of x-ray unit which delineates the whole jaw as a continuous picture. Osteomyelitis and foreign bodies are also better detected with this type of radiologic study. In some patients, posterior pharyngeal and nasopharyngeal x-rays must be taken to see portions of the upper airway that could not be visualized by direct observation.

If a swelling of the parotid gland is present intraorally, a sialogram may be able to demonstrate either a tumor or other disease process which might be in the deep part of the parotid. If central nervous system lesions are present, skull x-rays, CAT scans or brain scans may be indicated.

Plan

Once the diagnosis has been made, further steps can be taken depending upon the proficiency of the physician involved. Almost all fractures should be treated by a specialist who deals with these problems frequently. Immobilization with arch bars, interdental wires, or direct bone fixation can be a difficult technical task and should not be attempted by someone who is not familiar with these particular techniques. Most mandibular fractures are in ambulatory patients who do not require immediate care, but occasionally the primary physician may see a severe traumatic disruption of the bony continuity of the mandible which is causing bleeding into the throat, inability to swallow, and marked difficulty with respiration due to retroposition of the tongue from lack of support of the bony structures. In these acute stiuations, when transportation of the patient could lead to a respiratory arrest, a tracheostomy often is required to maintain an airway. Trying to intubate these patients is fraught with hazard and is extremely difficult. When the patient is transported by ambulance he should be placed in a prone position with the jaw dependent so that secretions can drain from the oral cavity and the tongue is then in a forward dependent position and does not obstruct the hypopharynx.

Dislocation of the mandible can be repositioned if certain basic steps are followed. Initially, the physician's two thumbs may be placed on the posterior molars, and with a firm but not overexcessive downward pressure the jaw may be relocated. If this is not easily done due to excessive pain, then intraarticular injections of Xylocaine, accompanied by intramuscular or intravenous muscle relaxants, will make the procedure much easier. After the jaw is relocated into the joint space, the patient should be instructed not to yawn or open the mouth fully for several days.

If ankylosis of the joint has occurred to a significant degree, an oral surgeon should be consulted, since open surgery of the ramus in which osteotomies with Silastic interposition or even condylectomies may be required. If the coronoid process seems to be abutting against the zygomatic arch, coronoidectomies may have to be done.

Many dental problems causing trismus can be repaired by a competent dentist. If a hematoma or fibrosis has occurred in the jaw musculature, a forced opening of the mandible may be required. This can be done with graduated bite blocks and gentle manipulation, or in more serious instances, as in radiotherypy fibrosis, actual separation of the fibrotic segment may be required under a general anesthetic.

In infectious processes, antibiotics are essential in their total treatment. Cultures will direct the physician toward the appropriate antibiotic, but in most cases wide spectrum antibiotics need to be started immediately and one cannot wait for culture and sensitivities to return from the laboratory 1–2 days after taken. Peritonsillar and retromolar abscesses can be drained by simple incisions and evacuation of the pus when they have localized. If the infection has gone beyond the peritonsillar space and extended into the pterygomandibular space, a full understanding of the deep anatomy is necessary. The abscess may extend into the deep fascial planes and may actually involve the carotid sheath and its contents, causing disastrous consequences if left untreated. Drainage of a deep cervical abscess should be attempted by a head and neck surgeon who is quite familiar with the anatomy of the area so that damage to nerves and major blood vessels is not perpetrated on the patient. The primary physician, if unfamiliar with surgical techniques, can aspirate an abscess intraorally in order to decrease trismus enough so that the mouth can be opened wide enough to admit a knife blade for incision.

If tetanus has been diagnosed, the main treatment is to use tetanus immunoglobulin of human extraction. Since tetanus is diagnosed on clinical grounds, this therapy should be instituted when serious consequences from the disease are suspected. Tetanus toxoid should be given for most wounds if the patient has not been immunized in the last 5 years. Tetracycline and erythromycin may have some effect on this disease but the immunoglobulin treatment is still the primary therapy of choice.

When no physical evidence to determine the etiology of trismus can be found, it must be assumed that an hysterical reaction is occurring. If the patient is using trismus to obtain a secondary gain, then great difficulty in dealing with this problem may occur. Most patients will have relief from their symptoms if assured that no serious problem is occurring, and with supportive help their symptoms usually can be contained. It is rare that trismus can be so severe that psychiatric consultation is necessary, but as in any physical problem, the primary physician must realize his limitations in dealing with the situation and refer the patient on to the appropriate specialist when he feels that the patient would receive better care.

Bibliography

1. Dengman, R. O., and Natirg, P. *Surgery of Facial Fractures*. W. B. Saunders, Philadelphia, 1969.
2. Guralnick, W., and Kahern, L. Surgical treatment of mandibular hypomobility. *J. Oral Surg.* 34: 343–348, 1976.
3. Mathog, P. H. Maxillofacial trauma. *Otolaryngol. Clin. North Am.*, June, 1976.
4. Smith, M., and Mayall, R. Tetanus oral surgery. *Oral Surg.* 41: 451–455, 1976.
5. Thoma, K. H. *Oral Surgery*, vol 2. C. V. Mosby, St. Louis, 1969.

Chapter 7

Lesions of the Oral Cavity

Robert O. Greer, Jr.

ULCERATED LESIONS—SINGLE, PAINFUL

Traumatic Ulcer

Subjective Complaints

The patient with a traumatic ulcer will complain of an isolated intraoral "sore" with pain and/or tenderness in the area of the lesion. The patient can usually identify lesional etiology (i.e., a broken tooth). Lesions can occur on any mucosal surface, but are most common on the tongue, lips, buccal mucosa, and gingiva. Short-term (no more than 3 weeks) tenderness may be found in these areas.

Objective Findings

Mucosal ulcers of less than 3 weeks' duration are usually identified. Lesional borders may be slightly raised, with a peripheral red halo. The center of the lesion is frequently filled with yellow to brown necrotic debris. The surface may be crusty, especially in the areas on the lips which are not continually bathed in saliva. The traumatic ulcer will often conform to the shape of the initiating agent (i.e., broken tooth, broken prosthetic appliance, trauma from atheletic injury, or trauma from an automobile accident). Occasionally a small amount of purulent material can be identified on the surface of the ulcer; mild lymphadenitis from contamination of the lesion by oral microorganisms may result.

Assessment

Carefully identify the etiology or elicit the cause of injury. Most traumatic ulcers become painless after 3–4 days and heal within 10–14 days. Occasionally lesions will persist for several weeks if repeated trauma occurs. The differential diagnosis should include squamous cell carcinoma, intraoral chancre, ulcer secondary to systemic disease, herpes simplex ulcer, and recurrent aphthous ulcer.

Plan

Debride the ulcer thoroughly. Examine the surface extensively for induration (a common feature of squamous cell carcinoma, but not traumatic ulcer). Remove or restore the etiologic agent if it is a fractured tooth. Application of a topical protective emollient such as Orabase (before bedtime and after meals) may provide some symptomatic relief. Triamcinolone (Kenalog in Orabase) should not be used without ruling out a viral etiology, since steroid preparations can enhance viral activity. Smears from herpetic ulcers will show cells with ballooning degeneration and multinucleated giant cells. Persistent ulcers not responding to the foregoing regimen should be surgically excised, closed primarily, and submitted for microscopic tissue examination.

Recurrent Aphthous Ulcer

Subjective Complaints

Patients characteristically complain of shallow painful mucosal ulcers ranging in diameter from 0.5 to 3 cm. Lesions are usually confined to the freely movable mucosa of the lips, buccal mucosa, tongue, soft palate, and mucobuccal fold.

Objective Findings

The initial lesions of recurrent aphthous ulcers may be macular or papular, but ultimately they ulcerate and become rimmed by a persistent red halo. Recurrent aphthous ulcers usually present as a single mucosal lesion as opposed to the crop or cluster form presentation of herpetic lesions. The mature aphthous lesion is a nonspecific ulcer which is frequently difficult to differentiate from squamous cell carcinoma, systemic ulcers, herpetic ulcers, or ulcerated vesiculobullous diseases such as erosive lichen planus, benign mucous membrane pemphigoid, or a syphilitic ulcer.

Assessment

Mucosal trauma must be evaluated in an attempt to rule out traumatic ulcer. A serology and a smear for giant cell inclusions will be helpful in eliminating a syphilitic lesion and recurrent herpes simplex. Lymphadenopathy is a nonspecific finding that can accompany any of the lesions listed. There is no age specificity for recurrent aphthous lesions.

Plan

Most recurrent intraoral aphthae resolve in 7–14 days without treatment. An oral suspension of uncoated Achromycin crystals, 250 mg per teaspoon in 5 ml of water, to be flushed over the lesion for 2–3 minutes may be helpful. Triamcinolone acetonide emollient may be helpful after meals and prior to going to bed (herpetic lesions must have been ruled out via a smear for giant cell inclusions, prior to this steroid application). Occasional analgesics are useful for pain.

Syphilis (Oral Chancre)

Subjective Complaints

Subjective symptomatology includes a solitary painful mucosal ulcer (usually on the lips or tongue). Tender lymph nodes are a common complaint in the early stages of the disease.

Objective Findings

Inspection will generally reveal a crateriform ulcer with a shiny center that is devoid of necrotic material. The borders may be indurated. Chancres may last for periods ranging from 2 weeks to 2 months, therefore, a differential diagnosis should include squamous cell carcinoma, persistent traumatic ulcer, herpetic ulceration, and recurrent aphthous ulcer. Definitive diagnosis is quite difficult on the basis of clinical observation alone.

Assessment

The history of a mucosal ulceration is of course not specific for syphilis, nor is lymphadenopathy. Numerous screening tests may assist in establishing a diagnosis including a Kahn, Wassermann, or reactive plasma reagin test. If these are positive, a fluorescent treponemal antibody test may prove helpful. Biopsy and microscopic tissue examination are rarely diagnostic; however, microscopic findings of vasculitis and endarteritis may be highly suggestive.

Plan

Syphilis can be managed by systemic pencillin in its early stages. Secondary lesions (macules, papules, and papillomatous lesions) and gummatous ulcerations can occur as secondary and tertiary phases, respectively; however, intraoral mucous patches and gummas are relatively uncommon findings today.

Ulcers Secondary to Systemic Disease

Subjective Complaints

Nonspecific painful ulcerations on any oral mucosal surface.

Objective Findings

Examination will reveal a painful, well demarcated, shallow ulcer with an erythematous halo. Lymphadenitis is nearly always present. A thorough history and screening tests are necessary to rule out syphilitic disease, aphthous ulcers, and herpetic ulcers. Biopsy is necessary to diagnose squamous mucosal neoplasia. Antineoplastic chemotherapeutic agents frequently cause oral mucosal and gastrointestinal ulceration. A thorough drug history is therefore mandatory in the cancer patient.

Assessment

The frequency of oral mucosal ulcerations secondary to non-neoplastic systemic disease is limited. Such ulcers most often occur in uncontrolled diabetes, anemia, and uremia.

Plan

Depending on history, a thorough hematologic and chemistry workup, evaluation of renal function, and glucose tolerance test may be warranted.

Squamous Cell Carcinoma (Ulcer)— Single, Painless

Subjective Complaints

Persistent ulceration of the oral mucosa. The most common sites are the lips, tongue, and floor of mouth. The patients are commonly heavy smokers or alcohol abusers.

Objective Findings

Classic clinical findings include a solitary crateriform lesion with an elevated, rolled, indurated border. The ulcer is usually devoid of necrotic debris. The ulcer base usually appears red and granular due to the lack of keratinization. Occasionally when a large lesion occurs on the tongue, detectable alteration in speech patterns may be discerned. The lateral border of the tongue is the most frequent site of intraoral occurrence. Superficial cervical, submaxillary, or submental lymphadenopathy may be present. Distant metastases can be observed in the lungs, liver, or other nodal sites in late stage disease.

Assessment

It is often difficult to distinguish squamous cell carcinoma from benign nonspecific ulcers, such as the type that occurs in herpes simplex, recurrent aphthous ulceration, or traumatic ulcer. As a rule, squamous cell carcinoma is much more persistent than the aforementioned, although it is rarely painful as an early lesion. The patient will commonly fit the classic pattern of being a male over 40 who smokes and/ or drinks heavily. By ruling out a history of trauma and obtaining a negative serology, one becomes even more suspicious that an isolated indurated oral ulcer may be squamous cell carcinoma.

Plan

As a general rule, when a suspicious ulcer is identified on the oral mucous membrane, it should be followed extremely closely to determine whether it is transient or persistent. Lesions that do not show signs of regressing within 10 days to 2 weeks require biopsy. If the clinician is extremely suspicious of the lesion on initial observation, there is no need for an observation period, and biopsy or referral are indicated at that juncture. It is always wise to use a Tumor Board approach to the management of oral malignancy. These lesions require a cooperative management approach often involving general practitioners of dentistry or medicine, otolaryngologists, chemotherapy, oncologists, and therapeutic radiologists. Squamous cell carcinomas require staging to include exact lesional size and extent, degree of infiltration of surrounding structures, lymph node involvement, and the presence or absence of distant metastases. The irradiated patient requires special consideration, and close cooperation between the dentist and physician is required to ensure meticulous oral hygiene and frequent applications of fluoride to minimize radiation caries. Frequent evaluation for postirradiation xerostomia or bony necrosis is also mandatory. Maxillofacial and social rehabilitation of the patient often require the efforts of a maxillofacial prosthodontist, speech therapist and psychiatric social worker.

MULTIPLE ULCERATED LESIONS

Herpes Simplex Ulceration— Multiple, Painful

Subjective Complaints

The most frequent complaint tends to be recurrent painful superficial ulcers of 7–14 days' duration on fixed oral mucous membrane that is tightly bound to periosteum (including the hard palate, alveolar ridge, and gingiva). Prior to ulceration, the lesions may have consisted of rather small, nontender, discrete gray or white vesicles without a halo.

Objective Findings

Initial lesion—small vesicles which ulcerate leaving punctate ulcers less than 1 mm in diameter. These punctate ulcers frequently coalesce to form a large solitary lesion. Tender submental, submaxillary, or cervical lymphadenopathy may be present. Herpetic lesions must be differentiated from recurrent aphthous ulcers, traumatic ulcers, squamous cell carcinoma, chancre, intraoral gumma, and ulcers secondary to systemic disease. Primary herpetic gingivostomatitis is a disease of childhood, secondary exacerbations are common in the adult. Lymphadenopathy is almost always present in the child, as is involvement of the labial mucosa; these findings are less common among adults with secondary herpetic lesions.

Assessment

The complaint of pain associated with an oral ulcer does not allow one to specifically identify the disorder involved, since nearly all oral ulcers ultimately become painful. Lymphadenitis also frequently accompanies oral ulcers. As a general rule, squamous cell carcinoma and other intraoral malignancies are not painful in their early stages. A chancre may be ruled out if a smear of the lesion is negative for spirochetal immobilization by syphilitic antiserum. Traumatic ulcer should be considered if a source of physical injury can be determined. Recurrent aphthous ulcers generally present a freely movable mucosa, as opposed to herpetic ulcers which occur on mucosa tightly bound to periosteum. A positive smear can be helpful in identifying herpetic lesions, if one can identify epithelial cells with ballooning degeneration and multinucleated giant cells microscopically.

Plan

Recurrent intraoral herpes simplex ulcers usually resolve in 8–14 days regardless of management. Kenalog in Orabase is contraindicated, since a corticosteroid may contribute to viral dissemination. Cryotherapy and photochemical activation have been tried, but have been largely unsuccessful, and may be dangerous. Debridement with application of a topical protective emollient (e.g., Orabase) may provide symptomatic relief. Longstanding,

persistent ulcers that do not resolve or that become indurated require biopsy to rule out neoplasia.

Gingival Ulcers, Multiple (Acute Necrotizing Ulcerative Gingivitis)

Subjective Complaints

Tender or intense generalized pain in the gingiva with fetid breath and intermittent gingival bleeding is the common symptomatic complaint.

Objective Findings

Clinical examination will generally reveal partial or complete destruction of the interdental papillae. A gray-white pseudomembrane with focal areas of ulceration and necrosis will often cover interdental papillae and marginal gingiva. Removal of the pseudomembrane leaves a raw bleeding surface. Patients frequently have regional lymphadenopathy and an elevated temperature. There is no apparent sex predilection for this disease that most often affects adolescents and young adults.

Assessment

One clinical manifestation of acute necrotizing ulcerative gingivitis (ANUG) (punched out interdental papillae) is frequently pathognomonic. Occasionally localized gingival candidiasis, diffuse gangrenous stomatitis associated with systemic disease or malignancy, and gingivitis associated with sickle cell anemia have to be considered in the differential diagnosis. A sickle cell hemoglobin electrophoresis preparation and smear for *Candida albicans* organisms will help eliminate two of the aforementioned. An oncologic and clinical laboratory workup may be necessary to rule out systemic or neoplastic disease.

Plan

The management of acute necrotizing ulcerative gingivitis involves eliminating etiologic agents (presently thought to be anaerobic fusiform and spirochetal organisms) and managing the underlying periodontal disease. Treatment involves careful scaling, curettement, and debridement of the area and rinsing or lavage with a solution of 3% hydrogen peroxide in saline (1:3) as many as 15 times daily. The administration of pencillin (500 mg q.i.d.) for 5–10 days may be necessary to effect regression of the disease.

Buccal Ulceration (Erosive Lichen Planus)

Subjective Complaints

The patient with erosive lichen planus will complain of a continual painful or burning sensation, most often in the buccal mucosa. The tongue, palate, lips, and gingiva may also be involved. Mucosa hemorrhage may also be identified.

Objective Findings

Eroded, hemorrhagic areas with necrotic centers are noted on mucous membrane surfaces. These central ulcerated areas may be surrounded by white keratotic foci (the reticular form of the disease), or bullae (the vesiculobullous form of the disease). Women are affected much more frequently than men. A pseudomembrane composed of necrotic cells and fibrin may cover the most severe areas of erosion. Patients are frequently tense or hyperactive, and emotional stress may be an initiating factor. Skin involvement is seen in 20–30% of the cases. Skin lesions often appear crusty or centrally striated.

Assessment

It is often difficult to delineate erosive lichen planus from pemphigus vulgaris, erythema multiforme, discoid lupus erythematosus, and benign mucous membrane pemphigoid. Tzank smears may prove helpful in identifying the acantholytic cells of pemphigus; an antinuclear antibody (ANA) determination, lupus erythematosus (LE) preparation, and evaluation for eosinophilia may be helpful in ruling out lupus erythematosus and erythema multiforme, although a microscopic tissue examination remains mandatory for definitive diagnosis.

Plan

No specific or uniformly successful management modality has been determined for erosive lichen planus. Symptomatic relief may be obtained by using vitamin A or topical steroids such as betamethasone. Occasional relief can be obtained by intralesional steroid injections.

Buccal or Labial Ulcerations (Erythema Multiforme)

Subjective Complaints

Symptoms include a sudden onset of oral mucosal ulcers, vesicles, or bullae. The bullae remain only a short time, passing rapidly to an ulcerative phase. Lesions are most common on the buccal mucosa and the lips. The lips often burn, fissure, and bleed readily.

Objective Findings

A denuded hemorrhagic surface covered by a pseudomembrane is a common finding. The patient may complain of pain, a foul oral discharge, and lympadenopathy. Frequently a recent herpes simplex infection or drug allergy can be documented. A history of previous attacks may be useful in supporting the diagnosis.

Assessment

No specific laboratory studies are useful. A biopsy may prove quite helpful although the histology is not always diagnostic. Similar oral lesions may be seen in pemphigus vulgaris, benign mucous membrane pemphigoid, allergic reactions, and herpetic gingivostomatitis. Biopsy with adjunctive immunofluorescent studies are necessary to definitively differentiate the latter diseases from erythema multiforme.

Plan

Erythema multiforme is usually self-limiting. Management, therefore, primarily involves supportive care. Some authorities recommend supportive antibiotic therapy or a steroid oral suspension used as a mouthwash. The management needs further evaluation.

MACULOPAPULAR LESIONS— NONPIGMENTED

Inflammatory Fibrous Hyperplasia (Denture Hyperplasia)

Subjective Complaints

This lesion is invariably located at the periphery of a denture border as nonpainful, asymptomatic, lobulated, redundant, or excess tissue.

Objective Findings

The redundant tissue is soft, flabby, or spongy and will frequntly blanch on digital pressure. The denture flange will fit reasonably well into an impression or soft tissue cleft within the lesion or along its edge. Tissue most frequently proliferates on either side of the denture flange. The anterior maxillary mucosa is most often involved. Mucosal erythema may be present and occasionally, following continued denture trauma, the mass will ulcerate.

Assessment

This is the most common of all exophytic oral lesions found at the edges of dentures. At times, the lesion will present as a pebbly, corrugated mass of tissue on the hard or soft palatal mucosa underneath a denture; in this case, it is called inflammatory *papillary* hyperplasia. The dentures *must be removed* for thorough inspection of mucosal surfaces. The remote possibility of a malignant neoplasm remains and may be considered in the differential diagnosis.

Plan

If the lesion is small, reduction of the denture flange by a dentist may allow it to subside in 3–4 weeks. If it is large and firm,

surgical excision and denture adjustment, rebasing, or refabrication are justified.

Buccal Nodular Lesions ("Irritation" Fibroma)

Subjective Complaints

The patient generally presents with a painless, asymptomatic, discrete, nodular swelling of the oral mucosa. The duration is usually unknown; the buccal mucosa is the most common site.

Objective Findings

A pink, sessile or pedunculated soft tissue nodule with a smooth contour can be identified. The lesion is frequently spongy to firm to palpation and well circumscribed. A history of trauma (such as cheek biting) may be elicited.

Assessment

The fibroma can easily be confused with other benign soft tissue tumors; it is in fact not a true tumor, but an inflammatory hyperplasia usually due to trauma or chronic irritation. Fibrolipoma, neurilemoma, rhabdomyoma, and leiomyoma must be entertained as differential diagnostic possibilities.

Plan

Excisional biopsy is the management modality of choice. If the etiology is determined to be contact mucosal trauma due to malocclusion, habitual cheek biting, or irritation from broken restorations or prosthetic appliances, corrective measures should be implemented by a dentist.

Gingival Nodules (Pyogenic Granuloma)

Subjective Complaints

An asymptomatic gingival nodule, papule, or polypoid mass with a hemorrhagic, granulomatous, or ulcerated necrotic surface is usually identified. The lesion most often involves the gingiva and bleeds readily when manipulated, a symptom that commonly brings the lesion to the patient's attention.

Objective Findings

The pyogenic granuloma is solitary, sessile, and granular to firm on palpation, depending on the degree of lesional fibrosis that has occurred. A hemorrhagic surface may be prominent. Erythema of the surrounding mucosa may also be present. Irritants such a calculus, overhanging margins of crowns, or silver amalgams or other composite dental restorations are often identified. Foreign material, fractured teeth, or chronic biting of the soft tissues are often identified as the initiating irritant.

Assessment

A host of other benign soft tissue lesions can have a clinical appearance similar to that of pyogenic granuloma. Traumatized fibroma, "denture hyperplasia," peripheral giant cell granuloma, and capillary hemangioma can readily mimic pyogenic granuloma clinically.

Plan

If the lesion is less than 4 mm in diameter, removal of the causative agent will often cause the lesion to regress. The vast majority require surgical excision and microscopic tissue examination for confirmation.

Gingival Nodule (Peripheral Giant Cell Granuloma)

Subjective Complaints

The lesions most frequently presents as a nodular to polypoid asymptomatic gingival soft tissue mass of unknown duration.

Objective Findings

Examination will reveal a nodular, well circumscribed, exophytic soft tissue growth that may feel hard to soft depending on the relative proportions of collagen and inflammatory component present. The lesion can be granular or have a necrotic surface if repeatedly traumatized. The tintorial quality ranges from pink to blue. The lesion frequently causes a radiographically evident cup or saucerization defect in the underlying bone. Because of this finding, a periapical radiograph can aid in establishing the diagnosis.

Assessment

An acceptable differential diagnosis should include pyogenic granuloma, since the two lesions are frequently identical on clincal examination. The peripheral giant cell granuloma will often appear dark blue, a feature that is rather uncommon with pyogenic granuloma. Traumatized fibroma and denture hyperplasia are also acceptable differential diagnoses; however, both lesions are generally much firmer than the peripheral giant cell granuloma.

Plan

Surgical excision is the treatment of choice. There is considerable reason to believe that this lesion arises from trauma or chronic irritation. Chronic irritants must therefore be removed. Patients with hyperparathyroidism will on occasion develop lesions that are clinically and histologically identical to peripheral giant cell granuloma (brown tumors). Serum calcium, alkaline phosphatase, phosphorus, and occasionally a bone scan and renal function studies are necessary to rule out the latter.

Lingual and Palatal Papilloma

Subjective Complaints

The most common finding is an exophytic, nontender soft tissue tag or growth on the mucosal surface. The lesion is most often found during a routine oral examination; few subjective findings can be delineated.

Objective Findings

Papillomas present as spongy, pedunculated or sessile, corrugated or cauliflower-like growth. The surface may have deep finger-like clefts. Seldom do papillomas attain a size larger than 3 cm in diameter. The most frequent sites are on the tongue, and soft palate and uvula. The surface is usually hyperkeratinized, imparting a white color.

Assessment

The most common lesions to mimic the papilloma are verruca vulgaris and verrucous carcinoma. Verruca vulgaris is common on the skin, but infrequent in the oral cavity. Verruca vulgaris also tends to be sessile, whereas papillomas are more often on a stalk. The two are easily separable on histologic grounds. Many pathologists in fact do not differentiate the two lesions. Verrucous carcinoma is nearly always a diffuse mucosal growth, much larger than 1 cm in diameter at the time of discovery. It tends to grow in a linear pattern along the mucosal surface, and ulceration is frequent. The patient with verrucous carcinoma will usually provide a history of tobacco use (especially the smokeless variety). Most patients are beyond the age of 65, much older than the typical patient with a papilloma.

Plan

The treatment of choice is surgical excision to include the stalk (if penduncu-lated) and a margin of normal tissue. The clinician should examine the skin surfaces for verruca vulgaris. If numerous skin lesions exist, they may be contributory to the oral disease, and should be eliminated as well.

Interdental Papilla Nodule (Peripheral Odontogenic Fibroma, Peripheral Fibroma with Calcification)

Subjective

This asymptomatic, polypoid gingival lesion is very often discovered by the pa-tient. A slight separation of adjacent teeth may frequently cause the patient to present to a dentist.

Objective

The peripheral odontogenic fibroma is almost exclusively seen on the free gingival interdental papilla. Most patients are between the ages of 5 and 25 with a peak incidence of 13. Females are more often affected than males. The lesion will normally be identified anterior to the molars. Radiographically, minimal bone resorption may be seen beneath the lesion. Early lesions are soft, vascular, and red, and bleed quite readily; older lesions are more firm. Irritation is a common cause; overextended margins of dental restorations or calculus are frequently identified as the etiologic agents.

Assessment

Inflammatory fibrous hyperplasia, pyogenic granuloma, and peripheral giant cell granuloma should be included in the differential diagnosis. If calcified foci can be palpated within the soft tissue overgrowth, the aforementioned disorders are less likely and the peripheral odontogenic fibroma should be the principal clinical diagnosis. Calcifications in this lesion probably represent osseous metaplasia.

Plan

The peripheral odontogenic fibroma should be excised, with special care to remove the lesion's origin in the periodontal ligament. Recurrence is a distinct management problem. Clinicopathologic features of 36 of these lesions have been examined critically on the Surgical Oral Pathology Service at the University of Colorado School of Dentistry. The recurrence rate can exceed 50%. The lesion has no malignant potential.

Lipoma

Subjective Complaints

The patient will complain of a slow-growing, painless mucosal mass. The patient may be aware that the lesion has a yellow color or that he is biting it.

Objective Findings

Inspection will reveal a nontender, soft, sessile or pedunculated polypoid mass. A distinct yellow color will be evident if the lesion is a superficial one. Lipomas are generally freely movable and solitary; however, multiple lesions have been documented. Most lipomas involve the buccal mucosa. There is no age or sex predilection.

Assessment

A differential diagnosis should include inflamed lymph node, dermoid cyst, and lymphoepithelial cyst. Intraoral inflamed lymph nodes are commonly painful or tender to palpation, unlike the lipoma. Aspiration should aid in differentiating lipoma from dermoid cyst or lymphoepithelial cyst. The latter lesions should have contents (fluid, proteinaceous debris, or keratin). If the lipoma is deeply situated in the tissues, it may be impossible to differentiate it from an irritation fibroma.

Plan

Most lipomas are adequately managed by surgical excision. Occasionally patients will refuse any treatment. Recurrence is exceptionally rare.

Squamous Cell Carcinoma (Macule or Papule)

Subjective Complaints

The patient with an exophytic macular or papular squamous cell carcinoma will usually present with an obvious intraoral mucosal elevation. These lesions are often painless and the only complaint is that the patient can identify a "spot" or mass.

Objective Findings

The clinician will be able to palpate a firm, nodular mass that is usually fixed to underlying tissues. Cervical, submental, or submaxillary lymphadenopathy may be present.

Assessment

The exophytic squamous cell carcinoma has to be differentiated from minor salivary gland tumors, common reactive lesions (such as pyogenic granuloma and peripheral giant cell granuloma), cysts, and odontogenic infections. Odontogenic infections are usually rubbery, fluctuant, painful, and hot. Pus will be identified on aspiration. Differentiation from reactive lesions is discussed elsewhere in this chapter.

Plan

Refer to Squamous Cell Carcinoma (Ulcer).

PIGMENTED MACULOPAPULAR LESIONS

Pigmented Oral Nodule (Nevus)

Subjective Complaints

The patient will present with an asymptomatic, pigmented intraoral macule or papule. It may have recently increased in size or been noticed for the first time, although present for years.

Objective Findings

A flat, nodular or polypoid, blue, black or brown soft tissue growth that is totally asymptomatic is the most common finding. There is no age, sex, or racial predilection. The palate and gingiva are the most frequent sites. The lesion does not blanch on digital pressure.

Assessment

Nodular nevi are usually firm; this tends to separate them from more compressible salivary gland retention cysts and hemangiomas, lesions that can also be pigmented. The mouth should be examined thoroughly for amalgam restorations, since the pigmented amalgam tattoo can resemble a nevus. The amalgam tattoo arises in association with previous restorative dental procedures and is frequently adjacent to a large amalgam restoration. Intraoral gingival pigmentation is common to Blacks and Hispanics, it tends to be diffusely present throughout the mucosa, and should not be confused with a nevus. The malignant counterpart of the nevus, melanoma, must always be considered in the differential diagnosis.

Plan

A nevus should be excised with adequate margins and should be carefully examined microscopically. There is no certain clinical means of differentiating a nevus from an early melanoma.

Melanoma

Subjective Complaints

The melanoma can present as a pigmented macule, pigmented nodule, or large exophytic pigmented mucosal mass. The lesion is painful if ulcerated and usually shows dramatic enlargement over a short span of time (quite noticeable to the patient). Bleeding may be a presenting symptom.

Objective Findings

A pigmented mucosal mass is usually identified. The most frequent site of occurrence is the anterior maxilla, or hard or soft palate. The tumor rapidly infiltrates adjacent and deeper tissue (including bone), causing tumor tissue to become firm and fixed when palpated. Lymphadenopathy may be present. Most intraoral melanomas occur during the 6th decade of life. When the lesion is solitary, asymptomatic, and flat, it is not always possible to differentiate it from a nevus or an amalgam tattoo.

Assessment

The rapidly enlarging pigmented exophytic melanoma is not easily confused with other pigmented mucosal lesions. The less ominous-appearing pigmented oral macule or nodule could easily represent a nevus, peripheral giant cell granuloma, amalgam tattoo, or hemangioma. When evaluating a pigmented lesion it is impor-

tant to determine if the lesion has been enlarging, and if so, for how long. A change in the degree of pigmentation, explained bleeding, or change in surface appearance is a suspicious sign. A high index of suspicion on the part of the clinician is often the key to diagnosis.

Plan

Surgical excision is characteristically the treatment of choice. If a primary care physician or dentist is at all suspicious of melanoma, it is mandatory to take measurements of the lesion and photograph it as well. Size is extremely important to clinical and pathologic staging. The pathologist and the person who will ultimately manage the disease process must know the extent of the initial disease. Melanomas have recently been subclassified into a variety of subtypes including a superficially spreading form and a vertical growth form. The prognosis is often dependent upon these subclassifications. Oral melanoma remains a neoplasm with an exceedingly poor overall prognosis.

Amalgam Tattoo

Subjective Complaints

The patient will present with an asymptomatic black, brown, or blue "spot" on the gingiva or edentulous alveolar mucosa. Recent amalgam (silver) restorations or a history of extensive dental restorative procedures in the past are common.

Objective Findings

Findings will include a flat, pigmented macule on the oral mucous membrane. Most lesions are less than 1 cm in diameter, and painless. Trauma to the mucosa by a rubber dam clamp or dental burr at the time of placement of a dental restoration may leave evidence of surface abrasion in the area of pigmentation. The foreign material (silver amalgam) that actually causes the pigmented area cannot be palpated within the tissues. Amalgam tattoos do not blanch upon digital pressure as do pigmented lesions such as hemangioma or mucocele. Satellite lesions such as those found in melanoma are uncommon.

Assessment

The amalgam tattoo cannot be differentiated from a nevus or melanoma. Palpation may be helpful as a differential diagnostic aid. If an amalgam restoration can be identified adjacent to an asymptomatic, pigmented lesion, it is good supportive evidence that the lesion is in fact an amalgam tattoo.

Plan

In general, amalgam tattoos require no treatment. If there is the least bit of suspicion that the lesion might be a melanoma or nevus, biopsy is justified. If the patient is unduly concerned about the lesion, removal is indicated as well.

LEUKOPLAKIC LESIONS

(The nonspecific term leukoplakia means white plaque. It may be used as a differential diagnosis for white lesions if the clinician understands that the term is a nonspecific one meaning white spot only and that it actually denotes no malignant or premalignant potential.)

Squamous Cell Carcinoma

Subjective Complaints

An asymptomatic white mucosal plaque is usually identified on routine examination or observed while brushing the teeth.

Objective Findings

This hyperkeratinized painless lesion cannot be scraped off with a tongue blade. The lesion may be speckled such that small, velvety red areas are dispersed throughout the broader white lesion. As a rule, lymph node involvement is late in this type of carcinoma. The vast majority of these lesions are discovered in individuals over 40 years of age. The most frequent sites are the tongue, lower lip mucosa, and mucosa of the floor of the mouth.

The borders may be distinct or indistinct and the surface can range from smooth to finely granular, mottled, or rough. Most patients elicit a lengthy history of tobacco or alcohol use. Occasionally the etiology can be determined by observing the lesion in the direct line of a pipestem or in the area where the patient holds a bolus of smokeless tobacco or snuff. Lymphadenopathy may signal the occurrence of metastatic spread.

Assessment

The primary procedure to perform when confronted with a white lesion is to determine whether it can be easily removed by scraping. A squamous cell carcinoma plaque cannot be removed. If the lesion can be removed by scraping, then it is most likely within the realm of a sloughing pseudomembranous disease. The true differential diagnosis is then narrowed to lesions such as hyperkeratosis from cheek biting, lichen planus, leukoedema, white sponge nevus, verrucous carcinoma, and papilloma. Cheek biting hyperkeratosis can usually be identified by carefully questioning the patient and discussing habits, especially those associated with stress. Lichen planus is generally a diffuse lesion found on several mucosal surfaces as opposed to the more solitary appearance of squamous cell carcinoma. In addition, lichen planus may undergo a more diagnostic vesicular or bullous phase, not seen with squamous cell carcinoma. Leukoedema is usually limited to the buccal mucosa and tends to disappear when the cheek mucosa is stretched. Verruca vulgaris and verrucous carcinoma (a squamous cell carcinoma variant) tend to be exophytic, corrugated, and quite elevated above the mucosal surface as solitary and diffuse lesions, respectively. Hyperkeratotic forms of squamous cell carcinoma are usually identified in adults over 40 years old.

Plan

The clinician must make every effort to identify a local etiology, since local irritation remains the most common cause of the white oral mucosal plaque. If the lesion fails to subside after 2 weeks of observation, surgical excision is justified. Large lesions may require extensive mucosal stripping and skin graft procedures. Tumor Board referral and management are the modalities of choice when a diagnosis of squamous cell carcinoma is rendered (see Ulcerative and Maculopapular Squamous Cell Carcinoma).

Leukoedema

Subjective Complaints

Asymptomatic diffuse, white, bilateral opalescence of buccal mucosa is usually observed during routine oral examination.

Objective Findings

Close inspection will reveal a dense, folded, milky opalescence, usually on the buccal mucosa. The white areas are not elevated above the surface. They are painless and cannot be removed with a tongue blade. These clinical findings are frequently seen in Blacks; however, careful inspection will show that the lesion can be identified in Whites as well. Stretching or tensing of the buccal mucosa will cause the whiteness to disappear. Occasionally the disorder occurs on oral mucosal surfaces other than buccal mucosa.

Assessment

Hyperkeratosis from cheek biting, lichen planus, and white sponge nevus should be included as differential diagnoses. White sponge nevus is hereditary and a disease of the young. Lichen planus can be painful if in the ulcerative or bullous state, unlike white sponge nevus. The constant cheek biter will usually elicit a history of trauma.

Plan

Leukoedema is merely an anatomic mucosal variation of normal. It is important to recognize the disorder and realize that no treatment is necessary.

Reticular Lichen Planus (also see Erosive Lichen Planus)

Subjective Complaints

Asymptomatic keratotic plaques on the oral mucous membrane are the typical finding. The patients tend to be of the nervous variety and may indicate that they also have lesions on their skin.

Objective Findings

Oral lesions present as reticular, white, lacelike striae. The buccal mucosa is most commonly involved although other mucous membrane surfaces are not immune to the disease. Lesions can also take on a patchy, circular, or annular form. They do not strip off when rubbed vigorously. There is no apparent relationship to tobacco use, nor is there a propensity for the disease among specific ethnic groups. Lesions tend to exacerbate during periods of emotional stress (commonly they undergo ulceration or progress to the bullous or erosive form of the disease). The reticular form is rarely painful; the bullous and erosive forms are characteristically painful. Skin lesions present as small flat papules which often coalesce to form larger flat plaques. Lesional borders are well delineated.

Assessment

Lichen planus can mimic traumatic hyperkeratosis, leukoedema, geographic tongue of the ectopic variety, and white sponge nevus. A thorough history usually is sufficient to identify traumatic hyperkeratosis. Leukoedema can be identified by putting tension on lesional sites. Under tension, the white plaques should disappear if they represent leukoedema. White sponge nevus tends to be elevated above the mucosal surface; it shows an inheritance pattern and has usually been present since birth. If erosive lichen planus and ectopic geographic tongue remain reasonable differential diagnoses, biopsy is necessary to distinguish between them.

Plan

The reticular hyperkeratotic form of lichen planus requires no treatment except for its identification (by microscopic tissue examination if necessary) and informing the patient. There are a few reports in the literature that suggest increased squamous epithelial malignancy in association with lichen planus. Periodic reexamination is therefore warranted. Lesions that progress to the painful, ulcerative or erosive phase of the disease may require applications of triamcinolone in a base (e.g., Kenalog in Orabase) applied at bedtime. Very severe cases have been treated with systemic cortisone; reported results have been quite variable.

White Sponge Nevus

Subjective Complaints

Lesions will most often be identified as rough, elevated, nonpainful areas on the oral mucous membrane.

Objective Findings

Diffuse, white, corrugated, hyperkeratinized areas are identified on the oral mucosa. These areas are often elevated above the mucosal surface and can take on a papillomatous appearance. The most common site is the buccal mucosa. The lesions are entirely asymptomatic. An autosomal dominance pattern can be established by pedigree studies or careful history. The lesions are generally present from birth, but may exacerbate at puberty. White sponge nevus cannot be scraped off with vigorous rubbing.

Assessment

Clinically, white sponge nevus has to be differentiated from leukoedema, traumatic hyperkeratosis, and lichen planus. Tension applied to the mucosa helps to support a clinical diagnosis of leukoedema, since the lesion will disappear when tension is applied. Leukoedema is not as rough or corrugated as white sponge nevus. Lichen planus is rarely identified in the childhood age group; white sponge nevus is common to this age group. In addition, a familial pattern is often documented in white sponge nevus, unlike lichen planus. The etiology can generally be determined for traumatic hyperkeratosis.

Plan

Accurate identification is usually all that is required. On rare occasions, the lesion can become traumatically ulcerated. Palliative procedures are justified in such cases.

HARD PALATE LEUKOPLAKIC LESIONS

Nicotine Stomatitis—Hard Palate, Nodules or Fissures, Nonpainful

Subjective Complaints

Variable red and white "parboiled" palatal mucosa is generally identified. The lesion is asymptomatic. Patients are frequently heavy pipe or cigarette smokers.

Objective Findings

Inspection will reveal marked clefting or fissuring of the palatal mucosa. The fissures tend to divide the mucosal surface into small, nodular white areas; each nodule will contain a central red area. The red focus represents the inflamed orifice of a minor salivary gland duct. Patients are uniformly heavy smokers and it is often easy to identify the exact hyperkeratotic area where the patient keeps his or her pipestem or holds the cigarette.

Assessment

Many lesions have a "dried river bed" appearance. If the smoking habit is discontinued, the disorder will usually abate rapidly.

Plan

Nicotine stomatitis seldom, if ever, becomes malignant. As with all white lesions, a high index of suspicion should be maintained, however. Ulceration is an ominous sign when seen in connection with this otherwise benign condition. Such a finding justifies biopsy.

OTHER LEUKOPLAKIC LESIONS

Mucosal Scar

Subjective Complaints

The patient will present with an asymptomatic white spot or linear hypertrophy in the area of previous surgery (usually an extraction site or site of trauma).

Objective Findings

Clinically, one can identify a white focus that is generally firm and does not rub off when scraped with a tongue blade. The lesion may be linear and resemble a healed incision; or nodular and hypertrophic in areas where the wound has healed by secondary intention.

Assessment

Oral scars are uncommon, but rarely represent a difficult diagnostic challenge. A thorough history is of paramount importance in establishing a diagnosis.

Plan

Generally no treatment is required, although occasionally adhesions (following major oral surgery) may have to be excised.

Candidiasis

Subjective Complaints

The patient with candidiasis will present with a chief complaint of mucosal soreness or burning, and a "film" of dead tissue in the mouth. The patient may be chronically debilitated from diseases such as diabetes, hypothyroidism, or cancer. A history of long-term broad spectrum antibiotic use or extended use of immunosup-

pressive agents is common. Patients are frequently denture wearers.

Objective Findings

Examination will reveal a white "milk curd-like" pseudomembrane that can be easily stripped or peeled off, leaving a raw, red, often bleeding surface. A large percentage of the patients have the lesion under an ill-fitting denture. Patients may have an associated angular cheilitis. Lesions of candidiasis often cause a generalized burning sensation throughout the mouth.

Assessment

The clinical pseudomembranous picture seen in these patients is rather specific. Occasionally, chemical burns and drug reactions can cause pseudomembranous sloughing. An exfoliative cytologic smear of the lesion often proves useful in establishing a diagnosis. Periodic acid-Schiff (PAS) staining will allow the clinician to identify the septate hyphae of *Candida albicans*. Cultures are less diagnostic.

Plan

Drug suspension or drug regulation in the chronically debilitated or cancer patient may be necessary. When candidiasis is demonstrated under an ill-fitting denture, reconstruction of the prosthesis may be necessary. In general, the lesions respond well to either a nystatin oral suspension or vaginal tablets used as oral troches.

Chemical Burn

Subjective Complaints

The most common chief complaint of the patient is a burning sensation in the mucosa adjacent to the site of a toothache. A history of local aspirin application to the mucosa can usually be obtained. A second common historical finding may be recent dental or medical application of a medicant to the mucosa.

Objective Findings

Examination will reveal a localized red mucositis in the case of a mild burn. In the case of a severe burn, a white necrotic focus can be identified. When the coagulated dead tissue is removed, a raw, bleeding, painful surface remains. Occasionally the lesions become secondarily infected, resulting in a hemorrhagic granulomatous mass with a purulent discharge.

Assessment

Adequate history should enable the clinician to arrive at a proper diagnosis.

Plan

The management modality of choice is application of a protective coating such as Orabase and initiation of a bland diet. If the lesion is painful, systemic analgesics may be prescribed. It is mandatory to have the offending tooth treated if it is in fact what stimulated the patient to apply aspirin to the mucosa. The patient should be informed that analgesic tablets such as aspirin work systemically and not topically.

INTRAORAL ABSCESSES AND SWELLINGS

Mucocele

Subjective Complaints

The patient will commonly complain of an intermittent mucosal swelling that ruptures and drains periodically. The lesion is painless, and usually has a blue color.

Objective Findings

The most common site is the lower lip mucosa. The lesion is usually a rounded or dome-shaped elevation that is freely movable, but cannot be moved independently of the mucosal layer. The mucocele cannot be emptied by digital pressure; aspiration will usually yield a viscous, clear fluid. The *ranula* represents a mucocele that oc-

curs in the floor of the mouth, generally involving a sublingual gland.

Assessment

The mucocele can mimic early mucoepidermoid carcinoma of salivary gland origin, hemangioma, or lymphangioma. On aspiration, all of the aforementioned will yield superficial pools of mucoid-appearing material. True salivary gland tumors are exceedingly rare on the lower lip; however, a palatal, buccal mucosa, or upper lip mucocele may be more problematic. Inclusion cysts and benign lymphoepithelial cysts can also resemble a mucocele clinically. Microscopic tissue examination is the only way to adequately differentiate these lesions.

Plan

All mucoceles should be completely removed surgically. The tissue must be excised in a manner that is least damaging to associated salivary gland acinar and ductal elements. Often all glandular elements that protrude into the incision are removed to avoid recurrence of the lesion.

Salivary Gland Neoplasm

Subjective Complaints

The classic history is one of a slowly expanding, nonpainful, nodular or polypoid soft tissue mass.

Objective Findings

A fluctuant or firm soft tissue nodule is usually identified. Salivary gland tumors are rarely seen on the lower lip. The two most frequently intraoral salivary gland tumors are the mixed tumor and mucoepidermoid carcinoma. Aspiration of both tumors may yield sticky fluid contents, although typically the lesions are solid. In their late stages, salivary gland tumors may be painful, firmly bound down to connective tissue structures, or ulcerated. Most salivary gland neoplasms occur in patients over 40.

Assessment

Advanced salivary gland tumors may contain discrete, soft, fluctuant areas. A lesion on the palatal mucosa, upper lip or buccal mucosa should be viewed with some suspicion, since the mucocele, the most common oral salivary gland lesion, is less common in these areas.

Plan

Wide surgical resection is the treatment of choice. It the lesion is diagnosed on the basis of an incisional biopsy, management parameters generally dictate a Tumor Board approach to management. Excisional biopsy is recommended.

Chronic Draining Alveolar Abscess

Subjective Complaints

Patients will frequently give a history of pain that started as a dull ache and progressed to a severe throbbing pain. The lesion will present as a swelling on the maxillary or mandibular alveolar ridge. A nonvital carious tooth can usually be identified in the area.

Objective Findings

A well circumscribed, soft tissue swelling that is warm, fluctuant, and tender to palpation can be identified. A sinus tract may be identified within the swelling or adjacent to it. When a sinus tract is identified, patients complain of little pain. The mucosal sinus may be red or bleed easily, and it is commonly surrounded by hemorrrhagic granulation tissue. Occasionally, after temporary emptying of the abscess, the sinus tract will heal and form a raised, firm, blue or red nodule. Radiographic examination is mandatory when one suspects a chronic draining alveolar abscess. Periapical films will reveal a poorly delineated radiolucency generally in the area of the root apex of the offending tooth. The lesion can vary in size, from small to quite large, often involving much of the jaw. Radiographs of the related tooth will frequently show such features as large restorations, narrowed pulp chambers or ca-

nals, or resorption of the root apex. The tooth may be painful to percussion; as a rule it will not respond to electrical pulp tests.

Assessment

It is important to realize that all abscesses involving teeth and extending into the soft tissue are not of pulpal origin. The lateral periodontal abscess, for instance, originates in a deep periodontal pocket, and is associated with periodontal disease, not pulpal disease. Adequate radiographs will usually show the absence of a periapical radiolucency and the presence of a periodontal pocket in lateral periodontal abscesses. In addition, the pulp of teeth with such lateral periodontal abscesses is nearly *always* vital. Sinus tract in the maxilla should be evaluated by paranasal sinus x-rays, and tissue from the tract should be biopsied to rule out oral antral fistula associated with carcinoma of maxillary sinus.

Plan

The acute abscess should be treated rather aggressively to alleviate the patient's pain as well as to ensure that no untoward sequelae (diffuse osteomyelitis) develop. Drainage may be established by opening the pulp chamber of the suspected tooth or by a trephination procedure, whereby an opening is made through the mucosa and bone to the abscess at the apex of the offending tooth. When a vestibular, palatal, or lingual space abscess has formed, a through-and-through drain may be placed in the abscess and frequently irrigated with a solution of hydrogen peroxide and saline. A sample of pus should be obtained for culture and sensitivity tests. In severe cases, antibiotic therapy may be indicated. It is generally considered unwise to extract a severely abscessed tooth unless the patient has been adequately treated with antibiotics. After drainage has been established, routine dental endodontic procedures may be performed. When there is a chronic abscess with a draining sinus, the origin of the lesion may be identified by placing a gutta-percha cone to the extent of the sinus and radiographing the area. Complete management of the acute and chronic draining alveolar abscess requires a thorough knowledge of dentistry, and management by a dentist or oral surgeon. Occasionally the lesion can progress to an oral antral communication (oroantral fistula) or diffuse osteomyelitis. Combined dental and medical management are more common when the disease progresses to this stage.

Hematoma

Subjective Complaints

A history of traumatic injury, accident, surgery, administration of local anesthetic, cheek biting or self-inflicted trauma will be elicited. The traumatized area will be tender and occasionally hemorrhagic.

Objective Findings

Hematomas can undergo early and late stage development. The early hematoma is warm, and digital pressure may cause the patient to experience a stinging sensation. The lesion is elevated above the mucosa, fluctuant to rubbery, and fairly well delineated from surrounding tissues. Most appear red or blue. The late hematoma will be harder, black, and painless. Early and late lesions can continue to leak or discharge blood at the periphery. If the lesion becomes secondarily infected, it may become quite granular.

Assessment

The hematoma must be differentiated from other pigmented lesions including mucocele, ranula, hemangioma, and lymphangioma. A history of sudden onset after recent traumatic injury strongly suggests a diagnosis of hematoma. The hematoma will not blanch on digital pressure as will the hemangioma or lymphangioma. Aspiration will usually reveal dark blue blood, if the lesion is an early one.

Plan

Hematomas are usually self-limiting lesions. Exceptions can be noted when the lesion arises from trauma to a large vessel.

Large vessel damage may require a pressure bandage or evacuation with an aspirating syringe. Occasionally surgery may be required to locate the offending vessel. An organizing hematoma is mandatory to healing of a tooth extraction site, and *should not be* removed during the immediate 48-hour postextraction period.

LESIONS OF THE TONGUE

Hairy Tongue

Subjective Complaints

The patient usually identifies a pigmented dorsal tongue surface. He or she may complain that it feels as if hairs are present on the tongue; the patient may also complain of a gagging sensation.

Objective Findings

The dorsal tongue surface is the site involved. The mucosal surface will show elongation of filiform papillae and an alteration in color. The most common color is black, but white, yellow, and brown pigmentation may also be encountered. Pain is not a common feature. A thorough history will often indicate that the patient is a habitual user of oxidizing agents in oral preparations. Excessive local use of antibiotics or antiseptics or poor oral hygiene with a subsequent accumulation of pigmented debris on the tongue surface, especially in heavy smokers or alcoholics, is a second common history.

Assessment

Few disorders mimic hairy tongue; recognizing the disorder is not a difficult diagnostic challenge.

Plan

Removal of the offending chemical agent (oxidizing oral rinses) or antibiotics will cause resolution of the disorder. Improved tongue-brushing techniques will help alleviate the disorder, especially if the etiology is poor oral hygiene. Extreme instances have been reported in which elongated papillae had to be sheared surgically to alleviate the condition.

Hemangioma

Subjective Complaints

The patient will present with a blue nodular swelling involving the lateral border of the tongue or the tongue dorsum. The lesion is most often congenital, but it may be initiated by an episode of trauma. Large lesions may cause speech difficulties.

Objective Findings

Most hemangiomas identified within the oral cavity are superficial and, therefore, appear as blue, red, or black lesions. Occasionally, deeply situated hemangiomas have no such tintorial qualities, and simply appear as nodules or swelling within the tongue. Oral hemangiomas most often involve the tongue; the next most common sites are the lips and buccal mucosa. The lesion will characteristically blanch and empty upon the application of digital presure. The lesion is not fluctuant.

Assessment

The hemangioma must be differentiated from the mucocele, ranula, and superficial cyst. Features that are useful in establishing this differentiation include the fact that the hemangioma is nonfluctuant and can be evacuated by pressure; the other lesions listed cannot be evacuated by pressure. A pulse may be detectable in a hemangioma; this finding is not seen with the mucocele, ranula, or cyst. The clinician can further establish a working diagnosis of hemangioma by aspiration of blood through a fine-gauge needle.

Plan

Surgery (including cryosurgery), sclerosing techniques, or both, are used in the treatment of hemangioma. Sodium psylliate injections can cause the lesion to fibrose, thus shrinking vascular spaces. Angiograms may be necessary to determine the extent of the lesion if it is large. The excision of a large lesion should not be attempted as an outpatient procedure; exsanguination remains a hazard.

Lymphangioma

Subjective Complaints

The most common finding is a painless swelling of the dorsal tongue surface or the lateral border of the tongue. Large lesions may cause speech difficulties. Like the hemangioma, the lymphangioma is often congenital.

Objective Findings

The lymphangioma is usually pink and not nearly as blue as the hemangioma. The surface is often corrugated or pebbly. Digital pressure will cause the lesion to blanch due to content evacuation. Aspiration can be quite helpful, often revealing yellow-gray contents as opposed to the red or blue contents of a hemangioma.

Assessment

The differential diagnosis of lymphangioma is essentially the same as that for hemangioma. Aspiration with a fine-gauge needle may help differentiate the two, based upon content appearance.

Plan

Surgical excision (including cryosurgery) remains the management modality of choice. Combination hemangioma/lymphangioma lesions have been identified. Operating room precautions should be taken in the case of lesions greater than 3 cm. As with hemangioma, it may require more than one surgical procedure to erradicate a lymphangioma.

Ventral Varicose Veins

Subjective Complaints

These lesions are identified as asymptomatic, distended vessels on the ventral tongue surface.

Objective Findings

Superficial, painless, red or blue distended and congested veins are easily identified.

Assessment

These lesions present little diagnostic challenge. Occasionally when there is marked distention of a venous channel, it can simulate other fluid-filled bluish lesions such as the mucocele, ranula, or hemangioma. Varicosities cannot easily be evacuated in a distal direction by digital pressure, because valves present in the normal segment of the vein will not allow retrograde blood flow.

Plan

Accurate clinical diagnosis is all that is required after a thorough differential diagnosis is entertained. They rarely bleed, but if that occurs, they may be electrocoagulated.

Geographic Tongue (Benign Migratory Glossitis)

Subjective Complaints

This condition is usually discovered as an asymptomatic tongue lesion. Occasionally it will cause the patient to complain of a burning sensation, tenderness, or pain within the tongue. Patients often indicate that the lesions "move from place to place on the tongue."

Objective Findings

This disease of unknown etiology results in irregularly shaped depapillated, circular lesions most often on the tongue dorsum, less frequently on the ventral tongue surface. Filiform papillae will desquamate for approximately a week; the area of desquamation will enlarge and then regress, resulting in a depapillated pattern that moves from week to week or month to month. Pain may be present if the depapillated areas are exceedingly large.

Assessment

Benign migratory glossitis is not a difficult diagnostic problem, although it can occasionally be confused with candidiasis or erosive lichen planus. A smear for *Candida albicans* organisms will help establish a diagnosis of candidiasis. With candidiasis a pseudomembrane can be stripped from the surface of the lesion, a feature not seen with geographic tongue. Erosive lichen planus can result in depapillated lesions on the tongue; unlike geographic tongue they are usually quite painful and do not migrate from week to week.

Plan

Psychologic influences have been implicated in the etiology of geographic tongue in recent years, especially stress. If stress can be eliminated, the disorder will sometimes regress. If burning and tenderness are constant symptoms, coating the denuded surface with triamcinolone in Orabase may relieve discomfort. Geographic tongue can occasionally occur ectopically on mucosal surfaces other than the tongue. Frequently when it occurs ectopically, biopsy is justified to establish a diagnosis.

Median Rhomboid Glossitis

Subjective Complaints

Patients will frequently complain of a visible "sore" on the dorsal tongue surface; however, the lesion is generally asymptomatic.

Objective Findings

Median rhomboid glossitis will present as a pale red to brown depapillated lesion on the dorsal surface of the tongue. The area can be smooth, nodular, or fissured. It is well delineated, painless, and quite often situated exactly in the middle of the tongue dorsum. The lesion has been reported most frequently in children, but can be found in all age groups.

Assessment

Median rhomboid glossitis has been confused with squamous cell carcinoma. The location of the lesion is the most helpful clinical finding used to differentiate the two. The midportion of the dorsal surface of the tongue is perhaps the most unlikely focus for squamous cell carcinoma in the entire oral cavity. Median rhomboid glossitis is rarely confused with other mucosal disorders.

Plan

In the majority of cases, no treatment is necessary. Occasionally the lesion can become ulcerated due to trauma; in such cases, symptomatic relief (application of a petroleum base) may be required

Reactive Lymphoid Aggregate (Accessory Tonsillar Tissue)

Subjective Complaints

An asymptomatic nodule on the tongue is the common finding.

Objective Findings

Smooth-surfaced papules and nodules on the posterolateral border of the tongue and posterior wall of the oropharynx can be identified. The lesions remain painless and asymptomatic.

Assessment

Lymphoid tissue is often abundant throughout the oral cavity. It can be confused with fatty deposits. Biopsy is often the only means of distinguishing the two.

Plan

The nodules represent no true pathologic reaction; their importance relates only to the differential diagnostic challenge.

Fissured Tongue

Subjective Complaints

Deep fissures or clefts can be identified disseminated throughout the dorsal tongue surface. These fissured areas are usually asymptomatic. If food debris accumulates in the fissures, inflammation may arise and the ridges of the clefts can occasionally become hemorrhagic and edematous.

Assessment

Fissured tongue is seen in about 5% of the population and affects both sexes equally. It is rarely confused with other disorders.

Plan

Fissured tongue requires no treatment other than proper oral hygiene instruction.

Lingual Thyroid Nodule

Subjective Complaints

An asymptomatic nodular enlargement of the tongue is usually encountered. Occasionally gagging is the presenting symptom.

Objective Findings

A nodular, spongy to firm mass is encountered on the posterolateral border of the tongue or the dorsal surface in the area of the primitive foramen cecum. The lesion is generally located posterior to the area in which median rhomboid glossitis is identified. The lingual thyroid may be the only functioning thyroid tissue in the body. Thorough inspection and palpation of the normal thyroid gland is mandatory.

Assessment

Thyroid uptake studies may be helpful in determining if the lesion is functional. Excisional biopsy should be undertaken with *extreme caution* in order to avoid total removal of a patient's thyroid tissue.

Plan

Thorough evaluation of thyroid function is mandatory prior to any surgical procedure. If the lesion proves to be the only functioning thyroid tissue, it should not be removed.

Granular Cell Myoblastoma

Subjective Complaints

A superficial, asymptomatic nodular swelling of the tongue is usually identified.

Objective Findings

The lateral and dorsal tongue surfaces are the most frequent sites involved. Lesions are usually small, slightly elevated, smooth-surfaced, and asymptomatic. The lesion may be freely movable within the tongue body. No age or sex predilection is encountered.

Assessment

The lesion does not usually interfere with mastication or speech. Since it is characteristically an asymptomatic nodule, it parallels the clinical presentation of several other asymptomatic tongue nodules including syphilis, squamous cell carcinoma, irritation fibroma, neurofibroma, and lipoma. The lipoma usually has a yellow color; neurofibroma is commonly associated with multiple neurofibromatosis, and skin lesions are common. The effective method of establishing a diagnosis is to biopsy the lesion. A VDRL should be ordered.

Plan

Treatment consists of excision, which is curative.

Bibliography

1. Dunlap, C., and Barker, B. *Oral Lesions: An Illustrated Quick-Reference Guide to Diagnosis and Treatment.* Hoyt Laboratories, Needham, Mass., 1975.
2. Greer, R. O. *Oral Pathology: A Clinicopathologic Approach to Instruction,* ed. 2. University of Colorado Medical Center Press, Boulder, Col., 1976.
3. Greer, R. O., and Carpenter, M. Surgical oral pathology at the University of Colorado School of Dentistry; a survey of 400 cases. *J. Colo. Dent. Assoc. 54:* 13–16, 1976.
4. Lumerman, H. *Essentials of Oral Pathology.* J. B. Lippincott Co., Philadelphia, 1975.
5. Silverman, S., and Galante, M. *Oral Cancer,* ed. 6. University of California Press, Berkeley, 1977.

Chapter 8
Disorders of the Oropharynx

Thomas Balkany

The oropharynx is a multistructured organ related to and interdependent on many adjacent structures. Most important clinically are its contiguity with the upper respiratory and digestive systems.

Structurally, the oropharynx is a musculomembranous tube, extending from the soft palate to the level of the epiglottis. It is derived from foregut endoderm, which adjoins the oral cavity ectoderm at the area of the circumvallate papillae of the tongue and the tonsillar pillars.

A concentration of lymphoid tissue is present at the entrance to the respiratory and digestive tracts called Waldeyer's ring. In the oropharynx this takes the form of the pharyngeal tonsils, the lingual tonsils, and scattered lymphoid follicles of the pharyngeal mucosa. This lymphoid tissue functions as a filtering mechanism to prevent deeper spread of infection which has penetrated the mucosal barrier of the upper airway. The physiologic reactions of Waldeyer's ring—inflammation, edema, hyperplasia—play a major role in the clinical manifestations of pharyngeal diseases.

Other important structures of the oropharynx include the posterior third of the tongue, the tonsillar pillars, and the adjoining deep fascial spaces of the neck.

The main functions of the oropharynx include respiration, deglutition, voice resonance, and speech articulation. Protective respiratory reflexes, including coughing and gagging, are mediated by the pharyngeal plexus of cranial nerves IX and X.

Swallowing is a complex act which requires both conscious and reflex motor activity. The peristaltic wave of deglutition begins in the oropharynx. The great majority of diseases of the oropharynx present with pain which may be acute or chronic and may be associated with fever, airway obstruction, or difficulty in swallowing. Sore throat may be the result of local disease or the earliest manifestation of systemic illness. Cancer and granulomatous and ulcerative diseases all occur in the pharynx.

ACUTE SORE THROAT

Subjective Complaints

Acute sore throat is among the most common complaints of people seeking medical care. Unlike most common disease complexes, the history is often not clinically helpful in diseases of the pharynx because of the similarity of symptoms, regardless of the underlying pathology.

The terms pharyngitis and tonsillitis are often used interchangeably. There is little difference between the presentation of the two; however, the former is a more frequently occurring and inclusive term denoting inflammation of any of the pharyngeal structures.

Acute sore throat is most commonly associated with upper respiratory tract infections. In systemic viral infections, sore throat is often associated with headache, myalgia, rhinorrhea, and cough.

A history of sore throat, fever, and chills following an upper respiratory tract infection is typical of secondary bacterial invasion of the oropharynx. The primary viral inflammation destroys ciliary function, increases mucosal exfoliation, and greatly predisposes to suppurative pharyngitis.

A historical search for underlying illness is important. This should include a review of the patient's general health, smoking and drinking habits, similar prior episodes, the state of dentition, allergic history, and any known systemic diseases such as diabetes mellitus which might predispose to infectious complications.

Pharyngitis often occurs suddenly with fever and chills. Pain is usually generalized in the throat and is worse with swallowing. Accumulation of viscous secretions produces a tendency toward coughing and emesis. Fetid breath is common and the tongue feels thick and coated.

Objective Findings

Physical examination is crucial in diagnosing the cause of sore throat. Most commonly in pharyngitis the pharynx appears red and edematous. White exudates may be present anywhere in the oropharynx. It is usually impossible to differentiate viral from bacterial pharyngitis on appearance alone.

White exudates may occur in any inflammatory disease of the pharynx. In addition to viral and bacterial pharyngitis, these may be symptoms of secondary syphilis or oral moniliasis (thrush). The differential diagnosis is described under Assessment.

Pharyngeal ulceration may be the result of local or systemic disease. The differential diagnosis includes blood dyscrasias, primary tumors, mucosal manifestations of primary dermatologic disorders, and simple localized inflammatory disease. Fever of 38.2°C or greater is an important sign of bacterial pharyngitis as is leukocytosis of 12,000 WBC per mm^3 or greater. Throat culture, of course, is helpful in establishing bacterial etiology of pharyngitis, but is not useful in the first 24 hours of illness.

The presence of pharyngeal exudate and systemic toxicity requires that the diagnosis of diphtheria and infectious mononucleosis be considered. In such cases, to a routine throat culture should be added culture with Loeffler's medium and tellurite agar and the Monospot test to objectively aid in diagnosis.

Gonococcal pharyngitis is being seen with increasing frequency. When suspected culture should be obtained with chocolate and Thayer-Martin medium. In cases of sepsis, rectal, urethral, and blood cultures are also indicated.

Assessment

Viruses responsible for pharyngitis are the same ones which cause laryngitis, croup, bronchitis, and the common cold. The site and degree of upper respiratory tract involvement are used in the classification of viral pharyngitis, since viral culture is not routinely available.

Viral pharyngitis associated with the common cold almost always occurs without fever or exudate. Conversely, exudative viral pharyngitis, which is most common in military populations, is a febrile illness. Pharyngitis due to adenovirus is often associated with conjunctivitis. When pharyngitis is associated with croup, myxovirus and parainfluenza virus are most often implicated.

Unlike viral pharyngitis, bacterial pharyngitis presents with a rapid onset of fever, malaise, headache, and abdominal pain. The presence of an exudate on the tonsils or tonsillar fossae is more common in bacterial pharyngitis but is not diagnostic of it. As mentioned, a fever of over 38.2°C and leukocytosis of 12,000 WBC per mm^3 are the most helpful objective findings in the first 24 hours. Unfortunately, the classic presentation develops in a minority of patients. It has been noted, for instance, that mild streptococcal pharyngitis commonly presents without exudate and that adenovirus pharyngitis may present with exudative pharyngitis, high fever, and leukocytosis.

The most important bacterial agent of pharyngitis is group A β-hemolytic Streptococcus. Contrary to popular belief, many other bacteria cause significant febrile pharyngitis and subsequent infectious complications. It is an unfortunate error to ignore these, as is done when throat cultures growing bacteria other than streptococci are discarded.

Antibiotic treatment of routine bacterial pharyngitis is usually recommended, although 75% of older children and adults are afebrile within 3 days of the onset of streptococcal pharyngitis without treatment. Untreated, other signs persist for another 2–3 days. The clinical illness is shortened by 24–48 hours with antibiotic treatment. The most important consideration is that if antibiotics are not used, streptococci are shed for up to 4 weeks in the majority of patients.

The presentation of streptococcal pharyngitis may vary in small children and infants. In this group streptococcal pharyngitis may begin insidiously with viral-like symptoms including rhinorrhea and low fever. Suppurative otitis media and lymphadenitis occur frequently.

Scarlet fever is indistinguishable from other streptococcal pharyngitis with the exception of the secondary rash. This rash usually occurs on the 2nd day of pharyngitis caused by scarlatinal strains of Streptococcus and is characterized by a diffuse, deep red erythema. The rash may occur anywhere, but most commonly inner arms and thighs and the trunk are involved. The face is usually flushed and red and circumoral pallor is common. The rash is caused by an erythrogenic toxin produced by the scarlatinal Streptococcus.

The complications of streptococcal

pharyngitis are suppurative, as in peritonsillar or pharyngeal abscess (see Chapter 12), and nonsuppurative. The most important nonsuppurative complications are acute rheumatic fever and acute glomerulonephritis. Recent investigations suggest that these complications are peculiar to the lower socioeconomic class and may reflect conditions such as poor nutrition and crowding.

Other causes of exudative pharyngitis are diphtheria and infectious mononucleosis. *Corynebacterium diphtheriae* most commonly localizes in the pharynx and is responsible for both local and systemic illness in nonimmunized people. The incubation period of diphtheria varies from 1 to 7 days. Typically, the onset is sudden with low fever, malaise, and sore throat. A thick exudate usually involves the tonsillar fossae and may spread from one side of the pharynx to the other. Extension to the larynx and trachea may be associated with respiratory obstruction. The exudate varies in color from dirty white to dark shades of gray, and bleeds when peeled off.

The diagnosis of diphtherial pharyngitis must precede laboratory confirmation for treatment to be successful. The presence of a marked exudate and signs of systemic toxicity indicate the need to obtain culture for diphtheria (Loeffler's medium and tellurite agar), direct smear for gram stain, and institution of therapy. Identification from direct smear is extremely difficult and absence of typical club-shaped bacilli arranged in palisades does not rule out the diagnosis.

The major systemic complications of diphtheria involve the cardiovascular and nervous systems. Myocarditis has been shown electrocardiographically in over 25% of patients with diphtheria, but is clinically less common. When myocarditis is present, the pulse is thready and rapid, heart failure with dyspnea ensues and is followed by cardiac enlargement and an S4 gallop. EKG may show T-wave flattening or inversion, bundle branch block, premature contractions, or atrial fibrillation. Myocarditis carries a grave prognosis.

Cranial or peripheral nerve paralysis may occur in diphtheria. Paralysis of the soft palate is the most common finding and is often manifest by nasal regurgitation during swallowing. Peripheral neuropathy usually involves the lower extremities with loss of tendon reflexes and weakness of dorsiflexion of the ankles.

Infectious mononucleosis is characterized by fever, pharyngitis, lymphadenopathy, lymphocytosis, and splenomegaly. The Epstein-Barr virus is thought to be the etiologic agent. Males are involved slightly more often than females, usually between 15 and 30 years of age. Epidemics have been reported and hospital personnel and medical students seem to be at high risk. Pathologically, lymph node involvement is characterized by proliferation of both lymphocytic and reticuloendothelial elements. Abnormal lymphocytes (Downey cells) are seen in peripheral blood smears. The spleen is tense and swollen. The incubation period is approximately 1 month. Onset is nonspecific with malaise, low fever, and sore throat. Anorexia and malaise may be particularly prominent. Petechiae of the palate are common during the first 2 weeks of illness.

Diagnosis is confirmed by the appearance of greater than 50% lymphocytes in peripheral smear with many atypical forms and by the heterophil or Monospot test. Liver function tests should be performed to rule out hepatic involvement. Complications of infectious mononucleosis include hepatic failure, splenic rupture, and myocarditis. The appearance of a diffuse erythematous rash following the administration of ampicillin is presumptive evidence of infectious mononucleosis.

Sore throat may also be caused by Vincent's angina, a localized infection of the tonsil or tonsillar fossa. It is usually due to a spirochete (*Fusobacterium necrophorum*) in combination with one of a variety of oral anaerobes. The lesion is quite painful but not associated with systemic signs. The typical appearance is that of a small ulceration or group of ulcerations covered with white exudate.

Systemic involvement with leukemia, uncontrolled diabetes, or agranulocytosis should be ruled out. Herpangina is an acute febrile illness of childhood caused by group A Coxsackie virus. Small vesicles occur on the tonsillar pillars and soft palate. This occurs most often during the summer and resolves spontaneously in a week or less.

Plan

Therapy should be specific for the individual cause of pharyngitis. If cultures are not obtained, all patients with severe pharyngitis should be considered to have streptococcal infection. It is estimated that one-half of all cases of severe pharyngitis are caused by streptococci.

Routine culturing of family members and close contacts of patients with proven streptococcal pharyngitis has been standard practice. There is, however, recent information indicating that practice to be cost-effective only in lower socioeconomic situations where crowding prevails.

Erythromycin is the drug of second choice. Some studies have shown better penetration into tonsil tissue with erythromycin than penicillin. Usual dosages are 10–20 mg per kg per day for 10 days.

When diphtheria is strongly suspected on clinical grounds, antitoxin should be administered immediately, prior to laboratory confirmation. Recommended dosage varies from 20,000 to 50,000 units intramuscularly. In severe cases, 50,000 units may be administered intravenously and 50,000 units intramuscularly. The antitoxin is made of horse serum, and history of sensitivity as well as conjunctival testing with dilute antitoxin (1:10) should be performed prior to administration. Penicillin G and erythromycin are both very active against the diphtheria bacillus and are used in moderately high dosage for 2 weeks.

When marked toxicity or laryngeal involvment is present in diphtheria, high dose steroid therapy has been used with success. Prednisone, 5 mg per kg per day, has been recommended. Severe laryngeal obstruction may require emergency tracheotomy. Bronchoscopy may be lifesaving when the exudate obstructs the lower trachea.

There is no specific therapy for infectious mononucleosis. Bedrest is required for icteric patients and those with splenic enlargement. Secondary bacterial infections should be treated with the appropriate antibiotic. Ampicillin is associated with a high incidence of dermatitis in mononucleosis patients and should be avoided.

Treatment of Vincent's angina includes topical irrigation with warm hydrogen peroxide/saline mixture and with systemic penicillin. Response is usually dramatic within the first 48 hours.

CHRONIC SORE THROAT

Subjective Complaints

The symptom of chronic sore throat often proves difficult to diagnose and treat effectively. This should not dissuade the physician from an aggressive search for treatable causes including infection, tumor, allergy, and irritants. Throat pain may originate in the oropharynx, or be referred from the cervical esophagus, larynx, hypopharynx, vallecula, nasopharynx, or deep neck structures. In the absence of physical findings, chronic sore throat should not be dismissed as chronic nonspecific pharyngitis and the search for an etiology subsequently abandoned. Time may reveal a previously occult neoplasm or site of inflammation.

The patient complaining of chronic sore throat often relates only nonspecific symptoms of mild pain with swallowing. Exacerbations may be caused by irritants such as cold, dry air, smoke, alcohol and acid foods. A careful history, however, may disclose a specific etiology. The patient may, for example, correlate his symptoms with bouts of purulent nasal discharge, suggesting flareups of chronic sinusitis or rhinitis. Correlation with sneezing or watery nasal discharge suggests an upper respiratory irritant or inhalant allergy. The pharynx may be affected by reflux of gastric secretions as well as nasal and sinus secretions. Symptoms of acid reflux from the stomach raise the possibility of throat pain secondary to laryngeal, esophageal, or hypopharyngeal irritation by gastric contents.

Mechanical irritation from a chronic cough may likewise result in chronic laryngitis and/or pharyngitis. Throat pain may result from desiccation of the mucous membranes of the upper airways. Desiccation may be due to mouth breathing, changes in the moisture of the inspired air (as with oxygen therapy or geographic change), loss of saliva (from radiation or diseases of the salivary glands), or structural changes of the nasal septum or turbinates resulting in increased nasal turbulence and subsequent decreased ability of the nose to warm and moisten inspired air.

Throat pain exacerbated by specific foods may suggest a food allergy, particularly if accompanied by itching of the throat or by gastrointestinal symptoms such as nausea, bloating, or diarrhea.

Localization of the pain may be useful in directing the physical examination to a particular structure such as the tonsils, the nasopharynx, the base of the tongue, or any other area where a specific inflammatory process may occur.

Chronic tonsillitis may present as constant or recurrent episodes of sore throat, often accompanied by low grade fever and malaise.

Throat pain referred from outside the oropharynx may be accompanied by localizing symptoms such as hoarseness, pain when speaking, pulmonary aspiration, pain with head or neck movement, or nasal obstruction. Symptoms of throat pain and weight loss in a heavy smoker and drinker should initiate a meticulous search for cancer.

Objective Findings

Examination of the oropharynx usually discloses the site of inflammation if not the cause. In cases of chronic tonsillitis, the tonsils may be either large or small, depending on the degree of edema, fibrosis, or atrophy they have undergone. They are generally cryptic and may be injected and tender to palpation. Unilateral tonsillar enlargement in an adult should be evaluated for masses suggestive of malignancy.

The lymphoid nodules in the posterior oropharynx may be hypertrophied and er-

ythematous, suggestive of chronic inflammation. Examination of the nose and nasopharynx may give further clues to the source of such inflammation. Tenderness of the adenoids is usually accompanied by hyperplasia and exudate and is suggestive of chronic adenoiditis. Thornwaldt's bursa, a midline embryologic remnant, may be subject to abscess and presents as sore throat with a nasopharyngeal mass. It is usually tender to palpation and visible to mirror examination. Retention cysts of the nasopharynx may become infected and present much the same way as Thornwaldt's abscess.

Palpation of the oropharynx may reveal a tender, elongated, styloid process medial to the tonsil. This finding constitutes a controversial source of chronic throat pain. The tongue and lingual tonsil may likewise be palpated to localize the pain. Indirect laryngoscopy is necessary to rule out cysts, neoplasms, inflammation, and structural deformities of the nasopharynx, vallecula, hypopharynx, and larynx. Palpation of the neck may disclose malignant or inflammatory adenopathy, thyroid disease, or tenderness of any of the cervical musculoskeletal structures.

If the physical examination is normal and the history nondiagnostic, a sedimentation rate and complete blood counts (CBC) serve as a rough screen for chronic inflammatory disorders. A soft tissue lateral x-ray of the neck may disclose soft tissue masses in the upper airways (such as Thornwaldt's abscess), cervical spine disease, an elongated styloid process or a radiopaque foreign body. A throat culture is often performed, but is usually not of diagnostic value in chronic sore throat (unless febrile episodes raise the possibility of recurrent streptococcal infections).

Assessment

History and physical examination may disclose a discrete etiology of chronic sore throat such as a tumor or infection. More often, however, history is nonspecific and physical examination reveals only erythematous, hypertrophied lymphoid nodules. This condition may be termed chronic hypertrophic or granular pharyngitis. Possible etiologies include undiscovered allergies, mechanical and chemical irritants, chronic infections of the posterior pharyngeal lymphoid nodules analogous to chronic tonsillitis, irritation from infected nasal and nasopharyngeal secretions, desiccation of the mucous membranes, or any combination of these factors. L-forms and Mycoplasma species have been cultured from homogenates of chronically infected tonsils where routine throat swabs have been negative. Unfortunately, though, response to specific antibiotic therapy has been disappointing.

Granulomatous diseases of the pharynx such as tuberculosis, tertiary syphilis, fungal infections, and brucellosis are rare and generally accompanied by widespread manifestations of the disease elsewhere.

Plan

Therapy is aimed at correction of specific etiologies where they are present and symptomatic relief where they are not. Chronic tonsillitis may be treated with tonsillectomy, if antibiotics and warm saline gargles fail to control the recurrences (this is a very rare indication for tonsillectomy). Adenoidectomy may likewise be used to treat chronic adenoiditis. Thornwaldt's abscess and nasopharyngeal cyst are amenable to marsupialization.

Allergic management may prove more elusive, particularly in chronic inhalant allergy where mucous membranes have undergone the chronic changes associated with repeated superinfections. Treatment consists of antihistamines, steroid nasal sprays, and avoidance of specific offending allergies, where possible. Hyposensitization injections may prove useful in inhalant allergies where conservative management has been unsuccessful. Local irrigation with normal saline helps clear crusts in purulent and atrophic pharyngitis. Granular pharyngitis, when not associated with a specific reversible etiology, may be treated by chemical or electrical cauterization. This treatment affords only temporary relief, however, and satisfactory long-term palliation may not be achieved despite aggressive therapy.

FEVER AND CHILLS FOLLOWING AN UPPER RESPIRATORY INFECTION (PHARYNGEAL ABSCESS)

Subjective Complaints

The fascial investitures of the muscles, bones, and organs of the neck divide it into a number of closed compartments. Suppuration in a compartment may result from direct invasion by pus or by liquefaction of a lymph node within the compartment draining an infected area elsewhere. The peritonsillar, retropharyngeal, parapharyngeal (also called pharyngomaxillary) and anterior visceral are among the spaces most commonly invaded during an upper respiratory infection.

Occasionally the familiar symptoms of an upper respiratory tract infection lead to spiking fever, chills, and systemic toxicity. Increasing local pain further heralds the onset of secondary bacterial infection and spread to a nondraining fascial space. The most common pharyngeal abscess is the periotonsillar abscess.

In the case of peritonsillar abscess, the symptoms of routine streptococcal or viral pharyngitis develop into severe odynophagia. The patient is not only unable to take liquids, he is often unable to swallow his own saliva, resulting in early dehyration.

The voice acquires a muffled quality, the so-called "hot potato voice." Trismus is generally present to some degree and may be severe. Fever, malaise, and systemic toxicity are the rule. Some relief is obtained if the abscess has drained spontaneously into the oropharynx, but more commonly the patient seeks medical attention before this occurs.

These classical symptoms are often obscured by administration of antibiotics. Presentation may be more gradual and may follow by a few days inadequate treatment of pharyngitis.

Retropharyngeal abscess, seen most often in children, presents with pain on swallowing. Respiratory embarrassment may occur as the process extends inferiorly toward the larynx. Trismus is classically absent, but may occur if the abscess has resulted by extension from the parapharyngeal space as often occurs in adults.

Asymptomatic retropharyngeal abscess is seen in the elderly and commonly results from tuberculosis of the spine. Lingual tonsil abscess and intratonsillar abscess present with extreme dysphagia unless the abscess has drained spontaneously.

Objective Findings

The objective findings are the key to diagnosing abscesses of the upper airway. Localization of swelling and pain guides the diagnosis and subsequent drainage. Peritonsillar abscess usually presents as a swelling of the anterior tonsillar pillar at its superior pole. The involved tonsil itself may or may not be enlarged relative to the opposite tonsil, but is displaced medially and may impinge on the edematous uvula. A common mistake is to confuse enlarged erythematous, exudative tonsils with peritonsillar abscess. The latter is not a severe case of tonsillitis, but an invasion of the space between the tonsillar capsule and the superior pharyngeal constrictor by pathogenic bacteria leading to suppuration in this closed space. The unilateral location of the swelling readily distinguishes peritonsillar abscess. Rarely, peritonsillar abscess may be bilateral. A masticator space abscess, usually of dental origin, may point lingually and be difficult to distinguish from a peritonsillar abscess. The history of preceding upper respiratory infection and lack of dental symptoms distinguish the peritonsillar abscess.

Retropharyngeal abscess is generally easily visualized as a swelling in the posterior oropharynx. Lateral soft tissue roentgenograms of the neck may disclose expansion of the posterior pharynx as well as vertebral exostosis or the presence of a foreign body. Laryngeal examination should be performed to assess inferior extension and potential for airway obstruction, especially when stridor is present.

Other upper airway abscesses are localized by careful physical examination. Parapharyngeal abscess may cause swelling of the peritonsillar, paratid, and submaxillary areas depending on avenue of spread. Rigidity of the neck and severe trismus help differentiate parapharyngeal from peritonsillar abscess. White blood cell count in the case of abscess is usually elevated beyond that seen with simple pharyngitis. Counts of 15,000–20,000 with a shift to the left are common.

Assessment

The etiology of pharyngeal and deep neck abscesses is direct or lymphatic invasion of fascial compartments by pathogenic bacteria. While most abscesses had previously been considered to be group A β-hemolytic streptococci, advances in anaerobic culturing techniques have revealed anaerobes to be present as sole pathogens or mixed with aerobes in the majority of cases. *Bacteroides melaninogenicus* and anaerobic streptococci are the most commonly cultured anaerobes.

While peritonsillar abscess is the most common fascial space infection, suppuration may also occur in a myriad of fascial compartments of the head and neck. Retropharyngeal, parapharyngeal, and anterior visceral space abscesses may all result from upper respiratory infections as well as from foreign body penetration. Although fascia is a strong barrier to the spread of infection, it may break down under the pressure of confined pus. Moreover, the compartments often interconnect, allowing great variation in the route of spread. An infection pointing in the pharynx may have originated from an infected tooth, a sinus infection, or a suppurating mandibular fracture.

The diagnosis of retropharyngeal abscess is today entertained by primary care physicians much more frequently than the entity is actually encountered. The possibilities of respiratory obstruction and/or direct mediastinal extension justify this caution. Retropharyngeal abscess resulting from upper respiratory infections is largely a pediatric disease, occurring most commonly in the 1st year of life. It generally results from suppuration of the nodes in the retropharyngeal space which drain areas of infected lymphoid tissue in the naso- and oropharynx. The retropharyngeal nodes undergo progressive atrophy from the age of 2 years until they are virtually absent by age 12. The lymphoid tissue they drain also shrinks progressively in late childhood and becomes less susceptible to infection, making retropharyngeal spread still less likely.

Plan

The treatment of abscess is incision and drainage. While abscesses occasionally respond to systemic antibiotics, the slower response and great possibility of persistence in spite of medical treatment make incision and drainage the treatment of choice.

Peritonsillar abscess is generally managed by aspiration of the peritonsillar space with an 18-gauge needle passed tangentially to the lateral margin of the superior pole of the tonsil where the bulging is greatest. Successful aspiration of pus confirms the diagnosis, obtains material for culture, relieves the pressure pain of the pus, and establishes a tract for further drainage. Unsuccessful needle aspiration may occur because of loculation of the pus inferiorly, incomplete liquefaction of the inflamed area (peritonsillar cellulitis) or incorrect diagnosis.

Alternately, the anterior tonsillar pillar may be opened with a no. 11 surgical blade in the same area, providing better drainage but more trauma and bleeding, and the possibility of pulmonary aspiration. Some caution must be exercised with this drainage, as the internal carotid artery normally lies just posterior and lateral to the tonsil. An aberrant carotid may be directly behind the superior constrictor which forms the posterior wall of the abscess cavity. The posterior oropharynx is often seen pulsating in the latter case, and palpation of the area further confirms the proximity of the internal carotid. Hot saline gargles speed the resolution of the process. Tonsillectomy has been carried out either

acutely or after the inflammation has resolved to prevent the otherwise common recurrence.

Tonsillectomy in the acute stage of peritonsillar abscess is practiced by many physicians. It reduces medical costs and patient discomfort.

Other pharyngeal abscesses are drained under general anesthesia with the patient intubated to avoid aspiration of pus. Systemic antibiotics are recommended until the process is resolved. Penicillin is the drug of choice, unless *Staphylococcus aureus* is suspected or encountered on culture. In these cases a penicillinase-resistant penicillin is used with the awareness that it is not as effective as penicillin against anaerobes and Streptococcus species. For this reason, penicillin may be used in combination with a semisynthetic penicillin for optimal coverage. Cephalosporins provide coverage of staphylococci and anerobes but achieve lower tissue concentrations in some areas. Clindamycin offers good coverage of *S. aureus* and anaerobes, but potential side effects, such as colitis, militate against its more frequent usage. Tetracycline and erythromycin are also less effective second-choice drugs. With the use of high dose systemic antibiotics, sequelae of deep neck abscesses following upper respiratory infection (e.g., metastatic abscesses, thrombosis of the internal jugular, and mediastinitis) have become uncommon.

Bibliography

1. Herzon, F. S. Infectious diseases of the head and neck. *Otolaryngol. Clin. North Am.*, 1977.
2. Levitt, G. W. The surgical treatment of deep neck infections. *Laryngoscope 81*: 403–411, 1971.
3. Sprinkle, P. M. Current status of Mycoplasmatales and bacterial variants in chronic otolaryngic disease. *Laryngoscope 82*: 737–747, 1972.
4. Templer, J. W. Inflammatory diseases of the oral pharynx. In *Otolaryngology: A Textbook*, edited by G. M. English, pp. 429–439. Harper & Row, Hagerstown, Md., 1977.

Chapter 9
Facial Skin Disorders

Matthew L. Wong

Facial skin disorders are among the most common problems seen in the head and neck region. The skin lesions are readily apparent and visible. The diagnosis may be extremely difficult, especially where related to drug eruptions. A thorough history is most important. A complete examination of the entire body is mandatory, as certain dermatoses have nonspecific appearances in the face but have characteristic body distributions.

Skin disorders are not stressed in most ear, nose and throat textbooks, and most dermatologic textbooks treat dermatoses by entities and systems, not by regions.

SUBJECTIVE COMPLAINTS

Skin disorders are different from other disorders of the body in that the lesion is readily seen. There may or may not be associated symptoms such as bleeding, pruritus, or pain. History is very important in the diagnosis of facial skin disorders. (Knowledge of possible etiologies is important in the subjective evaluation.)

Past Medical History. Asthma, hay fever, previous skin disorders (atopy, psoriasis, basal cell epithelioma, neurodermatitis, herpes simplex, etc.), systemic diseases (systemic lupus erythematosus, diabetes mellitus), and immune deficiencies. Patients with immune deficiency states are prone to infections and skin cancers.

Occupation/Association. Exposure to irritants, sensitizing chemicals.

Family History. Urticaria, atopic dermatitis, acne, rosacea, psoriasis, seborrheic dermatitis.

Age of Onset:

Infants. Superficial bacterial infection, herpes simplex, atopy.

Child. Warts, papular urticaria.

Adolescence. Acne.

Geriatric. Senile freckles, senile keratosis, carcinoma of the skin.

Seasonal/Travel. Contact dermatitis, photosensitivity.

Habits. Diet—allergy; smoking—carcinoma of the lip; contactant—contact dermatitis.

Pigmentary Changes. Malignant melanoma, senile freckles, Addison's disease, chloasma (melasma-patterned hyperpigmentation during pregnancy and on birth control pills).

Drug History. Very important, as drug eruptions are quite varied in appearance.

Allergic History. Atopic dermatitis.

Other Sites in the Body. Most skin reactions in the face can involve other sites, and sites of involvement are characteristic of certain diseases such as psoriasis, seborrheic dermatitis, and atopy.

Photosensitivity—Acute. Sunburn from prolonged exposure. If recurrent and not due to prolonged sun exposure, consider medication (phenothiazines, tetracyclines, and griseofulvins are among many medications that have photosensitivity as a side reaction). Porphyria can cause photodermatitis.

Growth Changes. Malignant neoplasms—squamous cell carcinoma, basal cell carcinoma, and malignant melanoma. Squamous cell and basal cell carcinomas are in the sun-exposed areas. Benign growths include warts, keloids, and keratoacanthoma (mimic a squamous cell carcinoma).

Scaly Lesion. Inquire about psoriasis, seborrheic dermatitis, secondary syphilis, and discoid and systemic lupus erythematosus.

Bullae/Vesicles. Must look for causes such as erythema multiforme, primary irritant and sensitization reactions (contact dermatitis), burns, pemphigus, herpes, and drug reactions.

Hives/Urticaria. Ask about mosquito or other insect bites, angioneurotic edema, food allergy, drug reactions, and contact dermatitis.

Syphilis. Chancre of the lips; macular papular eruptions in the secondary stage, and gummas of the tertiary stage.

Acute Conditions. Infections (as impetigo, folliculitis, cellulitis), contact dermatitis, dermatitis medicamentosa, acute photodermatitis, and herpes simplex.

Chronic Conditions. Can be persistent or recurring, as psoriasis, seborrheic dermatitis, atopy, and neurodermatitis.

Neck Mass. Tenderness—associated with acute infection. Nontender—large squamous cell carcinoma or other malignancy. Some malignant melanomas of the scalp metastasize to the regional lymph nodes while the primary site is still difficult to find on cursory examination (Table 9.1).

Table 9.1
Classification of Facial Skin Disorders

I. *Dermatitic skin*
   Atopic dermatitis
   Contact dermatitis, acute
   Exfoliative dermatitis
   Factitial dermatitis
   Lichen simplex chronicus (localized neurodermatitis)
   Nummular eczema
   Radiodermatitis, chronic
   Seborrheic dermatitis
II. *Growth change*
   Epithelioma, basal cell (always confirm by biopsy)
   Hemangioma
   Nevus
   Seborrheic keratosis
   Senile (or actinic) keratosis
   Verruca
III. *Infection*
   Folliculitis
   Furuncle
   Hidradenitis
   Impetigo
   Pyogenic granuloma
   Varicella
   Herpes simplex
   Zoster
IV. *Lesions, special type*
   Comedo, acne
   Insect bite
   Milium
   Purpura
   Urticaria
V. *Loss of tissue*
   Alopecia areata
   Excoriation
   Scleroderma
   Ulcer (determination of cause mandatory)
   Vitiligo
VI. *Scaling*
   Ichthyosis
   Lupus erythematosus, chronic discoid (further study mandatory)
   Psoriasis
   Seborrheic dermatitis
VII. *Vesicles, bullae*
   Erythema multiforme
   Primary irritant and sensitization reactions

OBJECTIVE FINDINGS

Regional Skin Lesions

Scalp

1. Seborrheic Dermatitis. Chronic scaly eruption, dry white yellowish scale (see Scaly Lesions, under Specific Skin Disorders).

2. Local Neurodermatitis. Chronic itchy lesion with pigmented lichenified skin, exaggerated skin lines overlying lichenified skin, and thick circumscribed scaly plaques.

3. Psoriasis. Chronic scaly eruption with a reddish hue (see Scaly Lesions, under Specific Skin Disorders).

Face

1. Acne. Papules to pustules, especially during adolescence.

2. Rosacea. Accentuation of normal facial flush, especially over central forehead, nose, malar prominence, and chin. Late change is *rhinophyma* with thickened oily skin due to sebaceous gland hypertropy. The nose is the most common site involved.

3. Senile Keratosis. Keratotic, discrete lesions with some brownish discoloration, in sun-exposed areas; can be macular or macularpapular.

4. Seborrheic Dermatitis. Chronic scaly eruption, up along alar and nasolabial groove and frown areas between the brows.

5. Sebaceous Cysts (more correctly termed epidermal inclusion cysts; true sebaceous cyst is rare). Cystic lesion in dermis and subcutaneous layers of the skin.

6. Epithelioma. Squamous cell and basal cell carcinoma (see Neoplasm, under Specific Skin Disorders).

7. Contact Dermatitis. Acute eruption from erythema to bullae on an erythematous swollen base, with severe pruritus.

8. Atopy. Pruritic exudative or lichenified eruption.

9. Photosensitivity or Photodermatitis. Erythema to swelling, vesicles and bullae with erythematous base; painful.

10. Chronic Discoid Lupus Erythematosus and Systemic Lupus Erythematosus. Red, asymptomatic, local plaque on the face in a butterfly distribution, scaly follicular plugging, atrophy, and telangiectasia. Often cannot distinguish the facial rash of chronic discoid from systemic lupus erythematosus without systemic involvement (joints, kidney) (see also Specific Skin Disorders).

Lip

1. Perleche. Inflammation at the corners of the mouth with accumulation of whitish epithelium resembling a pseudomembrane. Occurs in malnutrition and vitamin B deficiencies and oral moniliasis.

2. Herpes Simplex (Cold Sores). Ulcers with erythematous base; painful; start as ulcers.

3. Leukoplakia. Whitish areas, may be flat or raised. Flat leukoplakia has 5% incidence of malignant changes, and raised leukoplakia, especially with an erythematous base, has much higher incidence of malignant changes.

4. Carcinoma (Basal Cell and Squamous Cell) (see Neoplasm, under Specific Skin Disorders). Basal cell carcinoma occurs more on upper lip and squamous cell carcinoma more on lower lip.

5. Cheilitis. Inflammation of the lips as from lip biting, infection, and photodermatitis.

Ear

1. Localized Neurodermatitis. Involvement of auricle and postauricular area.

2. Seborrheic Dermatitis.

3. Contact Dermatitis.

4. Psoriasis.

5. Chronic Bacterial Infection. Pustule, folliculitis to cellulitis. If most of the auricle is erythematous, edematous, and very tender, this is perichondritis.

6. Discoid Lupus Erythematosus (see also Specific Skin Disorders, and Regional Skin Lesions, Face).

7. Carcinoma (Basal Cell and Squamous Cell).

Specific Skin Disorders

Dermatitis

1. Contact Dermatitis. Includes all dermatitis due to chemical substances, natural or synthetic, in contact with skin. The lesions are characteristically sharply demarcated and the spectrum of reaction ranges from faint transient erythema to massive bullae on an erythematous swollen base. Itching is an accompanying symptom. The incubation period varies greatly from as short as a week to longer. The most common sites are the face, neck, back of hand, forearms, male genitalia, and lower legs.

2. Atopic Dermatitis. The typical adult changes are thickening and lichenification due to rubbing and excoriation and may have partial depigmentation. In the infant, erythema, vesicular formation, and eczema are evident. The distribution is chiefly to the face, neck, antecubital fossa, hands, wrist, and popliteal fossa. Secondary bacterial and viral infections are the most common complications.

3. Neurodermatitis. Divided into circumscribed neurodermatitis (lichen simplex chronicus) and nummular dermatitis.

Circumscribed neurodermatitis shows typically accentuated skin lines and confluent papules characteristic of lichenification. Itching is an accompanying symptom. The most common sites in the head and neck are the occipital nuchal region, side of neck, scalp and external auditory canal.

Nummular dermatitis consists of round, nummular (coinlike) patches of oozing dermatitis, principally on back and extensor surfaces of the extremities. In the head and neck, the neck is the most common site.

Scaly Lesions

Most common of the scaly face lesions are psoriasis and seborrheic dermatitis.

1. Psoriasis. A chronic, recurrent scaling eruption. The scaling is silvery white, imbricated, and not readily detached. The plaques or papules are more or less raised and sharply marginated. Geographic distribution includes the scalp, elbows, knees, chest, back, and buttock.

2. Seborrheic Dermatitis. A chronic scaling eruption of yellowish, somewhat greasy adherent scales, in hairy areas rich in sebaceous glands and, in more extensive cases, the intertriginous areas. The common sites are scalp, eyebrow, nasal fold, retroauricular area, external auditory canal, and presternal and interscapular areas.

3. Other Facial Scaly Eruptions (include secondary syphilis). See Syphilis in this section and Discoid and Systemic Lupus Erythematosus under Regional Skin Disorders (Face), and in this section.

Neoplasm

1. Basal Cell Carcinoma (Epithelioma). Growth with waxy and pearly appearance, with central ulcer or dimple; slow-growing; lymph node spread is rare. Early ones can be difficult to distinguish from senile keratosis. Involves sun-exposed areas, and most commonly seen in face, auricle, and nose.

2. Squamous Cell Carcinoma. Small, reddish conical mass with ulceration. If large and friable, can have lymph node metastasis. Faster growth than basal cell carcinoma.

3. Keratoacanthoma (Molluscum Pseudocarcinoma). Benign, raised, umbilicated growth that resembles a fast-growing, well differentiated squamous cell carcinoma. It grows rapidly for 1–2 months (8–28 weeks) and then involves involution. Treatment is simple excision. Be careful not to mistake for a large aggressive squamous cell carcinoma.

4. Malignant Melanoma

Nodular type has pigmented nodules with satellitosis and varied coloration (brown to black); very aggressive, with early lymph node metastasis. Small nodular malignant melanoma has 75% cure rate, whereas those with lymph node metastasis have a 10–25% incidence of 5-year survival.

Superficial spreading melanomas are pigmented lesions that have hyperpigmented changes but no nodularity or satellitosis. They are characterized by centrifugal growth with regression of the older areas to a paler color. Look for any nodularity, as the prognosis and treatment are those for a nodular malignant melanoma and not superficial spreading melanoma.

Hutchinson's freckles. The most superficial form of malignant melanoma. It is also known as *lentigo maligna*. It is histologically malignant and resembles freckles that are growing. It has no nodularity, and has variegated color with a blue cast and irregularity in outline.

5. Wart. Occurs especially in the lip with a hyperkeratotic mass; it is nontender and nonpruritic.

6. Keloid/Hypertrophic Scars. Hypertrophic scar is a moderately raised, red, indurated enlargement of scar. Keloid is a marked, nodular enlargement and in ear lobe can be pedunculated. For reasons unknown, hypertrophic scars and keloids seldom form in the skin of the middle third of the face. They most commonly form in the ear, especially the ear lobe and the neck.

Infections

1. Pustules. As seen in acne.

2. Impetigo. A superficial pyoderma with a superficial vesicle that ruptures and is covered with a thick, yellowish crust. it is contagious and caused by *Staphylococcus aureus*.

3. Folliculitis. Infection along the hair follicles.

4. Cellulitis. Infection with swelling, erythema, and tenderness, and often accompanying fever. Most often are due to group A β-hemolytic streptococci but can occur with any organism.

5. Erysipelas (St. Anthony's Fire). An acute inflammation, due to *Streptococcus pyogenes*, with a sharply defined edematous, spreading, hot, erythematous area with or without vesicle or bullae formation.

Discoid and Systemic Lupus Erythematosus (see also Regional Skin Lesions, Face).

Chronic discoid lupus erythematosus and systemic lupus erythematosus are characterized by red, asymptomatic, local

plaques on the face in a butterfly distribution, scaly follicular plugging, atrophy,
and telangiectasia. Often cannot distinguish the facial rash of chronic discoid
from systemic lupus erythematosus without systemic involvement (joints, kidney).

Hives and Urticaria

Wheals with marked itching. The
wheals vary greatly in size, shape, and
amount of swelling. Angioneurotic edema
often involves lips and face over a larger
area. Insect bites will show accompanying
skin puncture mark.

Urticaria is divided into two types. The
acute form persists for less than 2 weeks,
often with massive initial onset and gradual subsidence. The cause is usually a
food, drug, or physical trauma. *Chronic*
urticaria persists recurrently for weeks,
months, or years. Obscure factors such as
chronic infection, gastrointestinal disease
or psychosomatic disturbances are etiologies.

Hirsutism

Congenitally, hair can be seen around
the upper lips of certain females. Male
type of hair development in females, especially around the lips, chin, and neck, is
caused by excess androgen secretion or
medication.

Pigmented Lesions

1. Nevi (Moles). Pigmented lesions
from flat to dome shapes, polypoid, and
even papillomatous. They can be amelan-
otic to brown or black and do not grow.

2. Addison's Disease. Diffuse darken-
ing of the skin.

3. Senile Freckles. Due to excess
amount of melanin in melanocyte of epi-
dermis and consist of yellowish or brownish macules on sun-exposed skin.

4. Chloasma (Melasma). Light brown
patches of irregular shape and size on the
skin of face, axilla, linea alba, groin, and
around nipple.

5. Malignant Melanoma (see Neoplasm).

Drug Eruptions or Dermatitis Medicamentosa

Usually abrupt onset of widespread
symmetrical erythematous eruption with
constitutional symptoms (malaise, arthral-
gia, headache, and fever). They are classified as:

1. Erythematous (sulfonamide, antihistamine, barbiturate).
2. Eczmatoid or lichenoid (gold, quinine).
3. Acneiform or pyodermic (steroid,
bromide).
4. Urticarial (penicillin, serum).
5. Bullous (iodide).
6. Fixed (barbiturate).
7. Exfoliative (gold, arsenical).
8. Nodose (sulfathiazole, salicylate).
9. Exanthematous eruption.
10. Photosensitization (phenothiazide,
cholorothiazide, tetracycline, griseofulvin).

Syphilis

1. Primary. Chancre is a painless superficial ulcer with firm indurated margins
and regional lymphadenopathy. In the
face, the lip is the most common site. It
appears 10–90 days after exposure.

2. Secondary. The lesions appear a few
weeks after chancre development and consist of nonpruritic macular, papular, pus-
tular, or follicular lesions, with maculopapular rash the most common. The skin
lesions are generalized and also involve
mucous membrane.

3. Tertiary. Lesions are (a) multiple
nodules that ulcerate or resolve by forming
atrophic pigmented scars, or (b) a solitary
gumma that starts as a painless subcutaneous nodule that eventually ulcerates.

ASSESSMENT

A thorough history and complete physical examination can often yield the diagnosis. It is important to examine the rest
of the body skin, as certain skin diseases
hve characteristic skin site involvements.

Infections. (1) complete blood count; (2)
culture and sensitivity is important; (3)

blood culture is done if evidence of sepsis.

Biopsy. All neoplastic lesions or suspicious neoplastic lesions or undiagnosed lesions are biopsied. Be sure to include in the biopsy a section of normal tissue.

Malignant Melanoma. Especially with lymph node enlargement, must have systemic workup of brain, liver, bone, and lung, as hematogenous spread occurs in over 15% of patients.

Squamous Cell or Basal Cell Carcinoma. If near the external auditory canal, eye, or nasal cavity, must have thorough evaluation of the contiguous structures. Once the carcinoma involves the ear, nose, sinuses, or eyes, the spread is rapid and aggressive.

Collagen Vascular Disease. Rheumatoid factors, antinuclear antibiotics, and LE preparation. Evaluation of joints and kidney function if systemic lupus erythematosus is suspected.

Syphilis. VDRL and other serologic tests if suspect.

Neurodermatitis. Psychiatric workup.

Atopic Dermatitis. Allergic workup.

Dermatitis Medicamentosa. Esosinophil count may be helpful; careful and repeat history must be taken and evaluated.

Male Type Hirsutism. Serum and urinary androgens.

Chronic Photodermatitis. Workup for porphyria, especially porphyria cutanea tarda.

Contact Dermatitis. Patch test with suspected agents. Inquire about (1) diffuse airborne contactants (insecticidal sprays, ragweed pollen, camphor, paints), and (2) local; cosmetics, metals (nickle, white gold alloys), plants (especially poison oak or ivy) and hatbands.

Immunodeficiencies. Recurrent infections, especially in infants and children, are suspect for immune deficiency disease. Must evaluate the immunoglobulins (especially IgG, IgA, and IgM) and B- and T-lymphocytes.

T-cell or lymphocytoid deficiency may result in tuberculosis, other fungal diseases, some viral and chronic gram-negative infections.

B-cell or plasmacytoid deficiency may result in extracellular pyogenic infections.

Patients on immunosuppressive therapy, especially transplant patients, are more susceptible to skin cancers and sarcomas.

Warts. In infants and children, facial warts are associated with higher incidence of laryngeal papilloma as well as with vaginal (venereal) warts in the mother.

Addison's Disease. Urinary 17-ketosteroids and 17-hydroxycorticosteroid, plasma cortisol, and ACTH levels.

PLAN

Nonspecific

Pruritus. Antihistamines such as chlorpheniramine, 4 mg b.i.d. to q.i.d., or Benadryl, 25–50 mg b.i.d. to q.i.d. sedative: phenobarbital, 15–30 mg b.i.d. to q.i.d., Valium, 5 mg b.i.d. to q.i.d. Corticosteroids: rarely.

Local Measures for Dermatoses

1. Acute. Lesions are recent, red, burning, itching, and blistering. Treat with a wet preparation such as NaCl or sodium bicarbonate and placed as a soak or wet dressing (wet to dry). Open dressing is preferred.

2. Subacute. Wet preparations as lotions and emulsions such as calamine, coal tar, or acne lotions.

3. Chronic. Wet preparation on a shake lotion, ointment, or cream.

Specific

Contact Dermatitis. Avoidance, local measures, corticosteroids rarely, and medication for pruritus. Topical preparation use include Synalar solution; neutral soap (e.g., Basis); Cordran Ointment, ½ strength, and Eucerin, equal parts; and salicylic acid, 2%, in Cordran ointment.

Atopic Dermatitis. Local measures, allergic workup and avoidance of allergens, and corticosteroids in severe cases.

Neurodermatitis. Topical steroid; avoid stress; recommend psychiatric care.

Infections. Antibiotics, as infections are usually due to staphylococcal organisms.

Penicillin or erythromycin is the drug of choice. For penicillin-resistant organism, dicloxacillin is used. For abscesses, incision and drainage along with antibiotics.

Drug Eruption or Dermatitis Medicamentosa. Diagnosis is important; cessation of offending drug; local treatment; antihistamines; and, rarely corticosteroids.

Psoriasis. Local treatment with tar or corticosteroid cream wrapped with Saran wrap; ultraviolet irradiation; systemic corticosteroid and systemic methotrexate in fulminant cases. Scalp psoriasis is treated with aerosol—HC, Baker's P & S liquid, or Anthralin preparations. Facial skin can be treated with Zetar emulsion, Cordran tape, Valisone ointment, or Kerolyt gel.

Seborrheic Dermatitis. Seborrhea of the scalp: Selenium sulfide or Selsun suspension, valisone, 0.1% lotion, or Sebizon lotion.

Seborrhea in non-hair-bearing area: 3–5% sulfur in hydrophilic ointment.

Seborrhea in intertriginous areas. astringent wet dressings followed by 3% iodochlorhydroxyquin and 1% hydrocortisone in an emulsion base.

Acne. Balanced diet; avoid exposure to oil and grease; eliminate all possible medication, especially bromides and iodides; treat with tetracycline, 250 mg q.d.; local measures as keratoplastic and keratolytic agents.

Urticaria/Hives. Antihistamine, epinephrine injections, and possible corticosteroid; avoidance of allergen.

Herpes Simplex. Avoid transfer to eye; local treatment with moist styptic pencil; analgesia and antipruritic agent as necessary.

Herpes Zoster. Locally, calamine lotion; analgesia and antipruritic medication as necessary. In elderly patient, workup for undiagnosed malignancy (lymphoma, leukemia, and other malignancies).

Systemic Lupus Erythematosus. Corticosteroid.

Discoid Lupus Erythematosus. Corticosteroid cream has been helpful; treat chronic infections with local and systemic antibiotics.

Rosacea. Avoid extremes of temperature; reduce emotional stress; and eliminate coffee, alcohol, and spicy foods. Topical therapy is similar to that for acne, with lotion containing sulfur and/or resorcin.

Porphyria. Protection from sun; abstinence from alcohol, estrogen, and iron salts, and sensitizing drugs as griseofulvin and barbiturates.

Acute Photodermatitis. Analgesia; hydration; cooling and soothing wet dressings; follow with lotions.

Addison's Disease. Corticosteroid replacement.

Hirsutism. Stop the androgenic drug, or workup and treatment for androgen-producing adrenal cortical neoplasm or hyperplasia.

Syphilis. Adequate penicillin therapy.

Warts. Surgical excision, liquid nitrogen, or keratolytic agents.

Cysts. Surgical removal.

Nevi. Watch, and early biopsy if growing or change in color. Avoid chronic irritation.

Senile Keratosis. Watch, avoid sun exposure or cover with sun screen lotion.

Keloids. Excision and intralesional injection with corticosteroid. Grenz (soft) x-ray therapy has been used by some. Requires 2000 rads (should be discouraged).

Hypertrophic Scars. Many will regress so wait for 9–12 months to see if regression occurs. If not, treat like keloid.

Keratoacanthoma. Proper diagnosis is the most important. They can be mistaken for large aggressive squamous cell carcinomas and thus excessive surgical excision may be performed. Local excision is all that is required for this disease.

Basal Cell Carcinoma. Total excision with a 5- to 8-mm margin; radiation therapy; local chemotherapy with 5-fluorouracil cream, or Mohs' chemosurgery. Small lesions may be treated by dermatologist with excision and curettage.

Squamous Cell Carcinoma. Total excision with at least a 1-cm margin. If there are palpable lymph nodes in region of drainage, a radical neck dissection is performed.

Malignant Melanoma. Nodular type: wide excision and regional lymph node dissection. Superficial spreading and Hutchinson's freckles: wide local excision.

Lesions with distant metastasis should be treated with chemotherapy, as well.

Bibliography

1. Andrade, R., Gumport, S. L., Popkin, G. L., Rees, and T. R. *Cancer of the Skin,* vols. 1 and 2. W. B. Saunders Co., Phildadelphia, 1976.
2. Arndt, K. A. *Manual of Dermatologic Theraputics.* Little, Brown and Co., Boston, 1974.
3. Behrman, H. T., Labow, T. A., and Rozen, J. H. *Common Skin Diseases,* ed. 2., Grune & Stratton, New York, 1971.
4. Fitzpatrick, T. B., Arndt, K. A., Clark, W. H., *et al. Dermatology in General Medicine,* McGraw-Hill Book Co., New York, 1971.
5. Korting, G. W., and Denk, R. *Differential Diagnosis in Dermatology.* W. B. Saunders Co., Philadelphia, 1976.
6. Mihm, M., Clark, W., and Fram, L. Clinical diagnosis, classification, and histogenic concepts of the early stages of cutaneous malignant melanoma. *N. Engl. J. Med. 284:* 1078–1082, 1971.
7. Whitlock, F. A. *Psychophysiological Aspects of Skin Disease.* W. B. Saunders Co., Philadelphia, 1976.

Chapter 10

Salivary Gland Disorders

Raymond P. Wood II

Dysfunction of the salivary glands is usually manifested in one of two ways: swelling of the gland, either diffuse or discrete, or by dry mouth (xerostomia). There may be accompanying pain and tenderness or overlying erythema. The history is important in suggesting certain disorders. The workup and treatment are usually straightforward. There is only one strong caveat—*never biopsy*, by needle or incision, discrete lesions of parotid glands or submaxillary gland. The only correct biopsy is *excisional*, by superficial parotidectomy or submaxillary gland resection. In this chapter, we will consider only diseases of the parotid and submaxillary glands. Minor salivary gland disorders are usually tumors (60–70%) and present as discrete submucosal intraoral swellings in the buccal mucosa or palate (although they can be anywhere in the oral cavity or pharynx). When suspected, they should be managed by excisional bippsy taking a margin of normal tissue.

HISTORY

Gland(s) Involved
  Single
  Multiple (parotids and/or submaxillary)
Nature of Enlargement
  Discrete
  Diffuse
Pattern of Enlargement
  Gradually increasing
  Intermittent swelling and recession
    Rapid—associated with eating
    Gradual—days, weeks, months
Lacrimal Gland Involvement
Pain
Erythema over Gland
Foul Discharge in Mouth
Facial Paralysis—usually with malignancy
Other Symptoms
  Xerostomia
  Xerophthalmia
  Joint pain and swelling
  Fever
  Weight loss
  Skin rash
  Malaise
Allergies
Medications (iodides, bromides, tranquilizers, etc.)

Alcohol Intake
Family History

SUBMAXILLARY GLAND

Owing to the size and location of the submaxillary glands, it is usually not possible to differentiate discrete from diffuse swelling of the gland. Because there are several lymph nodes located in the submaxillary triangle in close proximity to the gland with a consistency similar to that of the normal gland, it is not always possible to differentiate gland from lymph node, although the gland usually has a bosselated surface. The importance here is to rule out disorders which may produce submaxillary lymph node enlargement (infections—periodontal, floor of mouth—and tumors of the head and neck with metastases). This can be done only with a complete head and neck examination.

Intermittent Swelling—Rapid

Subjective Complaints. The usual history is that of swelling which occurs with eating. There may be mild tenderness associated. The swelling usually goes down over a period of hours. Occasionally, there may be pain and erythema of the area followed by relief associated with the release of foul-tasting fluid in the mouth.

Objective Findings. The gland may be minimally to moderately enlarged and is usually slightly tender to palpation. Bimanual palpation of the floor of the mouth may reveal the presence of a firm palpable mass.

Assessment. This history and findings are almost always associated with ductal obstruction. Although strictures do occur, ductal stones are far more common. Plain x-ray films of the floor of the mouth may be taken (occlusive views), and many stones are radiopaque (85% are). Sialograms may demonstrate the blockage, but not to be performed in an acutely inflamed state or will precipitate an acute sialadenitis.

Plan. If there is a stone in the Wharton's duct, the floor of the mouth around the duct is anesthetized with topical 10% lidocaine, and 2% lidocaine is injected along the duct. The ductal orifice is dilated with a lacrimal punctum dilator, and progressive dilation of the duct is carried out with lacrimal duct probes. If a stone is encountered, the probe is left in place and a small scissors used to incise along the probe to the stone, which is removed. Be sure not to push stone into gland proper. The cut duct edges are sutured open to the floor of the mouth. Recurrences are treated by excision of the gland.

Intermittent Enlargement—Gradual

(See Parotid Gland, Diffuse Swelling, Intermittent.) May occur alone or with parotid swelling.

Constant Enlargement

Subjective Complaints. Usually gradual, painless, unilateral gland enlargement.

Objective Findings. The gland feels firm and may be smooth or bosselated. The duct and ductal punctum are normal.

Assessment. The head and neck examination with special attention to the oral cavity fails to reveal any primary tumor. No nodes are palpable in the neck. Skin tests for tuberculosis and atypical mycobacterial infection should be done. A submaxillary gland sialogram may be done to help determine whether the mass is gland or adjacent lymph nodes, although it is not often helpful. The lesion is most likely tumor, 50% of which are malignant.

Plan. *Excisional biopsy* under general anesthesia is carried out. Frozen sections are obtained. In the absence of tumor, tissue sections are cultured along with any pus for routine and acid-fast bacteria and fungi.

PAROTID GLAND

Discrete Swelling

Subjective Complaints. The patient may be aware of a slowly growing discrete mass in the area of the parotid gland. There may be pain and facial nerve involvement.

Objective Findings. Palpation reveals a discrete mass in the gland, usually firm.

Remember that the gland extends from the level of the zygomatic arch to *below* the angle of the mandible and extends from just in front of the ear downward to beneath the ear lobe and over the upper sternocleidomastoid muscle anterior to the anterior border of the masseter muscle. Pain may be present and also weakness of part or all of the facial nerve. The external ear canal should be examined for evidence of otitis externa or tumor. The scalp should be examined for lesions, especially melanoma.

Assessment. Discrete lesions of the parotid are almost always tumors. It is usually not possible to rule out enlargement of lymph nodes associated with the gland unless a primary tumor of the scalp or external ear or ear canal can be demonstrated or external otitis is present. Lymphomas may also arise in nodes associated with the gland. Although radioactive isotope scans with gallium and technetium has been advocated, I think they add little to the management. The presence of pain or facial nerve involvement is almost *always* associated with a malignant tumor.

Plan. The important part of the plan is that *no* biopsy of the lesion is carried out *other than* excisional biopsy by superficial parotidectomy. Benign mixed tumors, the most common lesion, may be spread by incisional or needle biopsy. The whole specimen must be available to the pathologist. Needle biopsies of mixed tumors and lymphomas are worthless. Frozen sections are obtained. In uncommon malignant lesions, more extensive surgery requiring radical neck dissection and sacrifice of the facial nerve and surrounding structures may be necessary.

Diffuse Swelling, Intermittent, Rapid

(See Submaxillary Gland.) Stones in the parotid duct are reported to be one-tenth as common as submaxillary duct stones. The author has never seen one despite seeing many in the submaxillary duct.

Diffuse Swelling in Childhood

Subjective Complaints. The history may be either that of recent onset of mildly tender swelling of one or both parotid glands accompanied by upper respiratory infection (URI) or flu-like symptoms or of recurrent unilateral or bilateral, usually painless, swelling of the glands.

Objective Findings. There is visible and palpable enlargement of the gland or glands. There may be tenderness.

Assessment. When the enlargement is accompanied by systemic symptoms, the most common cause is *mumps* (viral parotitis). This can be confirmed by acute and convalescent serum viral antibody titers. Other considerations include cytomegalic inclusion virus disease (confirmed by urinary and salivary viral cultures) and diffuse infection with tuberculosis or atypical mycobacteria, confirmed by culture and skin tests.

The recurrent form is almost always *recurrent parotitis* of childhood, a disease of unknown etiology thought to be related to Sjögren's and Mikulicz' diseases. The diagnosis may be made by sialogram in which sialectasis is seen.

Plan. The treatment of these disorders is symptomatic, as no specific therapy exists except in the case of the mycobacterial infections. There, the appropriate antimicrobial therapy is based upon the culture results.

Diffuse Swelling in Adults

Subjective Complaints. The swelling may involve one or both glands. It may be rapid in onset or gradual. There may be pain or it may be painless. There may be erythema of the skin overlying the gland. There may be clear saliva or pus expressed from the ducts. Systemic symptoms may include fever, extreme malaise, xerostomia, xerophthalmia, joint pains, weight loss, night sweats, or nothing. The swelling may be described as intermittent over days to weeks.

Objective Findings. The affected glands may be nontender or very tender to the touch. Erythema of the skin may be present. The punctum of the duct may be inflamed and pus or clear saliva expressed. Cervical lymph nodes may be enlarged. Other salivary glands (submaxillary and sublingual) may be enlarged, as may the lacrimal glands.

Studies include CBC, chest x-ray, erythrocyte sedimentation rate, lupus prep, antinuclear antibodies, rheumatoid factor, serum calcium determination, culture of the saliva, and parotid sialograms.

Assessment. *Painless swelling* of the glands, sometimes intermittent, usually accompanied by xerostomia and xerophthalmia, is most likely *Mikulicz' disease or Sjögren's syndrome*. The difference between the two is that Mikulicz' disease is limited to the salivary and lacrimal glands, whereas Sjögren's syndrome has an associated collagen vascular disease (rheumatoid arthritis, lupus erythematosus, scleroderma) or other systemic disease such as lymphoma, sarcoidosis, etc. The sialogram in both disorders shows sialectasis. A helpful screening test is the Westergren sedimentation rate. If that is elevated, the other blood studies should be obtained. The serum calcium may be elevated in sarcoidosis. The chest x-ray may reveal mediastinal node involvement in sarcoid and lymphoma. Any enlarged cervical lymph nodes should be biopsied. Biopsy of the parotid gland or the oral minor salivary glands will reveal lymphocytic infiltration and ductal hyperplasia along with a decrease in the acinar cells.

Two other disorders of *painless swelling* unaccompanied by other symptoms include *fatty infiltration* of the gland and *acinar hypertrophy*. These may both be seen in alcoholics. The fatty infiltration may be associated with fatty infiltration of the liver. Fatty infiltration of the gland may also be seen in the recovery phase of acute starvation or protein-calorie malnutrition (kwashiorkor) as in fatty liver infiltration. The sialogram is normal in these cases. Biopsy of the gland establishes the diagnosis.

One condition which can mimic these disorders is *hypertrophy of the masseter muscles*. In this case, when the patient clenches his teeth the gland protrudes markedly. A sialogram (unusually unnecessary) shows the bilateral lateral displacement of the gland. Likewise, tumor of the masseter or underlying mandible may present with unilateral protrusion of the parotid. Mandible x-rays are helpful, as in palpation of the mandible and muscle.

Painful swelling of the gland which is unassociated with other symptoms may represent ductal obstruction (see Submaxillary Gland).

Painful swelling of the one parotid, with erythema over the gland and a red ductal orifice with pus expressed from the duct, is usually seen in very ill and frequently elderly patients. This is *acute suppurative* or *surgical parotitis*. Culture of the pus should be carried out. The most common organism is *Staphylococcus aureus*.

Plan. With the exception of acute suppurative parotitis, there is no specific treatment. In the other disorders, treatment of the underlying disease is indicated symptomatic treatment of the salivary gland disorder. In *acute suppurative parotitis*, after cultures are obtained, treatment including rehydration and intravenous treatment with antibiotic is begun. I prefer to use methicillin, 1 g every 4 hours, plus penicillin, 1 million units every 4 hours, for 24 hours. When the culture is reported, if Staphylococcus is the cause, the penicillin is stopped and the methicillin is continued at 1 g every 6 hours. Oral hygiene is prescribed using hydrogen peroxide, and sialogogues are used. If the gland continues to swell and the overlying skin becomes shiny and thinned, the gland is decompressed surgically. This must be done by a surgeon familiar with facial nerve surgery.

In the remaining disorders, occasionally the cosmetic effect of the enlarged gland is undesirable. In that case, a superficial parotidectomy is carried out. However, *no elective cosmetic surgery should be performed on patients with collagen vascular diseases or other serious underlying medical problems (diabetes, etc.) for any reason.*

Bibliography

1. English, G. M., and Hemenway, W. G. In *Otolaryngology*, edited by G. M. English. Harper & Row, Hagerstown, Md., 1976.
2. Rankow, R. M., and Polayes, I. M. *Diseases of the Salivary Glands*. W. B. Saunders Co., Philadelphia, 1977.

Chapter 11

Facial Trauma

Bruce B. Baker

SOFT TISSUE INJURIES

Facial Lacerations Generally

Subjective Complaint

"I cut my face."

Objective Findings

Taking of the vital signs reveals the cardiovascular-respiratory system to be either stable or unstable. Adequate ventilation confirms a patent airway and good respiratory effort. A quick overview of the general condition of the patient with respect to the presence of other injuries is appropriate. The history of the accident and subsequent events may give information (direction of the blow, nature of the instrument inflicting the damage, presence or absence of facial paralysis, loss of consciousness) that will establish or raise the index of suspicion of a given injury. Contusions, lacerations, and other forms of injury must be documented by diagrams, drawings, and photographs that indicate the location and length of lacerations, the absence of tissue, and a statement as to the functional integrity of the salivary ducts, eyelid motion, facial nerve function, vision, hearing, etc.

Appropriate radiographs may also help establish diagnoses or document injury by the presence of soft tissue swelling, subcutaneous air, air-fluid levels in the sinuses, and breaks in bony continuity.

Assessment

Resuscitation and stabilization of the patient with facial injuries assume top priority. First, finish with an alive patient! Second, one must rule out the presence of associated injuries. Facial injuries are of themselves seldom fatal, but associated injuries may be. One must rule out or in and treat appropriately any associated injuries such as ruptured spleens, head injuries, pelvic fractures. Careful attention should be directed to the possibility of a cervical spine injury. Blows severe enough to compromise the facial skeleton or render the patient unconscious may also injure the cervical vertebrae and/or the spinal cord.

When the initial concerns of resuscitation and the disposition of any associated injuries have been satisfied, one's attention should be directed to the facial injury. In addition to restoring the integrity of the skin, one must consider that structures below the skin surface may have been injured. One should test the function of each of these structures and deal with them accordingly. The three structures most frequently injured and overlooked are the facial nerve, Stensen's duct, and the levator palpebrae muscle of the upper lid. One should also consider that a penetrating object may not have entered at the anticipated angle or may have been deflected, injuring structures seemingly not directly in its line of flight.

Plan

First perform cardiopulmonary resuscitation according to the mnemonic "ABC" which stands for Airway (secure), Breathing (spontaneous or mechanical), and Circulation (establish). Once stable, the patient when indicated should then have a cross-table cervical lateral x-ray taken and read by the physician prior to any other x-rays or manipulation. Once this film confirms the absence of visible pathology, the remainder of the cervical spine series and then other appropriate views may be obtained. Consultation as required should be sought to resolve associated injuries. Once one has a stable patient in whom associated injuries are under control, repair of facial injuries is appropriate. This repair may occur almost immediately in the emergency room or it may be a matter of hours or days before the patient's condition allows facial repair.

Facial repair should be performed with instruments of the appropriate size and type. Most emergency rooms have "suture sets" woefully lacking from the viewpoint of facial surgery. The usual instruments for abdominal surgery are entirely unsatisfactory. Meticulous wound care should include "prepping" (the area will probably need to be anesthetized first), irrigating, and debriding of the wound. Debridement in the face should be most conservative. Skin edges should be trimmed and beveled. The principles of hemostasis, asepsis, and gentleness with tissues are still applicable. Repair should restore normal landmarks and function.

Appropriate tetanus prophylaxis should be administered and documented in the patient's record.

Scalp Lacerations

Subjective Complaint

"I gashed my head." The history of the type of injury and whether the patient lost consciousness is frequently quite valuable in evaluating these patients.

Objective Findings

Amnesia, confusion, and/or a depressed state of consciousness may be present in addition to other neurologic signs of intracranial injury. A thorough neurologic examination should be performed and recorded as a baseline should the patient's condition change.

Lacerations of the scalp tend to bleed profusely. Gentle palpation of the laceration with sterile gloves may reveal a fracture of the skull of either linear or depressed type. Scalp muscles may be divided depending upon the location of the laceration. Clear or bloody fluid may be noted behind the tympanic membranes or running down the victim's throat.

Assessment

Care should be taken that there is no underlying head or cervical injury. Neurologic examination and skull x-rays will be pursued as indicated. An echoencephalogram upon admission for patients suspected of having intracranial pathology can be useful to establish the midline and provide a basis for comparison should their condition deteriorate. Computerized axial tomography may provide a wealth of information when available.

Plan

Initial hemostasis may be obtained by pressure or putting hemostats on the galea and folding the hemostats away from the center of the laceration, thus pinching off the vessels. Individual vessels may need to be clamped if they persist or if the laceration does not extend through the galea. Debridement and removal of foreign bodies are appropriate, with care being taken to minimize damage to the hair follicles, and to approximate appropriate points on each side of the laceration. A 3-0 or 4-0 chromic suture is used to repair the periosteum (pericranium) of the skull and the galea. A 4-0 monofilament suture is used on the skin, though some advocate a through-and-through suture of wire to close all layers. Patients appreciate one's taking a few extra minutes to wash the blood out of their hair at the conclusion of the suturing. Scalp avulsions or those missing tissue may need to be grafted and should be referred to someone prepared to graft the area or swing a flap to provide coverage.

Some feel that any patient with a history of unconsciousness should be admitted for observation at least overnight. Others are more flexible, depending upon the patient's circumstances. Neurosurgical consultation should be obtained on patients with skull fractures or those suspected of having intracranial pathology.

Facial Lacerations

Subjective Complaints

Presence of a cut on the face in the malar, buccal, mental, preauricular, frontal, or mandibular areas. There may be a feeling of the face drooping in cases of facial nerve injury, which may be accompanied by epiphora or drooling.

Objective Findings

Visible laceration is present. There may or may not be a facial paralysis present. Saliva does not or does flow from the salivary ducts. A history of previous facial palsy is important.

Assessment

Documentation of the presence or absence of facial movement immediately after the accident and in the emergency room before local anesthesia or other medications alter facial nerve function, and testing, are of utmost importance. The management of a facial palsy of delayed onset might well differ from that of an immediate one. Should a facial palsy exist, the location of the lesion may be identified by further testing with the Schirmer test, the acoustic reflex, submandibular salivation testing, etc.

Continuity of salivary gland ducts may be further assessed by retrograde catheterization of the duct in question and the injection of saline or an appropriate dye to test for leaks in the system.

Whether the facial laceration should be repaired by the family physician or referred would depend upon the preferences of the patient and the patient's family, the degree of skill and experience of the physician involved, the type of laceration, and other miscellaneous circumstances. Those injuries involving avulsions, loss of tissue, and trapdoor-type lacerations probably should be referred to one experienced in such injuries, as a high degree of skill, much experience, and good fortune are necessary to produce good results in such injuries.

Plan

Most bleeding from lacerations in this area can be controlled by pressure alone. The ligation of individual bleeding vessels is quite appropriate, but the blind clamping of structures in the murky depths of a laceration is to be condemned for it often results in injury to the facial nerve or some other structure. The actual closure of such facial lacerations may be accomplished immediately, but if the wound is cleaned and dressed, little to nothing is lost with a delay of 24 hours or so should other injuries make such a delay advisable.

Facial nerve injuries are optimally repaired within 72 hours, as the distal end of the severed nerve will not stimulate after that period of time, a circumstance which may compound the difficulty in identifying the facial nerve. Facial nerve injuries should be referred to a physician experienced in their management.

Minor salivary ducts may be ligated if lacerated. Major ones are best repaired over a small catheter or polyethylene tube threaded retrograde through the duct and across the laceration to act as a stent. The stenting tube is then sutured in place and retained for a week or more if possible to try to minimize contracture and stenosis at the repair site.

Eyelid Lacerations

Subjective Complaint

"Cut my eye." The patient's opinion of his visual acuity is most helpful.

Objective Findings

A laceration of the eyelid is evident. It may involve the conjunctivae, the globe, the lid margin, the lower canaliculus. The patient may demonstrate inability to raise the upper lid. Epiphora may be present. Orbital x-rays may show an orbital fracture or foreign body.

Visual acuity is documented. The test used for this purpose should be recorded whether it be a wall chart, reading the newspaper, or just counting fingers. A history of trauma sufficient to break the orbital bones, or suggesting the presence of a foreign body, is important.

Assessment

Attention should be directed toward preserving vision. The minimum ophthalmologic examination should consist of a confirmation of the patient's visual acuity. Examination of the pupillary reflexes, extraocular movements, visual fields, and a funduscopic examination are prudent. A diligent search should be made for injuries to the globe itself or the extraocular muscles. Inability to raise the upper eyelid suggests division of the levator palpebrae muscle. Epiphora suggests obstruction or division of the lacrimal apparatus, as does a laceration close to the medial canthus. The use of a Wood's lamp and fluorescein dye will help demonstrate corneal abrasions. A routine history should help determine whether anything was traveling fast enough to penetrate the globe and should alert one to the possibility of fragments of glass or metal from windshields or hammer, being inside the globe and/or orbit. A point of entry may be visible, but orbital radiographs may help clarify the matter in questionable cases.

Plan

Injury to the globe or extraocular muscles, or decreased vision deserve ophthalmologic consultation.

Horizontal lacerations of the eyelids without loss of tissue may be closed using the general principles of soft tissue surgery. The author's preference is a 5-0 subcutaneous suture of proline or individual sutures of 6-0 silk. Vertical or oblique lacerations may be similarly managed.

In vertical ectropion secondary to scar retraction may be a problem, therefore occasionally a procedure such as a Z-plasty or other maneuver will be useful to break up the scar's contraction. Such techniques are generally best left to those familiar with them and/or to secondary procedures.

Lacerations of the lid margin and those involving tissue loss require a specialist's attention, as do injuries of the levator palpebrae muscle.

Nasal Injuries

Subjective Complaints

"Busted nose," cut on nose, nosebleed.

Objective Findings

The external laceration may extend to the nasal skeleton and lining in addition to the skin. Epistaxis may occur from either or both nostrils or drain down the throat. A thickened nasal septum is sometimes present. In severe injuries there may be an increased distance between the medial canthi. The nasal skeleton may be altered in its appearance. Radiographic examination may show nasal fractures or bony disruption in the area of the medial canthi. Clear fluid may run from the nose.

Assessment

External lacerations are of course readily visible. It is desirable to know which of the nasal layers are involved, for best results come from their individual reapproximation. Consideration should be given to the possibility of a nasal fracture and/or septal hematoma. The latter may be suspected when a thickened septum is seen, and aspiration of the hematoma provides definitive confirmation. Nasal fractures may be visible on x-ray, but one's clinical impression is more reliable.

Localization of the site of bleeding is the key to controlling epistaxis. This requires a light source (head mirror or head light) which can be projected intranasally, a suction equipped with a Frazier tip, and appropriate nasal instruments and supplies. Details on the control of epistaxis may be found elsewhere. (see Chapter 3), but it is desirable to obtain control of any bleeding before reduction of nasal fractures or the suturing of lacerations so that maneuvers to control bleeding do not disrupt repairs.

The presence of clear fluid running down the throat or out the nose should bring to mind the possibility of cerebrospinal fluid rhinorrhea. Radiographs of the cribriform plate may demonstrate a fracture.

Plan

The initial step should be to obtain hemostasis. During this process the septum is examined and any hematoma evacuated by incising the mucosa and perichondrium over the thickened portion of the septum with a no.11 blade after topical anesthesia is applied. The incision should be dependent in location and is left open. A drain may be placed for 24 hours if needed.

Repair of nasal fractures can be accomplished immediately after injury, but before swelling distorts the nose and face. If swelling prevents accurate assessment of facial configuration, reduction may be delayed for several days as the swelling resolves. In cases of nasal injury repaired in the operating room, one usually tries to reduce them at that time, warning the patient that further procedures may be necessary.

Repair of lacerations best proceeds from the inside out. The mucosa is repaired with an absorbable suture of 4-0 or 5-0 size. Cartilage is approximated by suturing adjacent edges of perichondrium or by transcartilaginous sutures if necessary. The skin is approximated with monofilament suture. Nasal packing, splinting, and dressing complete the repair.

Lip Lacerations

Subjective Complaints

"Split my lip," or "bit my lip."

Objective Findings

A laceration of either or both lips is present. The oral cavity may also be cut and there may be damage to the dentition. Maxillary or mandibular fractures may be present clinically or on x-ray examination.

Assessment

Lacerations of the lips tend to be either vertical ones involving the vermilion of the lip or through-and-through punctures with ragged edges that correspond to one or more of the patient's teeth. Since lip defects of from one-third to one-half of the width of the lip may be closed by direct approximation with satisfactory results, one should not hesitate to debride and trim the skin edges of lip lacerations to enhance the closure. Lacerations from the patient's own teeth are potentially quite bothersome as they represent a form of human bite, one of dirtiest wounds, frequently involve all layers of the lip, and frequently present as a "trapdoor" or "U"-shaped laceration corresponding to the dental arch. None of these characteristics is conducive to good results.

Plan

The essence of good lip repair is to precisely align the vermilion border of each side of the laceration so that the vermilion flows smoothly along. Few things detract more from a repair more than a telltale notch in the vermilion. The first stitch placed is one of 4-0 monofilament just adjacent to the border to insure its correct alignment throughout the repair. After this "key" suture is placed, the mucosa is loosely closed with a few chromic sutures, the muscle reapproximated with 4-0 chromic, and the skin closed with 5-0 or 6-0 monofilament sutures. Through and through lip lacerations are usually given antibiotic coverage postoperatively.

External Ear Injuries

Subjective Complaints

"Cut on my ear"; "bumped my ear"; or "poked my ear canal."

Objective Findings

Lacerations of the pinna are readily identified, but may involve the ear canal or tympanic membrane. A painful swelling may appear on the auricular cartilage, obscuring the fine architecture of that structure. It may be on either surface of the pinna.

Assessment

It is important to recognize and provide coverage for exposed cartilage as soon as possible to try to minimize the possibility of perichondritis. Recognition of external ear canal or tympanic membrane lacerations is most important and requires otoscopic examination. Frequently fresh or dried blood must be removed from the canal. On occasion it is necessary to anesthetize a painful ear canal to allow a satisfactory examination. An audiogram to document the level of hearing may be indicated in injuries to the canal, and most certainly is indicated prior to significant instrumentation of the canal or in injuries of the tympanic membrane. In certain circumstances approriate tuning fork tests will serve in lieu of an audiogram. Objects lacerating the tympanic membrane may dislocate the ossicles or cause other mischief in the middle ear. Hearing loss and vertigo would increase one's suspicion of middle ear damage.

The painful swelling following blunt trauma represents a hematoma between the auricular cartilage and the perichondrium. It is poorly absorbed in this location, and if not drained will organize, producing a "cauliflower ear," or tend to produce avascular necrosis of the adjacent cartilage and subsequent auricular deformity.

Plan

Injuries involving the external auditory canal (which tend to result in stenosis) and those involving the tympanic membrane should be promptly referred to the otolaryngologist.

Repair of the pinna may be performed by the family physician or referred, as circumstances suggest. Repair of the pinna is initiated by repositioning the cartilage, preferably by suturing the perichondrium, though one should not hesitate to employ transcartilaginous sutures if needed. It is useful to trim a margin of tissue from both sides of the laceration, then approximate fresh edge to fresh edge. This converts a dirty wound to a cleaner one. Once the cartilage is repositioned, each skin surface is closed. A rubber band drain may be employed if desired, to be pulled in 24–48 hours. The pinna is then dressed with a nonadherent dressing such as adaptic, sterile cotton soaked in sterile mineral oil and molded into the auricular folds and fossae to make a "cast," fluffs, gauze, and tape to complete the mastoid type dressing.

Hematomas may be aspirated with a large (18-gauge) needle if seen early. Sterile technique is imperative. A "mold" and dressing as described above are applied and the pinna is inspected in 24 hours. If there has been no reaccumulation the dressing is reapplied for several days. If the hematoma has reaccumulated, it may be reaspirated once or twice more if desired, or it may be opened with a blade, placing the incision in an inconspicuous plane of the pinna and using sterile technique. The walls are scraped, and a pressure dressing is reapplied. Repeat inspec-

tion to detect possible reaccumulation is necessary. Failure to evacuate the hematoma will usually result in an auricular deformity that is difficult to treat.

Both hematomas and lacerations involving the cartilage are usually given antibiotic coverage.

Intraoral Lacerations

Subjective Complaints

"Cut in mouth"; cut my tongue."

Objective Findings

Intraoral lacerations may be in the vicinity of a salivary gland duct or other structure. Facial palsy may be present. The palate should be inspected for tears or perforations.

Assessment

One should again consider what structures might be injured beneath the mucosal laceration, test their function, and repair them if needed. Opinions vary as to whether one should suture intraoral lacerations at all. Our general policy is to loosely approximate grossly displaced tissue with one-fourth to one-third the number of sutures used in a skin laceration of comparable length and shape. Old lacerations and those obviously severely contaminated are not sutured.

Tongue lacerations are difficult problems, particularly in children. Wide scars from secondary healing may interfere with tongue function, and delayed bleeding from the tongue in an uncooperative child can be a difficult problem.

Plan

Loosely approximate displaced intraoral tissue with one-third to one-fourth the number of sutures that would be used in a comparable skin laceration. A drain may be sewn in place for a day or so if deemed advisable. The suture material is chosen on the basis of how long it is desirable that the material remain. Chromic used intraorally requires four or five knots to be effective at all, and then may last from a few hours to a day or so. Silk is generally good for 3–7 days. Silk is used for stitches serving an important hemostatic function; it is preferred to a monofilament material because the latter, because of its inherent stiffness, tends to be irritating.

Perforations of the palate are best handled by a three-layer closure in experienced hands.

Tongue lacerations are closed with silk of 3-0 to 4-0 size with careful approximation of the mucosal edges and suture ligature of arterial bleeders. An acceptable alternative might be to hospitalize certain patients for observation for 24 hours so that any significant bleeding would be promptly discovered in an environment when appropriate measures could be taken quickly.

FACIAL SKELETAL INJURIES

Trauma to the Jaws

Subjective Complaints

"Hit in the jaw"; "hit in the face (or teeth)." Historically an account of the direction, force, and striking object can help one to suspect specific injuries, such as "My teeth don't fit together right," or "It hurts to chew," or "I can't close my teeth in front."

Objective Findings

A contusion or laceration may be present in the skin over the maxilla or mandible. There may be an open-bite deformity, technically defined as a deformity in which one or both tooth lines do not reach the occlusal plane, but evident as a failure of the incisors to come together, leaving a gap anteriorly between the maxillary and mandibular teeth. There may be a step deformity of the mandible or maxilla with accompanying mucosal tear or ecchymosis. A palpable defect in the maxillary sinus wall or alveolar ridges can be present. There may be instability of the mandible or maxilla as the fragments on each side of a fracture move when tested by the examiner. The student of occlusion may notice a disturbance in the relationship of the maxillary to the mandibular teeth. Teeth may be missing or broken.

Assessment

The aftermath of trauma to the facial skeleton requires one to distinguish between soft tissue, dental, and skeletal injury. Frequently the distinction is not at all clear-cut, and they frequently occur together. Soft tissue injuries have been considered earlier.

Malocclusion may result from soft tissue swelling, particularly at the temperomandibular joint, dislocation of an individual tooth or teeth, or a skeletal fracture of maxilla or mandible. Inspection and palpation of individual teeth with a tongue blade can frequently establish which tooth (or teeth) is the culprit. The symptom of pain is particularly helpful in locating the damaged area. By palpating the anterior sinus wall and buttress in addition to the mandible, one can often detect fracture lines not readily visible to the eye. Fractures accompanied by disruptions of the mucosa or significant displacement usually offer little diagnostic problem. By grasping the mandible in both hands and pushing and pulling, one may detect telltale crepitus or movement at a fracture site.

The open-bite deformity not present before trauma usually means a bilateral subcondylar fracture of the mandible. One should suspect this injury in a patient who falls straight forward onto his mentum or is stuck in a manner that would exert a similar force. Chewing is ineffective, and pain may be interpreted as otologic. It is possible to have this deformity as a result of an alveolar fracture alone or a midface fracture, but these are gross enough that they usually represent no problem in diagnosis.

Painful mastication may also reflect facial skeletal trauma or dental difficulties. Investigation in a manner similar to that described above will lead to the diagnosis.

The pain is a good localizer of the pathology. Patients with trismus or inability to open their jaws should be suspected of having a fracture of the zygomatic arch, vhich has been pushed in onto the coronoid process of the mandible, accounting for the patient's pain and difficulty.

Radiographic examination of the facial skeleton can be quite helpful. The exact views in a mandible series or a facial bone series differs from hospital to hospital, but each view is designed to demonstrate a particular area or bone. A special dental radiograph called a Panorex is most helpful as it can "straighten out" the mandible and provide a good view of that structure without superimposed shadows. The condylar and subcondylar areas are well visualized. Radiographs of the temperomandibular joint may be helpful.

Plan

Patients with facial fractures may have particular difficulty maintaining an airway. The fracture may mean loss of skeletal support for some soft tissue structures such as the tongue, which fall into the airway. Other factors can include difficulty in handling blood and secretions because of pain, foreign bodies in the airway such as dentures or teeth, and a decreased level of consciousness. First secure the airway and resuscitate the patient. Second, evaluate the patient for cervical or intracranial injury. Blows hard enough to fracture the facial skeleton may also damage the cervical spine or brain.

Facial fractures themselves are only rarely emergency matters. The patient is better served by completing a thorough preoperative evaluation of any general health problem as well as the injury itself. Facial fractures also merit a specialist's attention.

While the patient is being evaluated or awaiting transportation to the specialist, several interim measures can promote the patient's comfort and recovery. Adequate analgesia is appropriate when it is neurologically safe. Elevation of the head of the patient's bed and the application of ice flats to the injured areas will decrease swelling and pain. Provisions are made to help the patient handle secretions as needed. Immobilization of the fracture segments by a few interdental loops of wire or heavy silk or by a Barton bandage may make the patient much more comfortable. Transportation of facial fracture patients is generally safest in the prone position.

Diplopia

Subjective Complaints

Patient "sees double." Allow patient to explain his symptoms so that one is certain that the patient is speaking of seeing two images of the same object rather than blurred or decreased vision.

Objective Findings

Either decreased ocular movements or displacement of the globe are present. There may be a palpable fracture of the orbital rim or radiographically demonstrable fracture of the orbital floor. Other signs of periorbital or ocular injury may be present as ecchymosis, lacerations, puncture wound or lacerations of the globe, etc. The globe may exhibit enophthalmos, exophthalmos, or displacement in a vertical direction. Fractures involving the orbital floor may exhibit anesthesia in the distribution of the infraorbital nerve.

Assessment

First, distinguish between diplopia that is monocular and diplopia that is binocular. Cover each eye in succession and the diplopia of binocular type should go away. If it remains it is monocular diplopia. Second, one should be certain that the diplopia was produced by the trauma. Nontraumatic etiologies involve lesions of cranial nerves III, IV, or VI and are most commonly (1) a vascular lesion in the brainstem (look for other brainstem signs, especially in elderly patients), (2) an idiopathic palsy of the VIth nerve, or (3) some process raising intracranial pressure (headache and funduscopic examination), diabetes (urine and blood sugar and acetone determinations), multiple sclerosis, or myasthenia gravis. Third, with traumatic diplopia one must identify the origin of the displaced globe, restricted globe or compromised muscle and do what is necessary to correct it. Most instances of diplopia from facial fractures involve orbital floor fractures alone or are associated with other fractures.

Plan

Perform an ophthalmologic examination including visual acuity, pupillary response, tests of extraocular muscle function, and funduscopic examination. Patients with damage to the globe, damage to the extraocular muscles, or decreased visual acuity require ophthalmologic consultation promptly. Patients with orbital floor or other fractures accounting for their diplopia would most likely be served by ophthalmologic consultation prior to surgical correction of their fracture. Orbital fractures are repaired by multiple surgical specialists including the otolaryngologist, the plastic surgeon, and the ophthalmologist.

Periorbital Ecchymosis

Subjective Complaints

"I've got a black eye." A history of the trauma producing the bruising can be most helpful in assessing potential injury.

Objective Findings

Discoloration of the eyelids may be black, blue, green, or yellow, depending upon the interval since the traumatic episode. Subconjunctival hemorrhage is frequently present, as may be other signs of ocular damage such as a corneal abrasion; penetrating wound of the globe, conjunctivae, or adjacent structure; limited extraocular movements; enophthalmos; pupillary abnormalities; and deformities of the orbital rims or adjacent bones, including the nose. Radiographs may confirm fractures of the orbital floor or rim or of adjacent bones such as the nose or zygoma.

Assessment

Periorbital ecchymosis represents bleeding in the subcutaneous tissue from any of a number of common sources, as the loose skin of the eyelids offers little resistance to the spread of blood. The diagnostic challenge is to distinguish between those patients whose injury is limited to the soft tissue and those who have additional injury. The orbit, the nose, the sinuses, and the adjacent facial bones are all common sites for associated injuries. Injuries to the eyelids, globe, and other ocular structures should be suspected during the physical examination and history.

Blunt trauma to the globe may produce a hyphema or a silent rupture of the globe. The former may be recognized by a fluid level in the anterior chamber of the eye and the latter by the globe's softness to palpation.

A fracture of the infraorbital rim is most commonly in the form of the trimalar (tripod, zygomaticomaxillary complex) fracture, which has fractures at the infraorbital rim, the frontozygomatic suture line, and the lateral wall of the maxillary sinus. These fractures are frequently palpable and are readily demonstrable on appropriate x-rays.

The somewhat more subtle orbital floor or "blowout fracture" occurs with the orbital rim intact and is consequently harder to detect.

There may be herniation of the orbital fat or entrapment of the inferior extraocular muscles in the defect, producing limitation of movement of the globe (especially in an upward direction) with resultant diplopia and possibly enophthalmos. Diagnosis of this fracture requires a high index of suspicion. A Caldwell view of the maxillary sinuses, or tomograms, will confirm the diagnosis.

Plan

Tripod and "blowout fractures" are repaired by many different surgical specialists. Additionally patients with significant blunt trauma to the eye are best served by ophthalmologic consultation to document their preoperative ocular status and to provide for appropriate follow-up to detect potential late complications such as subluxation of the lens, retinal hemorrhage, or retinal detachment. Such referral would be wise in all patients with moderate or severe periorbital trauma whether there is a fracture or not. Not all patients with periorbital fractures require surgery, which is usually reserved for those with a persistent cosmetic defect or impaired function. Seldom is there a need to repair these fractures immediately. Nasal fractures can wait for the resolution of swelling, and zygomatic arch fractures are reduced to relieve trismus or improve cosmesis after a suitable period of observation.

Repair of orbital floor fractures with or without rim involvement entails releasing any trapped muscle and fat, reducing the fracture, and returning the orbital floor to its preinjury position by packing or wiring. Alternately, one may opt to insert a new floor of autogenous or synthetic material.

Compound Frontal Fractures

Subjective Complaints

"Hit in head above the eyes." There may be amnesia, loss of consciousness, headache, dizziness, fluid running down the throat or out the nose.

Objective Findings

A laceration will be present in the glabellar area or above the medial aspect of the eyebrows. Subcutaneous emphysema may be present. A depression or crack in the anterior sinus wall may be visible and/or palpable. Sometimes there is a concave deformity visible in the frontal sinus area. Epistaxis may occur. Supraorbital anesthesia may occur. Clear fluid may leak from the wound or run from the nose.

Assessment

The sin qua non of this injury is a fracture of the anterior sinus wall which communicates with the laceration. Evaluation of the injury should determine the integrity of the nasofrontal ducts, the integrity of the posterior sinus wall, and the presence or absence of a cerebrospinal fluid leak. Installation of a substance detectable in the nose after passing through the nasofrontal duct from the sinus is a useful operative technique to assess duct pat-

ency. Tomograms of the frontal sinuses help also to establish the status of the duct and the posterior sinus wall. Accurate assessment of the duct is most important because the sequela of an obstructed duct is sinusitis or likely mucocele with its potential complications of extradural or brain abscess, meningitis, orbital abscess or cellulitis, or exophthalmos.

Posterior sinus wall fractures are also of great moment. They may provide access for bacteria into the cranial cavity, or in the case of displaced ones cause dural tears, lacerations of the frontal lobe, or cerebrospinal fluid leaks.

Fluid running from the nose or sinus should be tested to confirm that it is CSF. Radioisotope studies may also be used to detect the site of leak in difficult cases.

Plan

These injuries should be managed by an otolaryngologist. Neurosurgical expertise is needed in cases of posterior wall involvement and/or cerebrospinal fluid leaks.

Emergency management of these patients should consist of establishing hemostasis, monitoring of the level of consciousness, performing an initial neurologic examination as a baseline, elevation of the head of the patient's bed, elementary wound care such as a sterile dressing, antibiotic coverage, and the collection of any fluid running out of the nose for later testing. The patient should be instructed to refrain from blowing his nose and coughing, and should sneeze only if unavoidable and then with his mouth open. A search for associated injuries should be conducted.

Once the necessary studies are completed, repair can proceed. Simple depressed fractures of the anterior sinus wall may be elevated through the fracture or via access holes drilled adjacent to the fragment. Care is taken to retain the periosteum on the bony fragments which are secured by suturing the periosteum or by using interosseous wiring.

Injuries in the area of the nasofrontal duct require confirmation of the patency of the duct. Compromised ducts require reconstruction (a procedure fraught with failure) or, more frequently, obliteration of the duct and sinus after complete removal of the sinus mucosa. These patients in particular deserve long-term follow-up to detect and deal with a mucocele should one develop.

The management of posterior wall fractures requires the cooperation of the neurosurgeon and otolaryngologist. Some prefer to approach these fractures solely through the frontal sinus. Others prefer to turn an adjacent bone flap for dual exposure. It is most important to ensure that mucous membrane has not been displaced intracranially, that dural tears and cerebrospinal fluid leaks have been repaired, and that foreign bodies are removed.

Treatment of any cosmetic defects may begin with the initial repair, but secondary procedures such as scar revision, dermabrasion, bone grafting, or cranioplasty may be necessary for optimal results in more extensive defects.

Bibliography

1. Chawla, H. B. *Simple Eye Diagnosis*, ed. 2., Churchill-Livingstone, New York, 1975.
2. Converse, J. M. *Surgical Treatment of Facial Injuries*, ed. 2, vols. 1 and 2. The Williams & Wilkins Co., Baltimore, 1974.
3. Dingman, R. O., and Natvig, P. *Surgery of Facial Fractures*. W. B. Saunders, Philadelphia, 1964.
4. English, G. M. Common injuries to the ear. *Primary Care 3*: 507–520, 1976.
5. Shumrick, D. A. Maxillofacial injuries. *Otolaryngol. Clin. North Am.*, (June): 221–233, 1969.

Chapter 12
Hypopharynx and Larynx

Matthew L. Wong

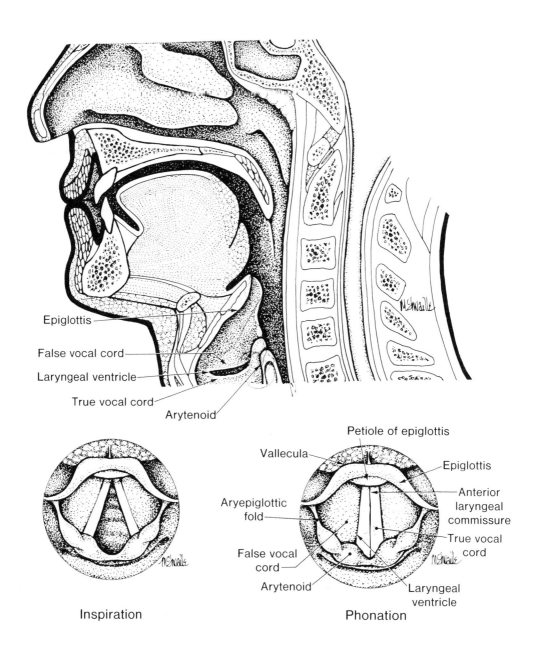

Epiglottis

False vocal cord

Laryngeal ventricle

True vocal cord

Arytenoid

Petiole of epiglottis

Vallecula

Epiglottis

Anterior laryngeal commissure

Aryepiglottic fold

True vocal cord

False vocal cord

Arytenoid

Laryngeal ventricle

Inspiration

Phonation

THROAT PAIN AND ODYNOPHAGIA

Definition

Throat pain is any discomfort of the pharynx and usually refers to the oropharynx, larynx, and hypopharynx, but can involve the inferior nasopharynx and the posterior portion of the oral cavity. Odynophagia is painful deglutition and can involve any area from posterior oral cavity to the cervical esophagus. So, in any complaint of throat pain and/or odynophagia, a complete evaluation must be made of the oral cavity, oropharynx, hypopharynx, larynx, and inferior nasopharynx. Commonly seen by primary care physicians, the patient with throat pain may ultimately be discovered to have a carcinoma of the hypopharynx.

Subjective Complaints

Throat pain with or without odynophagia can involve any of the above-described areas. Sharp knifelike pain is nonspecific but seen more with inflammatory lesions. Deep, boring, aching pain is either chronic mild inflammation or neoplasm. Sharp, brief, lancinating pain is neurologic as in glossopharyngeal neuralgia.

Acute. Sudden onset and short duration are usually inflammatory; occasionally a neoplasm with secondary infection will give acute symptoms.

Chronic. Usually neoplastic but can be chronic irritative or mild inflammatory (from chronic postnasal discharge).

Constant. Usually neoplastic but can be irritative and mild inflammatory (from chronic postnasal discharge).

Intermittent. Usually inflammatory, but early neoplastic disease can give intermittency.

Fever. Inflammatory.

Dysphagia. Neoplastic, inflammatory, and neurologic.

Weight Loss. Usually neoplastic.

Referred Otalgia. Any: source can be from nasopharynx to hypopharynx.

Neck Mass. Usually inflammatory if tender; neoplastic if nontender lymphadenopathy.

Cough. Chronic irritation from bronchitis and/or sinusitis. Tuberculosis and other granulomatous disease must be kept in mind.

Chronic Sinus Disease with Postnasal Discharge. Often a cause of chronic throat pain; usually in the morning and improves as the day progresses; worse when the postnasal discharge is purulent.

Dyspnea, Acute. Usually inflammatory; seen with peritonsillar, parapharyngeal and retropharyngeal abscess, and epiglottitis, floor of the mouth abscess, and Ludwig's angina. Rarely, a large neoplasm with secondary infection can obstruct the airway acutely.

Dyspnea, Chronic. Large neoplasm.

Trauma. Usually with acute trauma: either blunt or penetrating trauma, caustic ingestion, smoke inhalation, or hot food/liquid ingestion. Chronic trauma gives stenotic symptoms, except perichondritis of the larynx (with tenderness of the neck, sometimes with purulent discharge from the neck).

Age. Younger—usually inflammatory. Older—neoplastic, atrophic pharyngitis and laryngitis.

Radiation Therapy. Performed for neoplastic disease of the oral cavity, oropharynx, larynx, hypopharynx, and esophagus. Throat pain starts 3–4 weeks after the beginning of radiation therapy, is due to radiation mucositis and can last for 2–3 months. If occurring late after completion of radiation therapy, perichondritis or tumor persistence is suspected.

Systemic Diseases. Especially autoimmune diseases. Throat pain occurs in cricoarytenoid arthritis, most commonly seen with rheumatoid arthritis, but can occur with any autoimmune disease.

Neurologic. Except for neuralgia, throat pain and odynophagia are rare. More likely to cause dysphagia and aspiration.

Allergy. A common cause of chronic postnasal discharge.

Psychogenic. Rare, must rule out all organic causes.

Tobacco/Alcohol. Both are irritative and can cause chronic pharyngitis and laryngitis. Squamous cell carcinoma of the head and neck is closely linked to tobacco use—cigarette, pipe and cigar.

Objective Findings

Diffuse Pharyngitis. Most common cause of throat pain. There are two types. Viral pharyngitis is the more common; the pharynx is minimally erythematous or normal-appearing. In the bacterial variety, the pharynx is erythematous and usually with exudate.

Acute Tonsillitis. Marked inflammation of the tonsils. May have exudate and purulent material in the tonsillar crypts.

Peritonsillar Abscess/Cellulitis. A lateral extension of acute tonsillitis to peritonsillar tissues. The tonsillar pillars and ipsilateral soft palate are inflammed and swollen. The uvula is displaced to the opposite side. Fifty percent contain abscess and 50% are cellulitis. Aspiration in the proper area is important for diagnostic differentiation.

Parapharyngeal Abscess/Cellulitis. An extension of infection to parapharyngeal space. The origin is pharyngeal or dental. The lateral pharyngeal tissues are inflammed and swollen. The tonsils and surrounding pillars are displaced medially and not as swollen as peritonsillar abscess. Cervical lymphadenopathy is common. Infection can extend from base of skull to mediastinum.

Retropharyngeal Abscess. Usually occurs in children under 2 years of age and is secondary to suppuration of retropharyngeal lymph node. Because of the median raphe of the constrictor muscles, the swelling occurs only on one side of the pharynx and can extend from nasopharynx to posterior hypopharynx. Bilateral swelling means involvement of prevertebral space. It is best to avoid spontaneous rupture or uncontrolled aspiration, as aspiration pneumonitis and lung abscess may result.

Floor of Mouth Infection. Marked inflammation and swelling of the floor of the mouth. In severe cases, swelling at the base of the tongue results in airway obstruction. The floor of mouth is very tender on palpation and cervical lymphadenopathy is common.

Membranous Pharyngitis

1. Nonspecific bacterial pharyngitis or viral pharyngitis: the most common type.
2. Diphtheritic pharyngitis: has a dirty white or gray membrane that is adherent and when detached bleeds easily.
3. Vincent's angina: acute membranous pharyngitis that involves tonsils, both fauces, soft palate, and gums. The membrane is gray and separates easily.
4. Candidiasis: the most common fungal pharyngitis and may be membranous with white patches in the fauces, gums, tonsil, and buccal mucosa. Discomfort is minimal. Microscopic examination of the exudate will reveal the yeast.

Acute Laryngitis. This is an extension of acute pharyngitis. The entire larynx is mildly inflamed in viral and moderately inflamed in bacterial laryngitis.

Chronic Pharyngitis. Findings can be minimal. If from sinuses and postnasal discharge, the vertical lymphoid streaking can be seen in the posterior oropharynx. If from bronchitis, larynx and vocal cord also show chronic inflammation.

Chronic Laryngitis. The vocal cords have normal mobility. It is secondary to irritative and chronic inflammation. The findings are minimal with thickened, white vocal cords. Smoking, postnasal discharge, chronic sinusitis, and chronic bronchitis are the common causes.

Atrophic Laryngitis. This is the end stage of chronic laryngitis and is seen in the elderly. The mucosa is atrophic, with dryness and some inflammation. Dry, crusted exudate may be seen.

Tuberculosis. May occur any place in the pharynx, from oropharynx to larynx; is uncommon and almost always associated with pulmonary tuberculosis. The lesions ulcerate and tend to coalesce and are very painful.

Herpes of Pharynx and Larynx. Extremely rare. Groups of ulcerative lesions with erythematous bases are seen. Lesions are painful.

Perichondritis. Persistent tenderness and swelling of the larynx. The external neck is tender to palpation over the thyroid cartilages, with swelling of the laryngeal structures and loss of anatomic definition.

Trauma. In acute trauma, external neck examination shows swelling and tenderness of the neck, and thyroid cartilage prominence may be flattened or lost. The thyroid cartilage may be displaced laterally from the cricoid or trachea. Mirror examination may show hematoma, swelling, mucosal lacerations, exposed cartilage, vocal cord paralysis, and displacement of epiglottis posteriorly and the arytenoids anteriorly.

Chronic trauma will result in deformed laryngeal contour with loss of normal laryngeal crepitance and movement. Mirror examination may show stenosis, displacement of epiglottis posteriorly and arytneoids anteriorly, and vocal cord paralysis.

Cricoarytenoid Arthritis. Of rheumatoid arthritis patients, 25% will have cricoarytenoid arthritis. In acute phase, there is inflammation and some decrease in motion of this joint. Late changes include lack of tenderness but fixation of cricoarytenoid joints.

Carcinoma. Most common are the squamous cell carcinomas. They are exophytic or deeply infiltrating masses and are friable. They can occur in any place—oral cavity, oropharynx, hypopharynx, and larynx. Large carcinomas usually have lymph node metastasis.

Radiation Mucositis. Diffuse erythema and inflammation with moderate tenderness, sometimes with exudation.

Psychogenic. No abnormalities are seen.

Assessment

Thorough examination of the oral cavity, oropharynx, and hypopharynx is necessary. Good *indirect nasopharyngoscopy* and *laryngoscopy* are mandatory and often yield the diagnosis. Palpation of the tonsils and base of tongue must be done.

Inflammatory Diseases. Proper culture and sensitivities must be obtained. Culture and examination of the membrane under microscope yields the diagnosis. Heterophil titers are used to diagnose infectious mononucleosis.

Sinuses x-rays are helpful in those with chronic nonspecific pharyngitis and laryngitis to search for chronic sinus disease.

Chronic bronchitis and possible tuberculosis or other granulomatous disease must have chest x-rays. Skin tests should be done. Bronchoscopy and mediastinoscopy may be necessary.

All suspicious *neoplastic lesions* must be biopsied. Except oral cavity lesions, all other neoplastic lesions must be examined under general anesthesia so the full extent can be appreciated. In lesions of the hypopharynx and larynx, a direct laryngoscopy must be performed.

Patients with suspected *cricoarytenoid arthritis* should have autoimmune disease workup with erythrocyte sedimentation rate, rheumatoid factor, antinuclear antibodies, and LE preparation.

Trauma. Acute: Evaluate for airway obstruction, CNS and cervical vertebral injuries, chest and abdominal injuries *first*. Soft tissue x-rays and xeroradiography of the neck are helpful. Direct laryngoscopy is performed. Arteriography is useful in suspected major vessel injuries.

Chronic: Pain is not the usual symptom. Soft tissue x-rays and xeroradiography of the neck, dye contrast or air tomogram of the laryngopharynx, and direct laryngoscopy are necessary. Where there is severe airway obstruction, dye contrast laryngograms should *not* be done, as this will precipitate acute airway obstruction.

Allergy. Suspicious allergic basis must have allergy workup.

Psychogenic. Only after thorough evaluation for organic disease. Psychiatric care is helpful.

Plan

Acute Diffuse Pharyngitis. Viral etiology is treated with rest, adequate liquids, and analgesia.

Bacterial etiology is treated with specific antibiotics. Since the organism is usually a gram-positive variety (group A, β-hemolytic streptococcus and *Streptococcus pneumoniae*), penicillin, 250 mg *q.i.d.*, or erythromycin, 250 mg *q.i.d.*, for 7–10 days will suffice. Analgesia and an antipyretic are used as necessary.

Acute Tonsillitis. Viral etiology is treated with analgesia and antipyretics, and adequate hydration.

Bacterial tonsillitis: This is usually from group A β-hemolytic streptococcus. Penicillin or erythromycin will be sufficient. Cultures must be taken, as viral and bacterial tonsillitis cannot always be distinguished clinically. Tonsillectomy is not recommended for the occasional acute tonsillitis. If this occurs more often than three to four times per year, tonsillectomy may be considered.

Peritonsillar Abscess/Cellulitis. Half are abscess and half are cellulitis. Aspiration of the most fluctuant area is made. If there is no purulent material with a no. 18 needle aspiration in the most likely site, incision and drainage are not indicated. If purulent material is aspirated, incision and drainage are performed. This is done with local anesthesia.

There are then two treatment plans: The first is immediate tonsillectomy. After the diagnosis is made, the aspirate is cultured and the patient is hospitalized and given the antibiotic intravenously, and tonsillectomies are performed under general anesthesia, after 12–24 hours of treatment.

The second treatment plan is incision and drainage of the abscess. Antibiotics are given for 7–10 days, and a delayed tonsillectomy is performed 4–6 weeks later, after resolution of the inflammation. Tonsillectomy should be performed in all patients with peritonsillar abscess/cellulitis, as 25–30% will subsequently develop another peritonsillar abscess or cellulitis. This can be a serious problem, leading to severe airway obstruction and sepsis.

Parapharyngeal Abscess/Cellulitis. This is a serious form of infection. There is no natural barrier to this infection; it can spread to the base of the skull or down to the mediastinum. The patient must be hospitalized. Culture may be difficult to obtain as there is no fluctuant area. Intravenous broad spectrum antibiotic coverage is used with methicillin and ampicillin in dosages of 4 million to 6 million units per day, in divided doses. Airway obstruction must be watched and tracheotomy is performed as indicated. If the infection is small, intravenous antibiotics is all that is necessary. If the infection is extensive, incision and drainage via upper external neck incision (Mosher procedure) is necessary.

Retropharyngeal Abscess. The inflammation and swelling is in the oropharynx. This is usually in the infant and young child. The patient is admitted to the hos-

pital. The incision and drainage must be performed in the operating room under general anesthesia. With a gentle and proper intubation, the abscess is not ruptured. A ruptured abscess can seed the tracheobronchial tree, leading to pneumonitis and lung abscesses. The patient is given intravenous and later oral antibiotics for 7–10 days. Ampicillin is the drug of choice, since the bacteria is usually *D. pneumococcus* or *Haemophilus influenzae*.

Floor of Mouth Infection. Patient must be admitted to the hospital. Broad spectrum antibiotics are given intravenously, usually ampicillin. Watch for airway obstruction. If infection is small, this therapy will be sufficient. If large, incision and drainage are necessary. If the infection is above the mylohyoid (minimal neck induration), the incision and drainage are through the mouth. If the infection extends into the upper neck (below the mylohyoid), drainage is via external neck approach. Tracheotomy must be performed if there is impending airway obstruction.

Membranous Pharyngitis

1. Viral pharyngitis can cause a membranous exudate. This is self-limiting; treatment is with proper hydration, analgesia, and antipyretics.

2. Exudative bacterial pharyngitis is usually due to β-hemolytic streptococcus. Penicillin is the antibiotic of choice. Keep up hydration; use antipyretics and analgesia as necessary.

3. Diphtheritic pharyngitis: Recognition is important; this is a rare disease in this country. Treatment is antitoxin (20,000 to 100,000 units) after culture and gram stain have been performed. An antibiotic is used for any secondary infections. Penicillin is the most commonly used drug.

4. Vincent's angina: May be membranous and involves a gram-negative fusiform bacillus and a spirillum (*Spirochaeta denticola*). Treatment is systemic and local mouth care with debriding mouthwashes, such as Amoson or peroxide. Penicillin is the antibiotic of choice, and antipyretics and analgesia are used as necessary.

5. Candidiasis is recognized easily and confirmed by examination of the smear for the yeast. Treatment is with nystatin

mouthwashes of 100,000 units per ml. Gentian violet can also be used to paint the lesions. Must check for the causes such as prolonged antibiotic therapy or undiagnosed diabetes mellitus.

Acute Laryngitis. Can be an extension of pharyngitis and is viral or bacterial. Treat the same as for acute pharyngitis, with the addition of voice rest for 1 week. Steam inhalations are helpful.

Chronic Pharyngitis. If sinusitis and postnasal discharge are the source, systemic decongestant is given, usually Sudafed. If there is secondary bacterial infection, a 7- to 10-day course of broad spectrum antibiotic is used—ampicillin or tetracycline. Contributing factors of tobacco and alcohol must be stopped. Similarly, chronic bronchitis must be treated.

Chronic Laryngitis. Usually secondary to irritative and chronic mild inflammation (same as for chronic pharyngitis). If suspicious at all for neoplasm, do direct laryngoscopy and biopsy.

Atrophic Laryngitis. End stage of chronic laryngitis; humidification is helpful, and antibiotic is for secondary infection.

Herpes of Pharynx and Larynx. Analgesia medications; antibiotic if secondary infection.

Tuberculosis. Almost always from a pulmonary source. The treatment is chemotherapy, as for pulmonary disease.

Cricoarytenoid Arthritis. If this is acute, anti-inflammatory agents such as aspirin or Butazolidin are used. This condition must be followed closely to prevent the late sequelae of cricoarytenoid joint fixation. If both joints are fixed, the vocal cords are medially placed and severe airway obstruction can develop; tracheotomy is then necessary.

Carcinoma. The treatment plan depends on the site, size, and evidence of regional and distant metastasis. Small lesions usually have no nodal or distant metastasis, and treatment can be tumoricidal radiation therapy or complete surgical excision. Large lesions usually involve nodal spread, and treatment is a combination of radiation therapy (preoperative or postoperative), surgical excision with possible radical neck dissection, and adjuvant chemotherapy.

Radiation Mucositis. Plenty of analgesia; push fluids to prevent dehydration; broad spectrum antibiotic if secondary infection; and avoid alcohol and smoking. Will resolve in several weeks to several months.

Perichondritis. The most common cause is radiation therapy for neoplasms. A trial of high dose intravenous antibiotics and steroids is warranted; if unresponsive, a laryngectomy may be necessary.

Trauma. Acute trauma: If minimal and with mild to moderate edema and hematoma, observe. If there are fractures of laryngeal cartilage, large laceration and hematoma, vocal cord avulsion, cricoarytenoid joint dislocation, and posterior displacement of epiglottis, open reduction of the injury is mandatory. Tracheotomy is performed for airway obstruction and in conjunction with open reduction of the larynx.

DYSPHAGIA

Definition

Dysphagia is difficulty in swallowing. It can be, but is not necessarily, painful (odynophagia = painful deglutition). The site can be anywhere, including the oral cavity, oropharynx, hypopharynx, and esophagus.

Subjective Complaints

Acute. Usually inflammatory. Also neurologic, traumatic, and foreign body (especially fish bone).

Chronic. Neoplastic, neurologic, obstructive (stricture).

Intermittent. Inflammatory, irritative.

Persistent. Neoplastic, irritative (especially from postnasal discharges), neurologic, obstructive (stricture).

Fever. Usually inflammatory; rarely, caustic ingestion will cause necrosis of esophagus and mediastinitis.

Weight Loss. Neoplastic; severe stenosis with impaired nutrition.

Referred Otalgia. Any: inflammatory,

neoplastic.

Hoarseness. Any: inflammatory, neoplastic, neurologic, stricture, and stenosis.

Neck Masses. Tender lymph nodes—inflammatory. Nontender lymph nodes—neoplastic.

Retained Secretions. Neoplastic, neurologic.

Aspiration. Usually neurologic; also large neoplastic lesions.

Regurgitation of Food or Retained Undigested Food. Zenker's diverticulum, neoplasm.

Dyspnea. Severe inflammation—acute epiglottitis. Neoplastic—very large and extensive laryngeal involvement.

Trauma. Blunt or penetrating trauma to the neck; ingestion of caustic agents.

Tobacco/Alcohol History. Usually neoplastic; can be chronic irritative.

CNS Disorders. Usually neurologic basis, especially brainstem cerebral vascular disease, multiple sclerosis, and other demyelinating diseases; rarely, brainstem and cerebellopontine angle tumors.

Achalasia (Cardiospasm). Will cause dysphagia and is due to failure of relaxation of distal esophagus.

Gastrointestinal Problems. Reflux esophagitis with or without hiatal hernia can cause esophagitis or strictures. Occasionally reflux esophagitis will cause a lump in throat sensation mimicking globus hystericus.

Nervous and Psychiatric Disorder. Dysphagia nervosa; globus hystericus.

Collagen Diseases. Scleroderma involves the esophagus primarily. Dermatomyositis involves the pharynx.

Dysphagia Lusoria. Dysphagia due to compression of the esophagus from either (1) right subclavian artery arising abnormally from the thoracic aorta and passing behind or in front of the esophagus, or (2) a double aortic arch. Aberrant right subclavian artery compresses the esophagus and causes dysphagia only, whereas a double aortic arch compresses both the trachea and esophagus, giving dyspnea and dysphagia.

Objective Findings

Acute pharyngitis, acute tonsillitis, peritonsillar abscess/cellulitis, parapharyngeal abscess/cellulitis, and floor of mouth infections can all cause dysphagia (see Throat Pain.).

Acute Epiglottitis. Actually, acute inflammation of the supraglottis. The entire area is markedly swollen and inflamed, with very narrowed airway (see Stridor).

Acute Laryngitis. Diffuse erythema of not only larynx but also hypopharynx. Can be viral or bacterial. Viral laryngitis gives mild erythema and bacterial laryngitis gives moderate erythema and edema; exudate is uncommon.

Esophagitis. Distal esophageal causes (neoplasms, strictures, and reflux of gastric juice) cannot be seen. May see pooling and retention of saliva in hypopharynx. *Jackson's sign* is pooling of saliva in pyriform sinus.

Referred Globus Hystericus. Normal examination.

Caustic Ingestion. Acute burns in oral cavity, oropharynx, hypopharynx, and esophagus. Caustic lye burns are coagulative, and strong acid burns are liquefactive and more likely to be through and through. Crystalline lye agent gives contiguous burns. Liquid lyes almost always involve the esophagus.

Neoplastic Lesions. Usually squamous cell carcinoma; rarely, sarcomas and mixed tumors of minor salivary glands.

Squamous cell carcinomas are exophytic friable tumors or can be ulcerative with friable surrounding tumor masses. To cause dysphagia, carcinoma of the base of tongue, oropharynx, larynx, and hypopharynx must be large and usually have neck lymph node metastasis.

Carcinomas of the esophagus, except those of the cervical esophagus, are not seen except for the indirect evidence of retained secretions at the cervical esophageal inlet.

Esophageal Structures. Not seen except for retained secretions.

Zenker's Diverticulum. Retained secretion in the hypopharynx, and may see undigested food.

Achalasia. May see retained secretion in hypopharynx.

Collagen Vascular Disease. Scleroderma involvement of the esophagus is not seen, but other evidence of scleroderma is the clue. Same with dermatomyositis.

Neurologic. Neurologic disease, especially those of the brainstem. Brainstem disease will commonly be associated with other cranial neuropathies. The oropharyngeal gag reflex is decreased (IXth nerve); hemiatrophy of the tongue (XIIth nerve); loss of normal symmetrical soft palate elevation (pharyngeal plexus of Xth nerve); vocal cord paralysis (Xth nerve); and sternocleidomastoid muscle atrophy or lack of trapezius or sternocleidomastoid muscle movement (XIth nerve). The cranial nerves IX to XII are the more commonly involved ones; but nerves V, VI, VII, and VIII can be affected. Multiple sclerosis and other demyelinating diseases may have associated cranial neuropathies but also have long tract signs.

A large number of neurologic dysphagias are due to neuromuscular incoordination of the swallowing mechanisms. No abnormalities are noted on examination but are seen with ciné or video pharyngoesophagogram.

Trauma. Acute: Edema, hematoma, lacerations of the hypopharynx with/without laryngeal trauma (see Throat Pain).

Chronic: Associated with stenosis of the hypopharynx and larynx.

Trauma to the esophagus from external causes is rare as this structure is well protected.

Vascular Anomalies. Retained secretions may be seen in the hypopharynx; the patient is usually an infant or young child. Good subglottic visualization by indirect laryngoscopy will show extrinsic compression of the anterior tracheal wall, suggesting double aortic arches.

Psychiatric Disorders. No organic abnormality.

Assessment

A *complete physical examination* with a good neurologic examination and a good indirect laryngoscopy is mandatory.

A *ciné/video contrast pharyngoesophagogram* is performed in all cases of dysphagia. Esophageal lesions can be diagnosed by this method. A ciné or video study is performed with the contrast pharyngoesophagogram, as the dysphagia secondary to neuromuscular dysfunction cannot be diagnosed by any other means. No esophagoscopy must be performed before a contrast esophagogram. Without an esophagogram to demonstrate lesions, there is a much higher incidence of esophageal perforation with esophagoscopy.

An *acid upper GI study* is helpful if one suspects a reflux esophagitis or lump in throat sensation secondary to acid reflux esophagitis.

Direct laryngoscopy is performed if one sees or is strongly suspicious of a larynx and hypopharyngeal cause.

Esophagoscopy is helpful and needs to be performed in neoplastic lesions and strictures. Neuromuscular dysfunction and scleroderma of esophagus need not be esophagoscoped. In patients with caustic ingestion, the direct laryngoscopy and esophagoscopy help determine the degree and extent of burns. The endoscopic instruments must not be passed through an area of severe or circumferential burns, as perforations can result. Zenker's diverticula should be examined by esophagoscopy before excision to rule out a carcinoma in the diverticulum.

For vascular anomalies, a *contrast esophagogram* is helpful in the diagnosis of an aberrant right subclavian artery. *Bronchoscopy* is helpful in the diagnosis of double aortic arches. As indicated, arteriograms are used to distinguish the type and extent of vascular anomalies.

For acute inflammation, complete blood count with differential, proper cultures, and sensitives are determined.

For collagen vascular diseases, LE preparations, rheumatoid factor, antinuclear antibodies, erythrocyte sedimentation rates (Westergren method), etc., should be obtained as indicated.

Neurologic consultation must be obtained in those patients with suspected neurologic causes of dysphagia.

Psychiatric consultation is helpful with dysphagia nervosa and other causes of psychogenic dysphagia.

Plan

Acute pharyngitis, acute tonsillitis, peritonsillar abscess/cellulitis, parapharyngeal abscess/cellulitis, floor of mouth infections, and acute and chronic laryngitis: see Throat Pain.

Acute Epiglottitis. Hospitalize; intravenous antibiotic—ampicillin as *H. influenzae* is the most common organism in the child. Watch for airway obstruction, as 50% of these patients will require either endotracheal intubation or tracheotomy for airway obstruction. This disease is of brief duration, seldom lasting over 1 week.

Esophagitis. Reflux esophagitis is treated with antacid and anticholinergic medications. In those with accompanying large hiatal hernia, a repair of the hiatal hernia may be necessary.

Esophageal Strictures. These are treated with serial dilations. Severe strictures without response to dilations are treated with surgical resection and colon interposition or other gastroesophageal procedures.

Globus Hystericus. These symptoms from acid reflux are relieved if the acid gastric reflux is treated.

Caustic Ingestion. Determination of the extent. Burns confined to the oral cavity and orophraynx are self-limiting, and treatment is with an antibiotic suspension to prevent secondary infection; analgesia; and proper nutritional intake.

1. Esophageal burn: Hospitalize and give intravenous feedings until able to tolerate oral feedings. Broad spectrum antibiotics such as ampicillin suspension are used to prevent secondary bacterial infections and given for a course of 7–10 days. A 1-week course of corticosteroids is used to prevent strictures. In those with severe burns, a string is passed into the stomach to facilitate later dilations.

Patients with chronic esophageal strictures are tested with serial dilations and followed-up for the rest of their lives. In those with very severe strictures where dilations are not helpful, resection of the stricture and colon interposition or gastric pull-up procedures are used.

2. Burns of the hypopharynx and larynx: Mild burns will respond to antibiotics to prevent secondary bacterial infections. Severe burns: Antibiotics and 1 week of corticosteroids should be used to prevent strictures and secondary bacterial infection. Chronic strictures of the larynx and hypopharynx are among the most difficult problems to treat, and there are no satisfactory methods.

Neoplasms. Carcinomas of the base of the tongue, oropharynx, larynx, and hypopharynx which cause dysphagia are large and often extensive. The treatment will usually consist of radiation therapy pre- and postoperatively, wide surgical resection with radical neck dissection (if clinical lymph node spread is present or highly suspected), and adjuvant chemotherapy.

Carcinomas of the esophagus are treated with wide resection and reconstruction with colon or other intestinal interposition, if resectable; and radiation therapy alone if unresectable.

Minor salivary gland tumors and granular cell myoblastomas (rare) may be treated with local resections.

Zenker's Diverticulum. The cause is chronic spasm of the cricopharyngeus muscle and secondary pharyngeal diverticular outpouching. The definitive treatment is diverticulectomy and cricopharyngeal myotomy. In the elderly debilitated patients, the diverticulum is sutured high in the neck for dependent gravity drainage. This can be done under local anesthesia.

Cricopharyngeal Muscle Spasm. This can lead to Zenker's diverticulum, but in the earlier stage only the spasm exists. A cricopharyngeal myotomy will relieve this problem.

Collagen Vascular Disease. Scleroderma of the esophagus is treated medically with corticosteroids. If significant dysphagia is present, dilation is used. Similarly, dermatomyositis is treated medically with corticosteroids.

Neurologic. The primary neurologic process is treated and the dysphagia may or may not resolve. In those with brainstem infarctions, the extensive disorder of the deglutition precludes simple management. Occasionally, a spastic cricopharyngeus muscle may be treated with a myotomy. Commonly, chronic aspiration is the more serious problem, therefore esophagotomy or gastrostomy is performed.

Similarly, dysphagia due to multiple sclerosis and other demyelinating diseases are treated as for the primary diseases.

Achalasia can be treated with methacholine (5–10 mg subcutaneously). Esophagocardiomyotomy is necessary in 20–25% of cases.

Dysphagia secondary to neuromuscular incoordination may respond to periodic dilation.

Trauma. Acute trauma (see Throat Pain).

Chronic traumatic changes: Dysphagia may be a part of the entire deformity complex (see Throat Pain).

Vascular Anomalies. These are treated with thoracic and cardiovascular surgery to alleviate the problems.

Psychogenic Dysphagia. Psychiatric care.

HOARSENESS

Definition

Hoarseness is any unnatural deepening and harsh quality of the voice. Only the normal true vocal cords can produce the sharp and crisp qualities of the human voice.

Subjective Complaints

Acute. Inflammatory is most common; vocal cord paralysis and trauma are less likely causes.

Chronic. Any: Inflammatory, irritative, neoplastic, or neurologic disorder (vocal cord paralysis).

Persistent. Any: neoplastic, neurologic (vocal cord paralysis), inflammatory, and irritative (vocal cord polyps, nodules, and chronic laryngitis).

Intermittent. Inflammatory.

Fever. Inflammatory.

Upper Respiratory Infections or Viral Infections. Often precede acute laryngitis.

Weight Loss. Neoplastic.

Referred Otalgia. Neoplastic from hypopharynx; rarely, acute laryngitis will give referred ear pain.

Neck Mass. Tender lymphadenopathy is inflammatory. Nontender lymphade-

nopathy is neoplastic. Thyroid mass is important in unilateral ipsilateral vocal cord paralysis, as the mass can be a thyroid carcinoma.

Cough. Acute: accompanying acute laryngitis and pharyngitis with an acute bronchitis. Chronic: irritative phenomena from the coughing and sputum of chronic bronchitis.

Tuberculosis. Laryngeal involvement occurs in 5% of pulmonary tuberculosis cases. Other pulmonary granulomatous disease can involve the larynx.

Chronic Sinusitis and Postnasal Discharge. The secretion is irritating to the larynx and the hypopharynx. The hoarseness is worse in the morning and improves with the day, and worse when the postnasal discharge is thicker and purulent. This is often associated with throat pain.

Tobacco/Alcohol. Squamous cell carcinoma rarely occurs in those individuals who have not been moderate to heavy smokers. Tobacco is the most evident cause of squamous cell carcinoma of the larynx. Alcohol is a contributing factor. Chronic laryngitis, vocal cord polyps, and nodules can also be caused by these agents.

Dyspnea. Associated conditions are very large laryngeal or hypopharyngeal carcinoma, bilateral vocal cord paralysis, and large laryngeal cysts and internal laryngoceles.

Trauma. Blunt and penetrating trauma to the neck can cause laryngeal hematoma, vocal cord avulsion, and arytenoid dislocations. Endotracheal tube intubation and rigid bronchoscopy can cause cricoarytenoid dislocation and posterior commissure granuloma and ulcerations.

Voice Abuse. Acute: acute laryngitis with or without vocal cord hematoma.

Chronic: vocal cord polyps and nodules develop; this is the most common cause of childhood chronic hoarseness.

Metabolic Diseases. Hypothyroidism can produce myxedema of the vocal cords.

Granulomatous Disease. Tuberculosis and other granulomatous disease can involve the larynx and most commonly the posterior commissures.

Syphilis. Involves the larynx, especially

the posterior commissure.

Vocal Cord Paralysis. Unilaterally, the symptom is hoarseness without dyspnea. Bilateral vocal cord paralysis results in severe dyspnea and some hoarseness of a mild nature as the vocal cords are almost in apposition. Once diagnosis of vocal cord paralysis is made, the etiology must be sought. Central nervous system disorders account for 10%. They include CNS hemorrhage in the neonate, vascular occlusive disease of the vertebral-basilar arteries, brainstem tumors and, rarely, cerebellopontine angle tumors. Peripheral causes account for 90% of the etiologies. They can occur from any head and neck region to the chest. The hidden areas include: thyroid, chest, mediastinum, cardiac, and esophageal lesions. Diabetes mellitus and other causes of polyneuropathy must be sought.

Psychogenic. Rare, and only where organic abnormalities are ruled out. Spastic dysphonia and dysphonia plicae ventricularis have strong psychogenic components.

Objective Findings

Indirect laryngoscopy is performed with laryngeal mirror examination (most commonly used), fiberoptic laryngoscope, or Ward-Berci indirect laryngoscope.

Acute Laryngitis. This is the most common cause of hoarseness and usually follows an upper respiratory infection. The laryngeal mucosa is inflamed. The vocal cords are erythematous and edematous but have normal mobility.

Chronic Diffuse Laryngitis. This is the second most common cause of hoarseness and the most common cause of persistent hoarseness. Smoking is the most common cause in the adult. The findings are thickened, white vocal cords with normal mobility. A variant is pachyderma laryngis, in which the chronic inflammatory changes involve more the posterior larynx.

Vocal Cord Polyps and Nodules. These are variants of chronic laryngitis, and the most common cause is tobacco; but voice abuse, chronic bronchitis, and postnasal discharges are other causes. The polyps are localized edematous tissues in the vocal cord, and nodules are hyperkeratotic nodular tissues. They are most often found at the junction of the anterior and mid-third of the vocal cord. The vocal cords are normally mobile.

Vocal Cord Paralysis. The immobile vocal cord or cords are in a paramedian position (2 mm from the midline). It can be unilateral (most common) or bilateral. Accompanying larngeal and hypopharyngeal neoplastic diseases can be found, or the larynx and hypopharynx can be normal. If the larynx is normal, systemic workup for the etiology must be made.

Neoplastic Lesions. The most common is squamous cell carcinoma. It can be exophytic or a deeply infiltrating growth. Often there is a surrounding edema. In large hypopharyngeal lesions, the edema can obscure the tumor, therefore marked edema of the laryngopharynx points to a carcinoma. The laryngeal carcinoma can be small to very extensive. In order for hypopharyngeal carcinoma to produce hoarseness, it must be large and have spread to the larynx.

Rarely, a fibroma, chondroma, or granular cell myoblastoma can produce hoarseness.

Trauma. Acute: Blunt and penetrating neck trauma can cause lacerations, edema, swelling, hematoma, avulsion of the vocal cords, and arytenoid dislocations. Endotracheal intubations and rigid bronchoscopy can cause dislocation of the arytenoid and granuloma formations in the posterior commisure.

Chronic: This is also from blunt or penetrating trauma with late fibrotic changes and often stenosis. The anatomy is distorted. The vocal cords can be displaced and fixed, and the laryngeal lumen can be distorted and stenotic.

Cricoarytenoid Arthritis and Fixation. Cricoarytenoid arthritis is an acute process with inflammation of the cricoarytenoid joint. Of the patients with rheumatoid arthritis, 25% will have this, and a lesser percentage from other collagen vascular disease. The vocal cords have impaired mobility and the cricoarytenoid joint is quite erythematous. In the late changes, there is cricoarytenoid joint fixation with the vocal cord in the paramedian position.

Granulomatous Diseases. Granulation tissue or chronic inflammation of the posterior commissure is often from tuberculosis and other granulomatous involvement of the larynx.

Syphilis. Also involves the posterior commissure with its gummatous reactions.

Hypothyroidism. Myxedema of the larynx can occur with a thickened, myxedematous deposition in the larynx and the vocal cords.

Spastic Dysphonia. Tense voice with overadduction of vocal cords.

Dysphonia Plicae Ventricularis. The false vocal cords meet before the true vocal cord and produce a harsh, breathy voice.

Assessment

A good *indirect laryngoscopy* must be performed in all patients complaining of hoarseness.

Direct laryngoscopy (DL) is performed either under general or local anesthesia. It is used for diagnostic and occasionally therapeutic purposes. Patients with acute laryngitis, chronic diffuse nonsuspicious laryngitis, and vocal cord polyps that resolve do not need a direct laryngoscopy. Direct laryngoscopy is always used for anyone with a suspicious neoplastic lesion. Direct laryngoscopy is therapeutic in patients with vocal cord polyps, nodules, and localized squamous cell carcinoma *in situ,* as the lesions are removed at the time of the direct laryngoscopy.

Laryngograms—contrast dye and air tomograms—are used for neoplastic and chronic laryngeal stenosis. The dye contrast gives better definition. Air tomograms of the larynx are used for those with large laryngeal neoplasms or severe stenosis in which the dye may precipitate an acute airway obstruction.

Soft tissue x-rays and xeroradiograms of the neck are useful, especially in neoplastic and traumatic cases.

Barium swallow is used for neoplasm if a second primary or extension of the laryngeal neoplasm is suspected.

Bronchoscopy and esophagoscopy are used in neoplastic cases where extension or a second neoplasm is suspected.

For airway obstruction, usually with very large laryngeal or laryngopharyngeal carcinomas and bilateral vocal cord paralysis, the indications for *tracheotomies* are the same as for any impending airway obstruction.

VDRL and other serologic tests are indicated if one suspects syphilis.

Sputum cultures and sensitivity tests are performed for tuberculosis, other granulomatous disease, and chronic bronchitis.

Thyroid function tests are performed for myxedema of the larynx.

For collagen vascular disease, especially rheumatoid arthritis, use rheumatoid factor, LE preparation, antinuclear antibodies, and erythrocyte sedimentation rate.

Sinus x-rays are obtained if chronic sinusitis or postnasal discharge is suspected as the cause of the hoarseness.

For neck mass, there is no place for early biopsy. Acute inflammatory lymphadenopathy will respond to systemic antibiotics. In those with carcinoma of the larynx or hypopharynx, the nontender lymph nodes are assumed to be metastatic. Indiscriminate biopsy results in higher rate of local tumor recurrence and distant metastases.

Pulmonary function tests are particularly important if one is contemplating conservative laryngeal surgery for a small carcinoma of the larynx. Assessment of the degree of obstruction is helpful in those with bilateral vocal cord paralysis.

Psychogenic or psychiatric consultations are helpful in psychogenic hoarseness.

Plan

Acute Laryngitis. Treat expectantly with antipyretic and analgesic agents, for the cause is a viral upper respiratory infection. If there is a secondary bacterial infection, antibiotics are used. Penicillin or erythromycin are the usual choices. Voice rest is necessary for 1–2 weeks.

Chronic Diffuse Laryngitis. Treat the source. Avoidance of tobacco and alcohol should be advised, as these are the most common causes. If the cause is chronic sinusitis and postnasal discharge, use systemic decongestant such as Sudafed and antibiotics if secondarily infected. Chronic bronchitis should be treated with expectorants and broad spectrum antibiotics like tetracycline if there is purulent sputum. Voice rest for 1–2 weeks is necessary.

Vocal Cord Polyps and Nodules. Treatment is similar to that for chronic diffuse laryngitis. An additional cause seen with vocal cord polyps and nodules, but not in chronic diffuse laryngitis, is voice abuse. Cessation of the voice abuse is mandatory. In those who use their voice for a living (politicians, singers), speech therapy helps to prevent recurrence of the polyps and nodules. If the nodules and polyps do not respond to medical treatment, do a direct laryngoscopy and removal.

Vocal Cord Paralysis. A thorough evaluation of the entire head and neck, cardiac, chest, mediastinum, and esophageal areas must be made to try to find the etiology. Treatment is directed at the various etiologies, if found. In over 25% of the cases, an etiology is not found for the vocal cord paralysis.

1. Unilateral paralysis (left greater than the right): Wait for 6 months to see if there is any spontaneous vocal cord function return or overcompensation by the opposite vocal cord. If none in 6 months and there is persistent hoarseness, bothersome weakness of voice, or aspiration, direct laryngoscopy and injection of paralyzed cord with Teflon will give good voice and cure the aspiration.

2. Bilateral vocal cord paralysis: If there is airway obstruction, do a tracheotomy. Wait 6 months to see if there is any spontaneous return of vocal cord function. If none, a permanent tracheotomy can be left in, and the patient will talk by (1) plugging the lumen of the tracheotomy tube or (2) installation of a one-way valve in the tracheotomy tube so that during expiration, part of the air is expired through the apposed vocal cords. Another choice is an arytenoidectomy and lateralization of the vocal cord. This results in a harsh voice, but the tracheotomy is removed.

Neoplastic Lesions. Small laryngeal carcinomas can be treated equally well with tumoricidal radiation therapy or surgery. Radiation therapy leaves a better voice. Large laryngeal tumors require combination of radiation therapy and total laryngectomy with radical neck dissection if there is evidence of neck node metastasis. Adjuvant chemotherapy may be useful.

Hypopharyngeal carcinomas causing hoarseness are large, therefore the treatment is combination therapy: radiation therapy pre- or postoperatively, pharyngolaryngectomy and radical neck dissection if there is evidence of neck node metastasis, and adjuvant chemotherapy.

The benign tumors of the larynx (rare) can be removed surgically without a total laryngectomy.

Trauma. Acute: Impending airway obstruction should have tracheotomy. If the trauma is mild with just edema and small hematoma, patient can be observed. If the trauma is moderate to severe, especially with large hematoma, lacerations, fractures of laryngeal cartilages, vocal cord avulsions, arytenoid dislocations, and epiglottis dislocations, open reduction must be performed to restore vocal cord function and prevent laryngeal stenosis.

Chronic: The problems are impaired vocal cord function and stenosis. This is a most difficult problem to treat and no surgical method is uniformly successful. It is better to treat the acute injuries aggressively than to try to treat a chronic stenotic useless larynx.

Cricoarytenoid Arthritis and Fixation. The arthritis is usually secondary to rheumatoid arthritis and treatment is aspirin, Butazolidin, or corticosteroids. Must follow patient for a long time to prevent cricoarytenoid fixation.

Cricoarytenoid fixation, if unilateral, requires no treatment. If bilateral, arytenoidectomy and lateralization are necessary.

Granulomatous Disease. The pulmonary aspect must be evaluated. Direct laryngoscopy with biopsy for histologic examination and tissue cultures must be performed. The treatment is chemotherapy, as for pulmonary disease.

Syphilis. Serologic testing is helpful, but direct laryngoscopy and biopsy for histologic examination must be performed. The treatment is adequate dose of penicillin or ampicillin.

Hypothyroidism. This is treated with thyroid replacement, and direct laryngoscopy is not performed.

Spastic Dysphonia. Aggressive speech therapy is helpful. In cases in which speech therapy response is not satisfactory, section of the recurrent laryngeal nerve has been successful.

Dysphonia Plicae Ventricularis. Speech therapy is often helpful. If this is without success, stripping of the false vocal cord is helpful.

STRIDOR

Definition

Stridor refers to any noisy respiration. Inspiratory stridor is any noisy respiration arising from above the true vocal cords and can be from nasal cavity to supraglottic area. Inspiratory and expiratory stridor comes from the true vocal cord area or immediately below. Expiratory stridor comes from below the vocal cords and is produced from the tracheobronchial tree.

The three types of stridor are produced from the same areas regardless of age, but the etiologies and findings differ with age.

Neonatal and Infant Stridor

Subjective Complaints

Most are congenital stridors and are evident soon after birth.

Laryngomalacia. The most common form of congenital stridor, accounting for 75%. It is inspiratory and changes with position; better in prone position and worse with crying and supine position.

Vocal Cord Paralysis. The second most frequent neonatal and infant stridor (10%). There is inspiratory and expiratory stridor with severe dyspnea.

Subglottic Stenosis/Hemangioma. The third most common cause of neonate and infant stridor. The stridor is inspiratory/expiratory. Severe airway obstruction oc-

curs in 50%, necessitating a tracheotomy. The stenosis versus the hemangioma can be distinguished only on examination.

Recurrent or intractable croup may herald a previously undiagnosed subglottic stenosis.

Vocal Cord Webs. This is fusion of the vocal cords at the anterior two-thirds Inspiratory/expiratory stridor and a weak voice are evident.

Laryngeal Cyst. A rare cause presenting with dyspnea and stridor. Hoarseness depends if vocal cord function is impaired, as the cyst does not arise from the vocal cords but usually from the supraglottic area, especially near the ventricle.

Fever. The congenital stridors seen in the neonate and infant are rarely febrile.

Acute. The congenital stridors are acute if present soon after birth but they are persistent.

Chronic. All congenital stridors are persistent and chronic.

Aspiration. Aspiration accompanying stridor is rare and is caused by congenital laryngeal cleft, an extremely rare deformity in which there is a cleft in the posterior aspect of the laryngeal and trachea, resulting in a common channel from the esophagus to the trachea. Tracheal esophageal fistula gives aspiration, pneumonitis, and feeding problems, but stridor is not usually accompanying.

Associated Neurologic Disorder: Associated neurologic problems may accompany vocal cord paralysis. Especially seen are other cranial neuropathies.

Prolonged Intubation and Tracheotomy. Prolonged endotracheal tube intubation can produce iatrogenic subglottic stenosis (2–5). Prolonged tracheotomy can result in tracheal stenosis or tracheomalacia. High tracheotomy can cause subglottic stenosis.

Vascular Anomalies. These may or may not be associated with dysphagia. The most common cause is double aortic arch.

Blowing. Internal laryngocele will enlarge with blowing.

Objective Findings

Laryngomalacia. The epiglottis and supraglottic structures are flabby, and on inspiration can be seen being sucked through the vocal cords.

Vocal Cord Paralysis. Both vocal cords are in a paramedian position and immobile.

Subglottic Stenosis/Hemangioma. The vocal cords are normal with normal function. In stenosis, there is fibrotic tissue just below the vocal cords. In the hemangioma, there is a reddish-purplish mass below the vocal cords.

Laryngeal Web. A web of either thick or thin tissue is between the true vocal cords and involves the anterior two-thirds of the true vocal cords.

Laryngeal Cysts and Internal Laryngocele. A cystic lesion can occur anywhere in the larynx, usually not from the true vocal cords. The most common sites are the ventricles and laryngeal surface of the supraglottic area. Internal laryngocele may be indistinguishable from cyst of larynx and may be accompanied by external laryngocele. The external laryngocele is compressible and is crepitant. It may change in size with Valsalva mavelver.

Vascular Anomalies. They are the result of abnormal arterial development. A double aortic arch or an aberrant innominate artery will cause anterior extrinsic compression of the trachea. Double aortic arch is accompanied by esophageal compression and dysphagia, while aberrant innominate artery is not accompanied by dysphagia.

Trauma

1. Blunt and penetrating: this is extremely uncommon in the neonate.

2. Prolonged intubation causes a subglottic stenosis in 2–5%. The stenotic area is fibrotic and often annular. The posterior commisure can also be fibrotic so that the vocal cords are fixed in a paramedian-intermediate position.

3. High tracheotomy (at level of first tracheal ring) causes subglottic stenosis, more in the anterior subglottic area.

4. Tracheal stenosis occurs at the treacheal stoma or tracheotomy cuff site. Tracheomalacia occurs with prolonged tracheotomy and causes expiration stridor due to collapse of tracheal wall on expiration.

Assessment

Airway evaluation must be made with all stridor, for impending airway obstruction. Increasing hypoxia and hypercapnia are indications for tracheotomy or endotracheal intubation. Careful ausculation over mouth, larynx, trachea, and lungs may help identify the level of stridor source.

Direct laryngoscopy must be performed for all congenital stridors, to make or confirm the diagnosis. A second congenital pathologic process occasionally occurs.

Barium swallow is used to help delineate tracheal-esophageal fistula, laryngeal cleft, and vascular anomalies (as double aortic arch).

Bronchoscopy is not used routinely but is necessary with expiratory stridor. Direct laryngoscopy can visualize only the upper 1 cm of trachea.

Arteriogram is used if one suspects vascular malformation and is contemplating surgical repair.

Blunt or penetrating traumas are treated the same way regardless of age. *Air tomograms* of the larynx and *direct laryngoscopy* are necessary.

Subglottic and tracheal stenosis can be evaluated by *(1) laryngotracheogram*—air tomogram and dye contrast, and *(2) direct laryngoscopy and bronchoscopy.*

Plan

Laryngomalacia. This is a self-limiting disease and the patient will outgrow it by the age of 2 years. Reassurance is offered to the parents that the noisy breathing will go away and the child is no danger. Occasionally, tracheotomy is required.

Vocal Cord Paralysis. Tracheotomy may be necessary. If there is no vocal cord function return, an arytenoidectomy and arytenoid lateralization may be performed when the child is much older. Laryngeal surgery in the infant and young child is very difficult and can result in impaired laryngeal growth.

Subglottic Stenosis. Tracheotomy is necessary in 50% of the cases. With time and growth of the larynx and subglottic area, most patients can be decannulated. Dilation and injection of the stenotic area with corticosteroids may be helpful.

Subglottic Hemangioma. Tracheotomy is necessary in 50%. Biopsy for diagnosis is contraindicated, as death can occur from uncontrolled bleeding into the lungs. Irradiation is contraindicated. At the age of 2 years, the hemangioma can be resected.

Laryngeal Web. Thin mucosal webs can be incised and cured. Incision of thick webs will lead to recurrence and more fibrosis. It is best in thick webs to wait until the child is 2 years old and treat with laryngofissure opening of the larynx, incision of the web, and placement of a laryngeal keel for 3 weeks. This is usually successful.

Laryngeal Cysts. Aspiration if small, or marsupialization if large via direct laryngoscopy. *Internal laryngoceles* can also be treated this way. *Internal with external laryngoceles* must be excised through an external neck approach.

Vascular Anomalies. These are treated by thoracotomy and corrective surgery.

Trauma

1. Iatrogenic subglottic stenosis: The best cure is prevention. Avoidance of prolonged intubation is the best. While there is no good answer as to the length of intubation necessary to cause subglottic stenosis, it is best to tracheotomize a patient after 1–2 weeks of intubation. The very small infant with a subglottic stenosis, may outgrow it with age and increase in laryngeal size during growth.

In a large child the stenosis will not be outgrown. The treatment with dilation and steroid injections has been dismal. Various surgical methods have been proposed with some, but not universal, success in relieving the subglottic stenosis.

2. High tracheotomy: This procedure causes chondritis and fibrosis of the cricoid area. All high tracheotomies must be converted as soon as possible to regular tracheotomy to prevent subglottic stenosis.

3. Tracheal stenosis: Tracheal stenosis from tracheotomy can be minimized by a soft and proper-sized tracheotomy tube and good care to prevent infection. In short tracheal stenotic segments, a primary re-section and anastomosis can be performed. Long tracheal stenosis is difficult to repair.

Childhood Stridor

Subjective Complaints

Croup or Acute Laryngotracheobronchitis. This is the most common form of childhood stridor. It is inspiratory and expiratory, with a barking, croupy type of cough. The age is 2–7 years, and is endemic, more during the winter. Hoarseness may be associated.

Acute Epiglottitis. A supraglottic infection due mostly to *H. influenzae*. Age range is similar to that of croup. The stridor is inspiratory and often is associated with a "hot potato" voice, but not hoarseness. The onset is rapid, over 2–4 hours.

Allergic Rhinitis. Causes chronic nasal obstruction and inspiratory stridor and may or may not be accompanied by enlarged adenoids. After enlarged adenoids, allergy is the next most common cause of chronic nasal obstruction.

Markedly Enlarged Tonsils and Adenoids. Can give inspiratory stridor. Pulmonary hypertension and cor pulmonale can result.

Foreign Body. Common in the child. The stridor is expiratory if it lodges in the tracheobronchial tree. Foreign body can occasionally lodge in the larynx giving an inspiratory/expiratory stridor. This can mimic a chronic or recurrent croup.

Fever. Inflammatory lesions, especially croup and acute epiglottitis. Rarely, an infection secondary to foreign body aspiration.

Acute. Inflammatory process and foreign body are the common causes of acute onset.

Chronic. Markedly enlarged tonsils and adenoids are chronic. Laryngeal cysts are chronic. Neoplasms are chronic but they are very rare in the child. Occasionally an undiagnosed foreign body gives persistent symptoms.

Trauma. Birth trauma can injure the recurrent laryngeal nerve and give vocal cord paralysis. Blunt and penetrating trauma to the neck is uncommon in the child. The more soft tissue and higher position of the larynx protect the child's larynx from trauma. Automobile accidents and falling are the most common injuries to the infant and child's neck.

Prolonged Intubation and Tracheotomy. Prolonged endotracheal tube intubation can produce iatrogenic subglottic stenosis (2–5%). Prolonged tracheotomy can result in tracheal stenosis or tracheomalacia. High tracheotomy can cause subglottic stenosis.

Objective Findings

Acute Laryngotracheobronchitis (Croup). Viral infection of the larynx, trachea, and bronchus with accompanying acute inflammation of all the involved areas. The subglottis, being the smallest area in the airway at this age, is most severely affected and gives rise to the stridor.

Acute Epiglottitis. An acute bacterial infection of the supraglottic larynx. The tissues are erythematous and edematous. The epiglottis and the aryepiglottic folds are markedly swollen so that the normal C-shape assumes an annular pattern. The airway below this is obstructed and the vocal cords, which are normal and mobile, cannot be seen.

Markedly Enlarged Tonsils and Adenoid Tissues. A markedly enlarged adenoid obstructs the entire nasopharynx. Markedly enlarged tonsils meet and touch in the midline in a noninflamed state on just routine examination.

Allergic Rhinitis. Nasal mucosa is boggy, edematous with bluish discoloration. Secondary bacterial infection may be present. Adenoids may be hypertrophied as a secondary lymphoid reaction to the allergic rhinitis.

Foreign Body. Usually lodges in the bronchus, right more than left because of the right's greater diameter and more vertical path. Occasionally, a foreign body can lodge between the vocal cords, giving inspiratory and expiratory stridor and minimally croup. A localized expiratory stridor is indicative of a bronchial foreign body.

Trauma

1. Blunt/penetrating: This is extremely uncommon in the child. Penetrating trauma is rare. Blunt trauma is more common; edema, hematoma, lacerations of mucosa, vocal cords avulsion, and arytenoid dislocations can be seen.

2. Prolonged intubation causes a subglottic stenosis in 2–5%. The stenotic area is fibrotic and often annular. The posterior commissure can also be fibrotic so that the vocal cords are fixed in a paramedian intermediate position.

3. High tracheotomy (at level of first tracheal ring) causes subglottic stenosis but more in the anterior subglottic area.

4. Tracheal stenosis occurs at the tracheal stoma or tracheotomy cuff site. Tracheomalacia occurs with prolonged tracheotomy and causes expiration stridor due to collapse of tracheal wall on expiration.

Assessment

With all stridor, evaluation must be made for impending airway obstruction. Hypoxia and hypercapnia are indications for tracheotomy or endotracheal intubation.

Croup. A direct laryngoscopy is not necessary and can precipitate a complete airway obstruction. Anteroposterior (AP) and lateral x-rays of the neck will show the narrowing of the subglottic area and no enlargement of the epiglottis. As with any infection, a complete blood count (CBC) is indicated. Recurrent or intractable croup must have direct laryngoscopy, as foreign body of the larynx and subglottic stenosis can mimic croup.

Acute Epiglottitis. If the child has impending airway obstruction, no diagnostic test is performed. He is taken quickly to the operating room. With endotracheal intubation or bronchoscope ready, a direct laryngoscopy is performed. If the diagnosis is confirmed, either intubation or a tracheotomy is performed. CBC, blood cultures, and cultures of the supraglottic areas are made.

Sometimes the diagnosis between croup and epiglottitis is unclear. If there is no impending airway obstruction, a lateral x-ray of the neck can evaluate the epiglottis. A gently performed indirect laryngoscopy can easily visualize the epiglottis. It is important that only the smallest laryngeal mirror is used and that the visualization is only for the epiglottis, not the vocal cords.

Markedly Enlarged Adenoids and Tonsils. Enlarged adenoids can be evaluated by lateral x-rays of the nasal and oropharynx or by palpation through the mouth. Arterial blood gases and cardiac catheterization for pulmonary hypertension are helpful. If the tonsils and adenoids are abnormal, an adenoidectomy and tonsillectomy are indicated.

Allergy Workup. This is done in all suspected allergy cases.

Foreign Body. All patients with suspected foreign body must have a direct laryngoscopy and bronchoscopy. Cultures are taken at the time of the endoscopy if there is a secondary bacterial infection. Intractable or recurrent croup and localized expiratory stridor must be evaluated for foreign body.

Trauma. Blunt or penetrating traumas are treated the same way, regardless of age. Air tomograms of the larynx and direct laryngoscopy are necessary. Contrast laryngograms can be performed in the older child if no impending airway obstruction.

Subglottic and Tracheal Stenosis. This can be evaluated by (1) laryngotracheogram—air tomogram and dye contrast—and (2) direct laryngoscopy and bronchoscopy.

Plan

Croup. This is treated with hydration, steam inhalation (warm or cool). Severe airway obstruction necessitating a tracheotomy occurs only in 3%. As this is a viral lesion, antibiotics are indicated only if there is evidence of secondary bacterial infection.

Epiglottitis. Fifty percent of the patients will require either endotracheal intubation or tracheotomy. Either method is acceptable. To perform endotracheal tube intubation, a skilled anesthesiologist must be available to put in the tube and replace if it dislodged. Similarly, to perform a tracheotomy a skilled head and neck surgeon is necessary to keep the mortality and morbidity to a minimum. Before any tracheotomy is performed, securing of the airway is necessary either with an intubation or with a ventilating bronchoscope. Tracheotomy in infants and children without a controlled airway results in very high mortality and morbidity.

Intravenous antibiotics are given. The organism is usually *H. influenzae,* so ampicillin is the drug of choice. This disease is of a short duration, rarely lasting over a week; therefore the tracheotomy or intubation can be decannulated quickly.

Foreign Body. All foreign bodies must be removed. A skilled endoscopist must perform it.

Markedly Enlarged Tonsils and Adenoids. If properly indicated, a tonsillectomy and adenoidectomy are performed.

Allergy. Allergic workup and treatment are necessary for suspected allergic disorders. Routine systemic decongestant is not helpful in those with allergic rhinnitis.

Trauma

1. Blunt/penetrating: Similar to adults, moderate to severe acute injury must be repaired as soon as possible with open reduction regardless of the age of the patient. Minimal injuries can be watched. This aggressive attitude prevents late vocal cord dysfunction and stenosis, which are very difficult to treat.

2. Iatrogenic subglottic stenosis: The best cure is prevention. Avoidance of prolonged intubation is the best. While there is no good answer as to the length of time intubation is necessary to cause subglottic stenosis, it is best to tracheotomize a patient after 1–2 weeks of intubation. The very small infant with a subglottic stenosis may outgrow it with age and the increase in laryngeal size with growth.

3. Subglottic stenosis in the large child and adult will not be outgrown. The treatment with dilation and steroid injections has been dismal. Various surgical methods

have been proposed with some, but not universal, success in relieving the subglottic stenosis.

4. High tracheotomy causes chondritis and fibrosis of the cricoid area. All high tracheotomies must be converted as soon as possible to regular tracheotomy to prevent subglottic stenosis.

5. Tracheal stenosis from tracheotomy can be minimized by a soft and proper-sized tracheotomy tube and good care to prevent infection. In short tracheal stenotic segments, a primary resection and anastomosis can be performed. Long tracheal stenosis is difficult to repair.

Adult Stridor

Subjective Complaints

Acute. Usually inflammatory, but can occur with neoplasms, bilateral vocal cord paralysis, and trauma. In those with large laryngeal neoplasms or longstanding bilateral abductor vocal cord paralysis, a mild laryngitis or other inflammatory process can precipitate acute airway obstruction.

Intermittent. Inflammatory.

Chronic/Persistent. Usually neoplastic or vocal cord paralysis; cysts of larynx and stenosis of larynx, subglottis, or trachea are other causes.

Fever. Inflammatory.

Dysphagia. Neoplastic and neurologic.

Weight Loss. Neoplastic.

Referred otalgia. Acute: inflammatory. Chronic: neoplastic lesion of the hypopharynx.

Neck Mass. Tenderness: inflammatory lymph nodes. Nontender: neoplastic; if sufficient to cause stridor, the neoplasm is quite large.

Throat Pain. Inflammatory and neoplastic.

Neurologic. Associated with vocal cord paralysis. Search for brainstem diseases, multiple sclerosis, and other demyelinating diseases.

Psychogenic. Rare; the psychiatric symptoms may be subtle and may require several visits to be aware of this etiology.

Trauma

1. Cricothyrotomy or high tracheotomy causes subglottic stenosis if not converted early to regular tracheotomy.

2. Prolonged intubation can cause subglottic stenosis. While no specific time of intubation will cause stenosis, the (1) duration, (2) trauma, and (3) number of times of intubation are factors in development of subglottic stenosis.

3. External trauma: blunt/penetrating.

4. Tracheotomy can cause tracheal stenosis or tracheomalacia.

Allergy. Asthma causes bilateral expiratory wheezes and stridor.

Tobacco/Alcohol. Excess prolonged tobacco usage of cigarettes, pipe, or cigars is the single most important factor in squamous cell carcinoma of the head and neck. Excess alcohol consumption is a factor as well.

Surgery. Previous surgery, especially thyroid surgery. The recurrent laryngeal nerve is most commonly injured with thyroid surgery but can be injured by improperly performed tracheotomy and any neck and chest surgery.

An ill-performed laryngofissure can produce laryngeal stenosis. The most common complication of a hemilaryngectomy is glottic stenosis.

Objective Findings

Nasopharynx/Nasal Cavity. Markedly enlarged adenoid tissues in a young adult may cause inspiratory stridor. Carcinoma of the nasopharynx may cause inspiratory stridor. Any cause of nasal obstruction can cause inspiratory stridor; these include septal deviation, allergic rhinitis, and hypertrophic rhinosinusitis.

Oral Cavity/Oropharynx. Enlarged tonsils, peritonsillar abscess/cellulitis, parapharyngeal abscess, floor of mouth infections, and large carcinomas of the base of tongue and oropharynx can cause inspiratory stridor and airway obstruction (see Throat Pain).

In order for tonsils to be considered markedly enlarged, they must be touching each other in the midline without acute inflammation.

Supraglottis

1. Cysts/internal laryngocele. Cysts are large, mucosal-covered cystic masses and can arise from anywhere in the supraglottic region. The internal laryngocele arises from the ventricular apices and is air-containing. It may have an accompanying external laryngocele, which is compressible, has crepitance, and may enlarge with Valsalva.

2. *Acute epiglottitis.* This is not a disease of the child only but also occurs in adults. The findings are similar with such marked inflammation and swelling of the supraglottic area that the epiglottis and aryepiglottic folds are markedly enlarged and assume an annular shape. The airway is markedly narrowed and the vocal cords are not to be seen.

3. *Neoplasm.* Squamous cell carcinomas are the most common. To cause stridor they are large and are either exophytic, friable masses or deeply infiltrating with marked surrounding edema. The vocal cords may be obscured.

Larynx

1. *Carcinoma.* A common laryngeal cause of stridor is carcinoma. They are large and resemble in appearance the above description in the supraglottic tumor. They can arise from the true vocal cords or be an extension from hypopharyngeal primary.

2. *Cricoarytenoid fixation.* Late sequelae of cricoarytenoid arthritis. The vocal cords are fixed on a paramedian position. On indirect laryngoscopy, it can not be differentiated from bilateral vocal cord paralysis. On direct laryngoscopy, cricoarytenoid joint is fixed.

3. *Vocal cord paralysis.* Bilateral vocal cord paralysis is required to give stridor. The vocal cords are immobile and in a paramedian position. The glottic aperture (space between the two vocal cords) is 2–4 mm.

4. *Subglottic stenosis.* Usually acquired in the adults, either from prolonged intubation or high tracheotomy. The vocal cords are normal-appearing and are usually normally mobile. Circumferential fibrotic tissues are seen below the vocal cords with airway lumen narrowing.

5. *Laryngeal trauma.* Acute: results from blunt or penetrating trauma and can have marked edema, hematoma, vocal cord avulsion, arytenoid dislocation, and posterior epiglottic displacement posterior.

Chronic: stenosis with marked distortion of anatomy and narrowing of larynx and pharynx; vocal cords may be immobile.

Psychogenic. Noisy inspiratory and expiratory breathing without any abnormalities.

Neurologic. Seen occasionally with vocal cord paralysis. Cranial nerves IX to XII are the most commonly involved cranial neuropathies, followed by V to VII involvement. Occasionally polyneuropathies may have bulbar involvement.

Thyroid. While thyroid carcinoma can cause vocal cord paralysis, this is usually unilateral. In the extensive carcinomas, bilateral vocal cord paralysis may be evident. Both carcinoma of the thyroid and markedly enlarged benign diseased thyroid glands can cause extrinsic compression of laryngeal and tracheal structures.

Neck Lymphadenopathy. Tender lymph nodes are inflammatory. Nontender lymphadenopathy is neoplastic until proven otherwise. (See Masses in the Neck).

Trachea. Carcinoma and benign tumors of the trachea are rare. Tracheal stenosis and tracheomalacia are complications of tracheotomy and can cause airway obstruction. In stenosis, the tracheal lumen is narrowed by fibrosis. In tracheomalacia, the lumen is narrowed because of the weak wall. On expiration, the tracheal wall collapses as a result of positive intrathoracic pressure.

Bronchus. Acute asthma is the most common cause of expiratory stridor from the bronchus.

Assessment

A well performed *indirect laryngoscopy* is important and often yields the diagnosis. *Tracheotomy* is indicated for any impending airway obstruction, regardless of the etiology. A rising pCO_2 or a dropping pO_2 are indications of impending obstruction.

For infections, complete blood count, proper cultures and sensitivities, and blood cultures are taken as indicated.

Lateral soft tissue x-rays of the neck and xeroradiograms are helpful, especially in trauma, neoplasm, and stenosis.

Laryngograms—dye contrast or air to-

mograms—are useful in neoplasm, trauma of the larynx, and stenosis. They help to delineate the extent of the disease. If there is significant airway compromise, only air tomography is used as the contrast dye can precipitate airway obstruction.

*Tracheogram—dye contrast or air tomogram—*is used for neoplasm, stenosis, and tracheomalacia.

Direct laryngoscopy is not necessary for acute inflammatory disease, but is mandatory for neoplastic diseases, trauma (acute or chronic), and stenosis.

Bronchoscopy is helpful if one suspects tracheal or bronchial pathology. Either rigid or fiberoptic bronchoscopy can be used, but the latter can be performed more easily with less discomfort to the patient, at the bedside or in the office.

Barium swallow and esophagoscopy are necessary for evaluation of the esophagus if one suspects esophageal extension of the neoplasm or a secondary esophageal neoplasm.

Arterial blood gas determinations are helpful in evaluating the extent of the obstruction by the stridor.

Pulmonary function tests with flow volume loop studies are helpful and can delineate the extent of extrathoracic and intrathoracic disease. This is invaluable in those patients with combined laryngeal and intrapulmonary diseases.

Allergy workup is indicated for patients with asthma and allergic rhinnitis.

Neurology workup (complete neurologic examination) is necessary for all patients with bilateral vocal cord paralysis. Bilateral vocal cord paralysis is less likely to be from a neoplastic lesion in the head and neck and thoracic region and more likely to be from a diffuse neurologic process (*e.g.,* myasthenia gravis).

Psychiatric evaluation is needed if there is suspicion of a psychogenic origin.

Thyroid evaluation, with thyroid function tests, radioactive iodine (RAI) uptake, and thyroid scan, is made if stridor is related to thyroid disorders, either benign enlargement or malignant lesions.

Neck node biopsies are rarely indicated in those with stridor. Inflammatory lymph nodes need not be biopsied. Nontender lymph nodes in patients with stridor usually indicate a carcinoma, and a lymph node biopsy compromises the treatment of the cancer.

Rheumatoid arthritis is associated with cricoarytenoid arthritis in 25%. *Autoimmune disease workup* includes rheumatoid factor, LE preparation, and antinuclear antibodies. On direct laryngoscopy, the cricoarytenoid joint is fixed (late sequela of cricoarytenoid arthritis).

Plan

Nasal Cavity/Nasopharynx. Mechanical obstruction of the nasal cavity by deviated nasal septum, polyps, and hypertrophied turbinates can be surgically corrected. Hypertrophic mucosal disease and allergic rhinitis can be treated with medication and with allergy workup and treatment. Enlarged adenoids are removed by an adenoidectomy. Carcinoma of the nasopharynx is treated by tumoricidal dose of radiation therapy to the primary tumor and neck nodes.

Oral Cavity/Oropharynx. Treatment of peritonsillar, parapharyngeal, and floor of mouth abscesses and cellulitis are described in the section on Throat Pain. Carcinoma of the base of tongue and oropharynx are treated with combination of radiation therapy, surgical excision, and radical neck dissection if lymph nodes are palpable, and adjuvant chemotherapy. Markedly enlarged tonsils are treated with tonsillectomy.

Supraglottis

1. Cysts and laryngocele: Cysts can best be managed by direct laryngoscopy and marsupialization. Internal laryngoceles can be likewise treated. If the laryngocele has both an internal and external component, an external neck approach is the procedure of choice.

2. Acute epiglottitis. Fifty percent will develop airway obstruction necessitating intubation or tracheotomy. High dose intravenous antibiotics (broad spectrum) are given. This disease is of short duration, seldom lasting over 1 week.

3. Carcinoma. Small supraglottic carcinomas rarely cause stridor. If they are small, either tumoricidal radiation therapy or conservation laryngectomy is used. If there is evidence of lymph node metastasis or a high statistical likelihood of metastasis, radical neck dissection may be performed. Usually the carcinomas are extensive, so the treatment is radiation therapy (pre- or postoperatively), total laryngectomy, radical neck dissection if lymph node spread, and adjuvant chemotherapy.

Larynx

1. Carcinoma. Treatment is the same as for supraglottic carcinoma. Usually the carcinoma is large if stridor is present.

2. Vocal cord paralysis. There must be bilateral vocal cord paralysis to give stridor. Tracheotomy is performed for airway obstruction. Then wait for 6 months for return of vocal cord function. If no return, can leave in tracheotomy indefinitely and patient still can talk. Alternative is arytenoidectomy and lateralization of one vocal cord. This allows decannulation of tracheotomy but leaves patient with a harsh, breathy voice.

3. Cricoarytenoid fixation. Treated the same way as bilateral vocal cord paralysis. The accompanying autoimmune disease (usually rheumatoid arthritis is treated with aspirin, Butazolidin, or corticosteroid).

4. Subglottic stenosis. A most difficult problem to treat. Can leave patient with permanent tracheotomy or perform some type of operation to open this area. Serial dilation of the stenotic area has been uniformly poor in opening up the stenotic area.

Trauma

1. Acute trauma: If minimal with just swelling, watch; if significant injury, open reduction is indicated.

2. Chronic trauma: Usually has marked stenosis and vocal cord dysfunction. Dilation is never successful. Surgical repair has limited success. It is best to avoid this problem with early reduction of acutely traumatized larynx.

Psychogenic Stridor. A more difficult problem to treat and best left to psychiatrist.

Neurologic Stridor. Stridor comes from bilateral vocal cord paralysis. Some neurologic processes may be treated. Myasthenia gravis can be treated, medically and/or with a thymectomy, and the vocal cords may return to normal function.

Thyroid. Carcinoma of thyroid with bilateral vocal cord paralysis is far advanced, with poor prognosis. Benign thyroid disease is usually in adenomatous goiter with large cysts, and a thyroid lobectomy will solve the airway obstruction problem. These patients should be on thyroid replacement therapy or else the remaining thyroid will enlarge and give similar problem. Rarely will Graves' disease represent with airway obstruction; if it does, suppressed and ablative therapy is used.

Trachea. Carcinoma of the trachea is rare and is treated by resection if small and by radiation if large and unresectable. All benign tracheal neoplasms are excised. Tracheal stenosis can be treated either by leaving in a permanent tracheotomy tube or by tracheal resection (Grillo method) if deemed resectable. Tracheomalacia is treated the same way as tracheal stenosis, with either resection or permanent tracheotomy.

Bronchus. Acute asthma is treated medically with epinephrine 1/1000 at 0.3–1 ml, given in divided doses subcutaneously. Aminophylline intravenously or by suppository may be needed. In some cases, intravenous steroids may be necessary.

Bibliography

Throat Pain and Odynophagia

1. Ballenger, J. *Diseases of Nose, Throat and Ear,* ed. 12. Lea & Febiger, Philadelphia, 1977.
2. DeWeese, D., and Sander, W. *Otolaryngology,* ed. 4. W. B. Saunders, Philadelphia, 1976.
3. English, G. *Otolaryngology.* Harper & Row, Hagerstown, Md., 1976.
4. Paparella, M., and Shumrick, D. *Otolaryngology,* vol. 3. W. B. Saunders, Philadelphia, 1976.
5. Strong, S. Diseases of the oral cavity and pharynx. *Orolaryngol. Clin. North Am.* 5: 2, 1972.

Dysphagia

1. Ballenger, J. *Diseases of Nose, Throat and Ear,* ed. 12, Parts II, III, and V. Lea & Febiger, Philadelphia, 1977.
2. Bockus, H. *Gastroenterology,* ed. 3, vols. 1 and 2. W. B. Saunders Co., Philadelphia, 1974 and 1976.
3. Chusid, J. G. *Correlative Neuroanatomy and Functional Neurology,* ed. 16. Lange Medical Publications, Los Altos, Calif., 1976.
4. English, G. *Otolaryngology.* Harper & Row, Hagerstown, Md., 1976.

5. Paparella, M., and Shumrick, D. *Otolaryngology,* vols. 1 and 3. W. B. Saunders Co., Philadelphia, 1973.

Hoarseness

1. Alberti, P., and Bryce, D. *Centennial Conference on Laryngeal Cancer.* Appleton-Century-Crofts, New York, 1976.
2. Ballenger, J. *Diseases of Nose, Throat and Ear,* ed. 12, Part III. Lea & Febiger, Philadelphia, 1977.
3. English, G. *Otolaryngology.* Harper & Row, Hagerstown, Md., 1976.
4. Montgomery, W. *Surgery of Upper Respiratory System,* vol. 2. Lea & Febiger, Philadelphia, 1973.
5. Ogura, J. Cancer of the head and neck. *Otolaryngol. Clin. North Am.* 2: 0, 1909.
6. Paparella, M., and Shumrick, D. *Otolaryngology,* vol. 3. W. B. Saunders Co., Philadelphia, 1973.
7. Sisson, G. Problems of the larynx. *Otolaryngol. Clin. North Am.* 3: 3, 1970.

Stridor

1. Ballenger, J. *Diseases of Nose, Throat and Ear,* ed. 12. Lea & Febiger, Philadelphia, 1977.
2. Hollinger, P. H., and Brown, W. Congenital webs, cysts, laryngoceles, and other anomalies of the larynx. *Ann. Otol. Rhinol. Laryngol.* 76: 744–752, 1967.
3. Jazbi, B. Pediatric otorhinolaryngology. *Otolaryngol. Clin. North Am.* 10: 1, 1977.
4. Montgomery, W. *Surgery of Upper Respiratory Tract,* vol. 2. Lea & Febiger, Philadelphia, 1973.
5. Paparella, M., and Shumrick, D. *Otolaryngology,* vol. 3. W. B. Saunders, Philadelphia, 1973.
6. Sisson, G. Problems of the larynx. *Otolaryngol. Clin. North Am.* 3: 3, 1970.
7. Wong, M., Finnegan, D., Kashima, H., et al. Vascularized hyoid repair for subglottic and upper tracheal stenosis. *Ann. Otol. Rhinol. Laryngol.* 87 (in press): 1978.

Chapter 13
Mass in the Neck

Raymond P. Wood II

In approaching the problem of a mass in the neck, one immediately encounters the fact that there are normally palpable masses in the neck (e.g., almost all children have multiple palpable lymph nodes). Furthermore, few areas are as subjective as the results of palpation, depending as it does upon the skill and previous experience of the examiner. The terms used in describing neck masses include "soft," "rubbery," "hard," "freely movable," "fixed," and even "relatively fixed" and "matted." Even the location of neck masses may be vague—"jugulodigastric," "high posterior triangle."

In terms of normalcy of neck masses, essentially all children below puberty have palpable neck nodes. However, nodes larger than 2 cm are distinctly abnormal. This arbitrary size is thus used as a criterion. Most adults will have persistence of at least one enlarged node from childhood, which they can often relate has been present. Its presence is often known by enlargement and regression during viral infections. Otherwise, the presence of a palpable neck node in an adult is pathologic.

Fortunately, there are some statistical guidelines as to the seriousness of palpable lumps in the neck. In children, 80% of palpable neck masses (over 2 cm) are *benign*. In adults, however, 50–80% of palpable masses are *malignant* and most of them are metastatic, usually from tumors of the head and neck.

Neck masses are described in location using the commonly described triangles of the neck. Their location also influences the likelihood of their being benign or malignant. We speak of midline masses (usually benign), anterior triangle masses (in front of the sternocleidomastoid muscles), submental triangle masses, submandibular triangle masses (either submaxillary gland or lymph nodes), and posterior triangle masses (usually malignant). Also included are supraclavicular masses (frequently metastatic disease from below the clavicles).

For the purposes of this discussion, we shall divide the masses into those of children and those of adults (although remembering that those common to one group *can* occur in the other) and we shall not discuss the supraclavicular lesions.

The evaluation of neck masses assumes the performance of a *complete* examination of the head and neck, following the taking of a complete history including general health, family history, drug history, any early radiation exposure, and history of exposure to infectious diseases such as tuberculosis.

History

Age of patient.
Place of birth and residence.
Exposure to infectious diseases, animals, birds, unpastuerized milk, etc.
Irradiation to head, neck, or thorax.
Duration of neck mass.
Growth of mass (constant and gradual, rapid, intermittent growth and shrinkage).
Pain.
Associated head and neck symptoms: pain, nasal obstruction, bleeding, ear pain, odynophagia, dysphagia, hoarseness.
Inflammation.
Recent infections, oral surgery, skin lesions.
General health: fever, night sweats, weight loss, malaise.
Family history: thyroid disease or surgery, tumors of the head and neck, endocrine disturbances.

Physical Examination

Skin and scalp lesions: infection, tumor.
Ears: *Pinnae and external auditory canals*: infection, tumor. *Middle ear*: tumor, mass behind tympanic membrane.
Nose (skin and mucous membranes): infection, tumor, obstruction of nasal passages, serosanguineous discharge.
Nasopharynx: tumor.
Oral cavity: periodontal infection, extraction sites, tumor of floor of mouth, tongue, buccal mucosa, retromolar trigone.
Oropharynx, tonsil: infection, tumor, unilateral enlargement, tonsillar pillar.
Hypopharynx: base of tongue (palpate), pharyngeal and larynx walls, epiglottis, aryepiglottic folds, pyriform sinuses (pooling of secretions), postcricoid area, false and true vocal cords.
Neck: palpation of all triangles; attention to submaxillary glands, tail of parotid, normal laryngeal crepitus, thyroid gland.

Neurologic examination: all cranial nerves with attention to V (especially infraorbital branch), VI, VII. Also palpate abdomen for liver and spleen and other nodal areas (axilla, groin, etc.)

Laboratory Studies

Minimum laboratory studies include, complete blood count (CBC), chest x-ray, and skin test for tuberculosis.

PEDIATRIC NECK MASSES

Midline Neck Masses—Children

Subjective Complaints

Most midline neck masses in children present as slowly growing, usually painless lumps. Occasionally there is a history of the mass having become tender and inflamed and perhaps draining. There are usually no systemic symptoms.

Objective Findings

The mass may be located anywhere from just beneath the chin to just above the sternal notch. The most usual location is in the area of the hyoid bone. Unless it has been infected, it will usually be unattached to the skin. It may feel cystic. Some of these masses will be attached to the isthmus of the thyroid gland.

Assessment

By far the most likely lesion in this area is a thyroglossal duct cyst. Because they are sometimes associated with absent thyroid in the usual location, a thyroid scan should be obtained. Also occurring in the midline are pyramidal thyroid lobes, which will be shown by the scan. Dermoids may present as midline lesions. Also an occasional submental lymph node may present in this way.

Plan

Thyroglossal duct cysts should be excised before they grow or become infected. It is necessary to prove the presence of functioning thyroid tissue in the normal location before excision. The important point about excision is that the midportion of the hyoid must be removed to prevent recurrence. Dermoids should be excised. Submental nodes may be watched if they don't exceed 2 cm in diameter. Occasionally, if an inflammatory node is suspected, a course of 7–10 days of antibiotics may be used.

Anterior Triangle Masses—Children

Subjective Complaints

The usual presentation is that of a slowly growing, painless, lateral neck mass. There may be rapid growth, which may or may not be associated with tenderness and overlying erythema. In some cases, there may be a history of intermittent drainage from a small sinus opening along the anterior border of the sternocleidomastoid muscle.

Objective Findings

Lateral neck masses in children may be cystic or solid. They usually lie deep to the sternocleidomastoid muscle and are freely movable. Inspection along the anterior border of the sternocleidomastoid muscle should be made for sinus openings. Also, the external auditory canal should be inspected carefully, as should the tonsillar fossa. Palpation of the thyroid gland and the lower deep jugular neck nodes should be performed. The remainder of the body should be examined for lymph nodes. A CBC, chest x-ray, and tuberculin skin tests are part of the workup. If the tuberculin test is weakly positive, skin tests for photochromogens and scotochromogens should be applied. Where low cervical lymph nodes in the area of the thyroid are found, a thyroid scan should be performed. In those patients in whom cervical sinus tracts are found, or those with external auditory canal sinus tracts, radiopaque dye contrast sinograms should be carried out.

Assessment

By far the most common lesions will be congenital. Second, will be infectious diseases, frequently chronic and often due to mycobacteria. Third, will be tumors of the thyroid gland. Also possible are lesions such as lymphomas, neuroblastomas, etc.

Plan

The treatment (and definitive diagnosis) is surgical excision. Where diagnosis is not certain, *tissue* from the mass should be sent for culture for routine fungus, and mycobacterial cultures. Pus should be examined by gram stain as well as crush preparation for sulfur granules. The finding of papillary thyroid carcinoma calls for near-total thyroidectomy and resection of any associated lymph nodes. The mycobacterial infections are treated with the appropriate antibiotic agents. Actinomycosis is very responsive to penicillin therapy. In the case of branchial cleft cysts, complete excision is necessary. Previous injection of any sinus tracts with methylene blue aids in complete removal of any tracts associated with the cyst.

Posterior Triangle Masses—Children

Subjective Complaints

Most posterior triangle masses present as discrete, slowly growing, painless masses.

Objective Findings

Examination of the scalp should be carried out to rule out melanoma and infectious lesions such as impetigo. If the lesions are seen in a child of Chinese origin, squamous cell carcinoma of the nasopharynx is a strong possibility, and an examination of the nasopharynx is indicated. Examination of the external ear canal should rule out external otitis. Other lymph node groups should be examined.

Assessment

In addition to examination of the nasopharynx under anesthesia and biopsy, x-ray examination of the base of the skull is indicated. The presence of other nodes in the body suggests lymphoma.

Plan

Infectious scalp lesions should be cultured and appropriate antibiotic therapy instituted. Any lesion resembling melanoma should be biopsied. If identified, a metastatic workup is carried out. If negative, wide resection of the primary and neck node dissection in continuity is carried out. If no lesions are found, direct biopsy of the nodes is necessary, with examination of frozen sections and culture of the node tissue.

ADULT NECK MASSES

Midline Masses—Adults

Most midline neck masses in adults are the same as those in children. The emphasis shifts toward thyroid carcinoma, however. Thyroglossal duct cysts are not uncommon in adults. The presentation and plan are the same.

Anterior Triangle Masses—Adults

Subjective Complaints

The location of the mass in the lateral neck is important. If high and in the submaxillary triangle, a history of recurrent swelling with eating is important (see Salivary Gland Disorders, Chapter 10). Slowly growing lesions in this region may be either submaxillary gland or associated lymph nodes. Most other lesions in the anterior triangle will be painless and slowly growing. A history of any oral lesions should be sought.

Objective Findings

The basic examination of nasopharynx, oropharynx, oral cavity, hypopharynx, and larynx are required. Biopsy of any suspicious obvious lesion is carried out. Masses high in the area of the mastoid tip and medial to the sternocleidomastoid should be checked to see if they move in an anterior-posterior direction and not in a superior-inferior direction. The presence of nodes low in the neck requires careful palpation of the thyroid gland.

Assessment

In adults, the most likely possibility will be metastatic tumor, usually from the head and neck. In the face of a negative clinical examination, x-ray studies of the sinuses, nasopharynx, hypopharynx (by ciné barium swallow), and larynx (by air contrast tomographic laryngogram and CAT scan) are indicated. These are followed by examination under anesthesia by direct nasopharyngoscopy, laryngoscopy, and bronchoesophagoscopy. The tonsils and base of the tongue are palpated. If no lesions are found, biopsy of the nasopharynx, tonsil, retromolar trigone, base of tongue, and pyriform sinus are carried out. If the lesion is fixed to the mandible in the submaxillary triangle, tomograms of the mandible are ordered. Any lesion of the upper neck which appears fixed to the carotid artery (in the absence of any visible primary lesion) where anterior-posterior movement, but not superior-inferior movement, is present requires carotid angiography to rule out chemodectoma (carotid body tumor).

Plan

The identification of a primary tumor (almost always a squamous cell carcinoma) will require the appropriate therapy of surgery and/or radiation therapy and usually chemotherapy. Submaxillary gland tumors are usually treated by wide resection. Infectious diseases such as actinomycosis and the mycobacterial infections, which are not uncommon in the submaxillary area, are treated with the appropriate antibiotics. Carotid body tumors should be resected and vascular anastomosis or graft carried out. Lymphomas must be biopsy-proven and the treatment is chemotherapy and/or irradiation.

Posterior Triangle Masses—Adults

The considerations are the same as for children, with nasopharyngeal carcinoma being a strong likelihood.

Bibliography

1. Altman, R. P., and Margileth, A. M. Cervical lymphadenopathy from atypical mycobacteria; diagnosis and surgical treatment. *J. Pediatr. Surg. 10:* 419–422, 1975.
2. Devine, K. D. The patient has a lump in the neck. *Postgrad. Med. 57:* 131–135, 1975.
3. *Information for Physicians—Irradiation Related Thyroid Cancer.* U. S. Department of Health, Education and Welfare, Publication No. (NIH) 77-1110. U. S. Government Printing Office, Washington, D. C., 1977.
4. Jaffe, B. F., and Jaffe, N. Head and neck tumors in children. *Pediatrics 51:* 731–740, 1973.
5. MacComb, W. S. Diagnosis and treatment of metastatic cervical cancerous nodes from an unknown primary site. *Am. J. Surg. 124:* 441–449, 1972.
6. Proctor, B., and Proctor, C. Congenital lesions of the head and neck. *Otolaryngol. Clin. North Am. 3:* 221–248, 1970.
7. Putney, F. J. The diagnosis of head and neck masses in children. *Otolaryngol. Clin. North Am. 3:* 277–299, 1970.
8. Winegar, L. K., and Griffin, W. The occult primary tumor. *Arch. Otolaryngol. 98:* 159, 1970.

Chapter 14
Disorders of Speech and Articulation

Darrel L. Teter

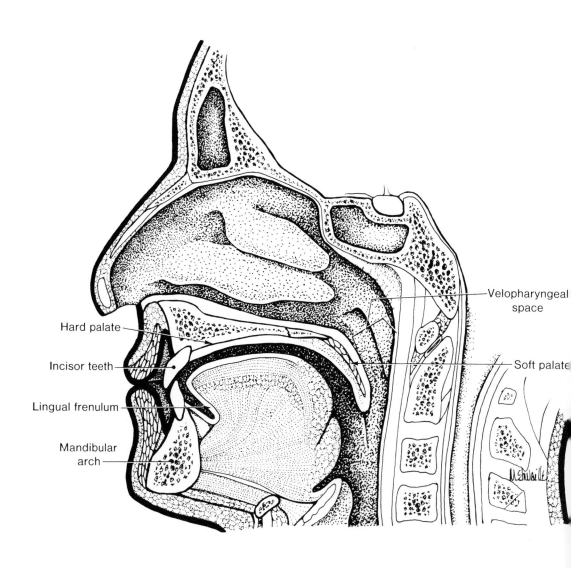

SPEECH AND LANGUAGE DELAY

It is not uncommon for the parent of a 2- to 3-year-old child to present to the physician the complaint that the child is not talking. Too often the response to the parent is, "Wait, he or she will talk when ready."

The process of developing speech and language is a complicated one essential to a normal existence. The acquisition of speech and language is linked to age readiness, requiring early intervention and management of the child with abnormal speech and language development.

Diagnostic Approach

Subjective Complaints

Speech and language delay is most commonly seen on a developmental basis and will often resolve itself with time and sufficient environmental stimulation. Several pertinent areas need be examined by the physician before determining the necessity and course of further evaluation.

1. Language and speech are more often delayed in males. A general "rule of thumb" places the male child 3–6 months behind the female.

2. Delay is more common in second children and markedly more common when the first child is female and the second is male. This most probably is due to several factors, including the fact that the normal sex differences are more noticeable when an older sister's language is being compared to a younger brother's developing language.

3. Often a youngster's speech and language will not develop in a normal manner because he or she has no need for language. If a child's immediate needs are all being anticipated and met without requiring structured verbal output, then there will be no need for structured verbal output and normal development will not occur. The child must receive language stimulation and be required to respond. He must also be rewarded for responding if language and speech are to develop.

Objective Findings

If it appears that the delay is developmental, more parental stimulation and pa-
tience should be suggested and the child's development should be reevaluated in 90 days. If, however, it appears that adequate stimulation is present and the child is more than 6 months delayed, then referrals for further evaluation are necessary. (For Language Developmental Chart see English, G. M.: *Otolaryngology*, Chapter 52, pp. 573–576, Harper & Row, 1976.)

Assessment

If familial or birth history suggests predisposition or high risk for hearing loss, then audiometrics are always indicated. In the hands of skilled personnel, very accurate audiometrics can be obtained from children as young as 7 months, without the use of highly sophisticated instrumentation.

If the subjective complaint is one of speech problems (poor articulation) the oral-peripheral mechanism should be evaluated to make certain that the mechanism is normal. The tongue should have sufficient range of motion to protrude through the teeth, to touch the lateral apex of the lips, and to curl and touch the alveolar ridge. If such a range is not possible, a paresis or a short lingual frenulum must be suspected and ruled out.

If the child is not developing normal expressive and/or receptive language, then referral should be to a competent speech and language pathologist.

Plan

Referral for audiometrics and speech and language evaluations should be made whenever it appears to the primary care physician that the delayed speech and language is not within normal developmental limits.

The audiometric evaluation will reveal whether auditory acuity is within normal limits for the acquisition of speech and language. The presence of any conductive hearing loss will necessitate medical and/or surgical intervention, and most probably otologic referral.

The presence of any significant sensorineural hearing loss will necessitate amplification in the form of a hearing aid and, perhaps, immediate placement for long-term language and educational needs.

Often, it is determined by a professional

evaluation that the child presents with specific delays, either in acquiring normal articulation or in acquiring and using expressive and receptive language. In such instances, the speech and language pathologist will design and institute the program best suited for the long-term needs of the child.

STUTTERING

One of the most perplexing and important questions facing the primary care physician arises when the parents of a child developing speech become concerned that he or she is going to stutter. Of all the speech problems possible, the one of most concern to the general population is stuttering.

Diagnostic Approach

Subjective Complaints

The problem arises when the child developing speech and language begins to repeat words or phrases. Many parents instantly become concerned that the child is going to develop into a stutterer. The presenting complaint is always, "He or she is starting to stutter." The universal response is, "Don't worry, it will go away." Such may not be good advice since the development of stuttering is, in part, dependent upon the family attitudes toward the child's developing speech. Several important facts concerning the normal dysfluencies of developing speech need to be known before advice can be given to the parents of a youngster.

1. Normal developmental dysfluencies occur in all children as they acquire speech.
2. Normal dysfluencies occur as the child (a) develops speech; (b) meets intense changes in his or her life; or (c) enters the educational system.
3. Normal dysfluencies can occur as word, sound, or phrase repetitions; as hesitations; or as sound prolongations. Dysfluencies may occur as often as 20% of the time.
4. Normal dysfluencies are not accompanied by any secondary characteristics

(such as head movements or facial grimaces).
5. When the family and/or child begins to react to the dysfluencies in a negative manner, then the reinforcement that occurs may lead to true pathology.

Objective Findings

When the complaint is heard that a child is beginning to "stutter," several areas of concern need to be reviewed:
1. What form is the dysfluency taking? Is the child repeating words or phrases, or is he or she prolonging words?
2. What percentage of the utterances are dysfluent? Is it occurring more than 25–30% of the time (more than 30 dysfluencies out of every 100 words or phrases)?
3. Is the child reacting to the dysfluencies? Are the family members beginning to react by asking the child to talk differently?
4. Has the child developed any secondary characteristics that accompany the dysfluencies?

If the primary care physician feels that the parental concerns center around normal developmental dysfluencies, then they can be counseled that with caution, the problem should resolve itself. If, however, they are unduly concerned, or the child is beginning to respond negatively to the dysfluencies, then referral to a qualified speech pathologist should be made.

Plan

The speech pathologist will review the situation and make a decision either to indirectly treat the child through family counseling, or to treat the child directly with therapy.

Indirect treatment through counseling will be recommended if:
1. The dysfluencies are within normal range of development.
2. No secondary characteristics are developing.
3. The child has shown no anxiety concerning his dysfluencies.

Under these circumstances, the parents will be counseled so that they do not negatively reinforce the dysfluencies and do attempt to establish an atmosphere conducive to good speech development. Such an atmosphere allows for expression of thoughts and ideas at the child's pace.

Direct treatment through therapy will be suggested if:

1. The child has developed secondary characteristics.

2. If the child's dysfluency rate exceeds the 20% expected dysfluency rate.

3. If parental counseling fails to produce a reduction in the amount of dysfluencies or in the anxiety level felt by the child and/or family.

ADULT APHASOID DISORDERS

On occasion, the physician will be presented with language disorders in an adult whose problem masks itself as a hearing problem or a problem of memory loss secondary to fatigue. It is of essence that measures be taken to ascertain if the complaint is one of a developing aphasia that could be related to involvement of the central nervous system.

Diagnostic Approach

Subjective Complaints

Often the physician may be presented with complaints such as: (1) "I can't understand the words people say to me," or (2) "I can't seem to recall the names of objects or individuals," or (3) "I try and say the name of something and another word comes out," or (4) "I get very confused when I must deal with numbers or abstract concepts."

When such subjective complaints are related, formal evaluation is immediately indicated.

Objective Findings

The patient complaining of receptive or expressive language problems should be referred for neurologic evaluation and for language evaluation. The referral should be made as quickly as possible and a definitive diagnosis of the neurologic and language status made as quickly as possible.

Plan

The neurologic evaluation should be done to rule out cortical involvement secondary to neoplastic disease, trauma, or occlusive or degenerative vascular disease. The language evaluation should be made to determine the specific areas of expressive and/or receptive involvement and the nature of the involvement. Such information is essential to providing immediate and long-term care for the patient with aphasoid disorders.

Bibliography

1. Bloodstein, O. *A Handbook of Stuttering.* Brooklyn College, Brooklyn, N. Y., 1975.
2. Eisenson, J. *Adult Aphasia, Assessment and Treatment.* Prentice-Hall, Inc., Englewood Cliffs, N. J., 1973.
3. English, G. M. *Otolaryngology,* Chapter 52. Harper & Row, Hagerstown, Md., 1976.
4. *If Your Child Stutters, A Guide for Parents.* Publication No. 11, Speech Foundation of America, Memphis.
5. Schuell, Jenkins, and Jiminez-Pabon. *Aphasia in Adults, Diagnosis, Prognosis and Treatment.* Harper & Row, New York, 1964.

Chapter 15
Enophthalmos

W. Bruce Wilson

Enophthalmos is a backward displacement of one or both eyes in relation to the surrounding bony orbit. As with proptosis, measurement can be made with an exophthalmometer.

This is a rarer condition than proptosis. In most cases the etiology is easier to uncover than in proptosis. History taking is important but it is more simplified than in proptosis. Age, sex and race do not afford any significant help in diagnosis. Since the major diagnoses are congenital eye or orbital malformation, orbital inflammation, trauma, radiation, and, rarely, tumors, the history is directed toward these entities. All are slow in development. Family history may help in regard to defining an orbital malformation.

Objective signs that are so helpful in proptosis are not of significant value here. In other words, retropulsion characteristics, lid signs, vascular signs and signs of cranial nerve compromise are not significantly different in any one of the diagnostic groups.

Associated systemic symptoms and signs are helpful only in orbital tumors that may lead to enophthalmos. Scirrhous breast carcinoma metastatic to the orbit may lead to enophthalmos. Intracranial tumors do not lead to enophthalmos.

Specific Etiologies

The eye may be congenitally small and therefore set deeper in the orbit, giving enophthalmos. This is uncommon. Even more rare would be an unusually deep orbit. A mild degree of this undoubtedly accounts for people who seem to have "deep-set eyes."

Any condition that causes an atrophy of orbital structures may give enophthalmos. This is most apt to occur with fat atrophy. Thus orbital infection or pseudotumor may lead to enophthalmos when the condition resolves. By history one would probably be able to reconstruct the cause (see Chapter 16, Proptosis). Facial hemiatrophy may be associated with enophthalmos. In this case, the associated facial changes make the diagnosis relatively straightforward. Occasionally orbital varices will produce mild enophthalmos after many episodes. Radiation destruction of orbital fat is another cause.

Tumors are rarely associated with enophthalmos. As mentioned above, a breast carcinoma might be the most likely. A longstanding benign tumor that had produced marked pressure in the orbit might lead to enophthalmos when it is surgically removed.

Trauma is perhaps the most common cause of enophthalmos. If enough tissue is lost by prolapse into a sinus, by loss of lid and orbit structures, or by surgical excision, enophthalmos may result. This is usually seen in cases of orbital floor fracture.

There are a few unusual, transient causes of enophthalmos. A simultaneous retractive action of all of the rectus muscles, as seen in pineal tumors, may produce retraction mystagmus. This is seen only when the patient tries to look away from center gaze.

Assessment

In enophthalmos associated with trauma about the eye, a sinus x-ray series or facial fracture views are ordered. Opacity or fluid level in the maxillary or ethmoid sinuses is evidence of fracture. In orbital floor fractures, entrapment of the inferior rectus muscle and damage to the infraorbital nerve may occur.

References

1. Duke-Elder System of Ophthalmology, Vol. XIII, pg. 1235 (enophthalmos).
2. Moss, H. M. Expanding lesions of the orbit. *Am. J. Ophthalmol.* 54: 761–770, 1962.
3. Pfeiffer, R. C. Traumatic enophthalmos. A. O. 30: 718–726, 1943.
4. Smigiel, M. R., and MacCarty, C. S. Exophthalmos; the more commonly encountered neurosurgical lesions. *Mayo Clin. Proc* 50: 345–355, 1975.
5. Wright, J. E., *et al.* Computerized axial tomography in the detection of orbital space occupying lesions. *Am. J. Ophthalmol.* 80: 78–84, 1975.
6. Zakharia, H. S. *et al.* Unilateral exophthalmos; aetiological study of 85 cases. *Br. J. Ophthalmol.* 56: 678–686, 1972.

Chapter 16
Proptosis

W. Bruce Wilson

The term proptosis as generally used is synonymous with exophthalmos. The term signifies that one or both eyes are displaced in a direction anterior to their normal position within the orbit. In addition to being proptotic the eye may be displaced up, down, medially, or laterally. The eye is rarely displaced in one of these directions without proptosis. Whether an eye is proptotic or not can usually be determined by a careful visual inspection of the relative position of the two eyes. An exophthalmometer can be used to obtain an objective measurement of a proptotic eye. An exophthalmometer is also valuable for determining bilateral proptosis and for following the clinical course of proptosis.

PLAN OF EVALUATION

There are several subjective and objective features of proptosis that one needs to consider when examining a given patient.

Subjective Considerations

Age, sex, and race are important. Some tumors are found almost entirely in childhood. Examples would be neuroblastoma, rhabdomyosarcoma, and medulloblastoma. Meningiomas are tumors of middle-aged white women. Nasopharyngeal carcinomas are more common in Chinese males.

One needs to inquire about the past history of a tumor that could have metastasized from a distant site or by direct extension. Skin, lung, breast, and central nervous system tumors are perhaps the most common. A history of hyperthyroidism may be helpful, since a patient may present in a euthyroid state and have thyroid orbitopathy. Trauma produces multiple complications that may lead to proptosis, e.g., bleeding, edema, and infection. Pregnancy may be associated with a relatively rapid enlargement of both meningiomas and pituitary adenomas. Intermittent proptosis suggests orbital varices. Bilateral proptosis is usually secondary to hyperthyroidism, orbit pseudotumor, or cavernous sinus disease. The rapid onset of proptosis suggests hematoma, edema, or infection. Occasionally thyroid orbitopathy and orbital pseudotumor present with the rapid progression of proptosis. In children rahbdomyosarcoma is often rapid in course. In adults metastatic tumors may change rapidly. If proptosis responds to steroids one would suspect orbital pseudotumor. Occasionally meningiomas and hemangiomas are somewhat responsive.

A family history of von Recklinghausen's disease or retinoblastoma of the eye may provide a clue to the etiology of the proptosis.

Objective Considerations

A clinical impression of the consistency of the "mass" may be obtained by retropulsing the eye into orbit. If the orbit is very soft it suggests a benign tumor or encephalocele. If the eye is very difficult to retropulse it is suggestive of a malignant lesion. Thyroid orbitopathy falls in between.

Lid signs are important from two aspects. Ecchymosis of the lids suggests dyscrasia or neuroblastoma. A mass involving the lid structures suggests a tumor in the anterior part of the orbit, such as a dermoid cyst, a lacrimal gland tumor, or a hemangioma. Orbital varices may be seen in the lower fornix when the lid is retracted.

Vascular signs are of importance because they suggest either collagen vascular disease, Graves' disease, cavernous sinus disease, or vascular tumors. The signs to look for are edema of the lids, edema of the conjunctiva, and dilated vessels of the conjunctiva. Pulsating proptosis would suggest a carotid cavernous sinus fistula or an encephalocele, primarily. An orbital bruit may be heard in the presence of a vascular tumor or a fistula.

A decrease in vision and the presence of diplopia are indicative of an infiltrating lesion. If a tumor is present it is more likely malignant. In the absence of visual loss and the presence of diplopia one would think of a benign orbital lesion.

Associated neurologic and systemic symptoms and signs need to be considered. Intracranial neurologic signs may suggest a tumor of the intracranial cavity or cavernous sinus disease. Ear, nose, and throat symptoms may suggest the possibility of disease in the sinus such as a mucocele or tumor. Pharyngeal signs may suggest a

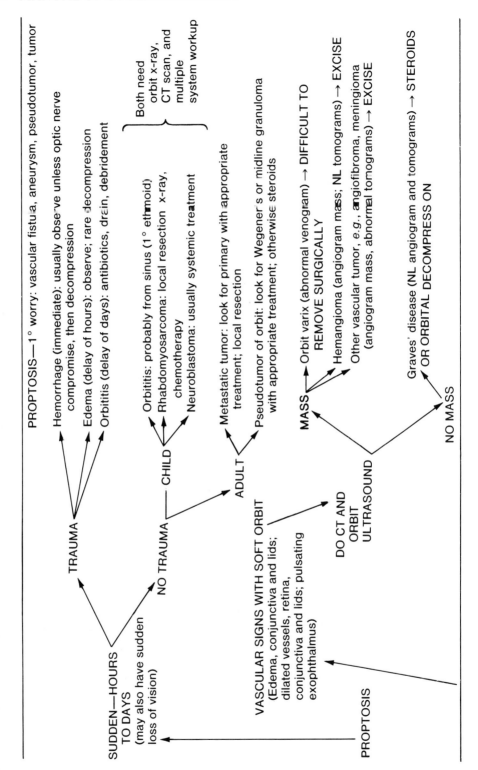

PROPTOSIS—1° worry: vascular fistula, aneurysm, pseudotumor, tumor

TRAUMA

Hemorrhage (immediate): usually observe unless optic nerve compromise, then decompression

Edema (delay of hours): observe; rare decompression

Orbititis (delay of days): antibiotics, drain, debridement

NO TRAUMA — CHILD

Orbititis: probably from sinus (1° ethmoid)

Rhabdomyosarcoma: local resection x-ray, chemotherapy

Neuroblastoma: usually systemic treatment

Both need orbit x-ray, CT scan, and multiple system workup

ADULT

Metastatic tumor: look for primary with appropriate treatment; local resection

Pseudotumor of orbit: look for Wegener's or midline granuloma with appropriate treatment; otherwise steroids

MASS

Orbit varix (abnormal venogram) → DIFFICULT TO REMOVE SURGICALLY

Hemangioma (angiogram mass; NL tomograms) → EXCISE

Other vascular tumor, e.g., angiofibroma, meningioma (angiogram mass, abnormal tomograms) → EXCISE

NO MASS

Graves' disease (NL angiogram and tomograms) → STEROIDS OR ORBITAL DECOMPRESS ON

SUDDEN—HOURS TO DAYS (may also have sudden loss of vision)

VASCULAR SIGNS WITH SOFT ORBIT (Edema, conjunctiva and lids; dilated vessels, retina, conjunctiva and lids; pulsating exophthalmus)

DO CT AND ORBIT ULTRASOUND

PROPTOSIS

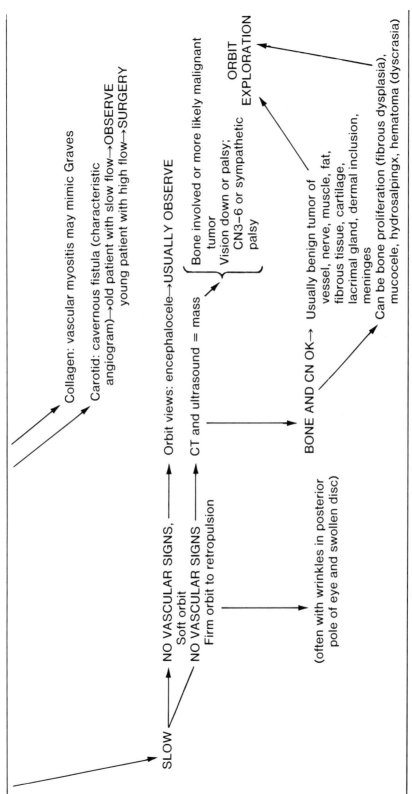

Figure 16.1.

nasopharyngeal tumor. Systemic signs may help one detect dyscrasia, histiocytosis, sarcoid, neuroblastoma, or tumors of the breast and lung that have involved the orbit.

All of the cases of proptosis in the following discussion are considered as unilateral. Less commonly, bilateral proptosis is seen. It may be congenital as in craniofacial dysostosis. Osteopathies may cause bilateral proptosis. Examples are fibrous dysplasia, osteitis deformans, infantile cortical hyperostosis, leontiasis ossea, osteopetrosis, and acromegaly. The most common cause would be hyperthyroidism. Occasionally nonspecific pseudotumor or specific pseudotumor (e.g., Wegener's granulomatosis) may cause bilateral changes as well as cavernous sinus disease. Rarely, neoplasia such as lymphoma or histiocytoma is a cause. Systemic amyloidosis has rarely been associated with changes in both orbits.

Radiographic Studies

Soft Tissue. Soft tissue studies may be helpful in the differential consideration of proptosis. Abnormal collections of calcium (often seen better with the CT scan than with conventional x-rays) would suggest old infection or trauma, or the possibility of a tumor (dermoid, retinoblastoma, meningioma). An air-fluid in a sinus would indicate trauma or infection in most cases. Occasionally an adjacent orbital tumor will exhibit this finding. Soft tissue studies may indicate a mass in the orbit with a distinct edge. This would suggest a tumor rather than pseudotumor. Free gas in the orbit suggests mucocele, wall fracture or, rarely, infection by gas-producing organisms.

Bone Studies. Dense, thick bone may be diagnostic of a dysplasia of bone causing the proptosis (fibrous dysplasia, Paget's disease, osteopetrosis, or Hurler's disease) or a tumor adjacent to bone (meningioma or hemangioma). Bone destruction almost always indicates a tumor (probably malignant) or infection of bone. Rarely, pseudotumor may do this. A mucocele may displace bone. Enlargement of normal orbital dimensions of foramina may indicate specific diagnoses: enlarged optic canal (optic glioma, craniopharyngioma, nasopharyngeal tumor, pituitary adenoma), enlarged superior orbital fissure (neurofibromatosis, meningioma), or enlarged lacrimal fossa (lacrimal gland tumor).

Vessel Studies. Arteriovenous malformations, aneurysms, carotid cavernous fistulas, and vascular tumors (meningioma, angiofibroma, or hemangioma) can be detected by carotid arteriography. Orbital venography is essential to establish the diagnosis of orbital varices or cavernous sinus thrombosis.

SPECIFIC EXAMPLES OF PROPTOSIS

Sudden Onset of Proptosis within a Few Hours of Trauma

Subjective Complaints

The proptosis comes on a few hours after relatively severe trauma, caused by a blunt object, and remains stable. Blurred vision and diplopia occur in association with the proptosis. The orbit feels very uncomfortable as if it were going to explode. The eyelids are quite black and blue.

Objective Findings

Examination indicates vision is moderately reduced but it is difficult to determine because of the swollen lids. The pupil on the side of the injury is mildly dilated and does not respond as well to light as the pupil on the other side. The eye moves but is somewhat limited in all directions. There is no specific restriction of one direction, which would suggest a cranial nerve palsy. Visual fields are full to a confrontation finger-counting method. The ophthalmoscopic examination of the eye does not reveal any obvious damage. Examination of the orbit and lids reveals the lids to be markedly swollen and ecchymotic. Retropulsion of the eye is very difficult to accomplish. The orbit seems very tense and it is painful to push on the eye.

Assessment

The history of sudden onset of proptosis following blunt trauma is suggestive of hemorrhage or edema in the orbit. The markedly swollen ecchymotic lids would be further evidence for this. The fact that the orbit is very tense and painful when one attempts to push the eye back in the orbit also would further suggest this possibility. The fact that the pupil is slightly dilated and does not respond as well as the other pupil to light indicates a concussion effect on the iris. The fact that the eye moves poorly in all directions and does not have loss of movement in one plane favors a mechanical limitation of movement within the orbit, e.g., edema or blood rather than a cranial nerve palsy. The differential between hemorrhage into the orbit and edema of the orbit would be primarily based on the fact that edema develops over a number of hours and hemorrhage is essentially immediate. Edema does not produce as tense an orbit as hemorrhage does. Additionally, pain is more severe with an orbital hemorrhage.

Plan

The workup would include skull and orbit x-rays and a blood count. The presence of fractures of the orbital walls would further complicate the problem of management. For example, a blowout fracture of the floor or medial wall of the orbit might entail surgery to correct that problem. However, the absence of fracture would allow the physician to concentrate on the question of whether to decompress the orbit and remove the hematoma, or alternatively, to observe the patient. Because most patients are very uncomfortable it is difficult to get the patient to cooperate well in order to obtain the best possible vision. The concern about severe ocular damage is largely alleviated if the eye examination is normal. If there is further question, tomograms of the optic nerve canal may be done to exclude the possibility of fracture in that area compromising the optic nerve. In general both hemorrhage and edema into the orbit may be managed by observation. In the event that optic nerve function is gradually decreasing in the face of edema and dilated veins of the optic nerve head, one may elect to decompress the orbit. There are four accepted approaches to decompression of the orbit. The more benign procedures would involve removal of the lateral wall, orbital floor, or ethmoid air cells. The transfrontal removal of the orbital roof is done by some but involves the possible complications of the neurosurgical procedure. It would be rare that adequate decompression could not be obtained by a combination of the benign approaches.

Sudden Onset of Proptosis 3 Days after Trauma

Subjective Complaints

Injury occurs 3 days before the sudden onset of proptosis. The proptosis develops over a period of 1 day. Part of the trauma may have been caused by a sharp instrument that perforated the lids. Intense pain is associated with the onset of proptosis. Pain had not been present in the first 2 days post-trauma. Vision was fairly suddenly reduced. The eye is painful to move or even to light touch. The patient feels generally ill as if he might have the flu.

Objective Findings

Vision is significantly reduced. The pupil is the same size as the other eye but reacts poorly to direct light. The other pupil, of the normal eye, reacts very briskly to direct light. This defines a defect in afferent transmission of the optic nerve on the proptotic side. Ocular mobility is almost zero. The patient will not attempt to move the eye in one direction or another. He complains of severe pain when asked to do this. It is difficult for the patient to count fingers in any of the four major quadrants of the visual field. The optic nerve is swollen with dilated veins. This indicates external pressure on the optic nerve. Examination of the orbit reveals the lids are very swollen and tender. They are also red. The conjuctiva is swollen. Even the slightest attempt to push the eye back into the orbit is painful and the patient does everything possible to resist this maneuver. The patient is not febrile in spite of his complaints of a flu-like feeling. Careful examination of the swollen lids reveals what appears to be a small puncture wound in the upper lid in the central area.

Assessment

The delay in development of sudden proptosis associated with severe pain, loss of vision, and other signs suggestive of infection points toward an orbital cellulitis. The swelling of the conjunctiva, while it may be found in hemorrhage or edema of the orbit, makes one particularly concerned about the possibility of infection. The marked swelling of the lid with redness in the absence of ecchymosis also would support this suggestion. The extreme tenderness of the eye and orbit are further indications of infection.

Plan

Orbit and optic canal x-ray views are obtained to be sure there is no fracture complicating the problem. In children fractures of the ethmoid sinus may be associated with orbital cellulitis. This is particularly true if this is associated with chronic infection in the sinus. The x-rays help exclude the possibility of a foreign body within the orbit. Most metallic foreign bodies are tolerated well within the orbit but organic material almost routinely causes infection. A CAT scan may help define a nonmetallic foreign body. A blood count is done and reveals an elevated white count of 10,000–15,000 WBC with a shift to the left. This further confirms the suspected cellulitis. The area of perforation may be probed to obtain purulent material. The abscess may be drained through the primary site of the penetrating injury. Further orbital surgery may not be necessary. Occasionally cellulitis or abscess or both lids will appear to make the eye proptotic. If the lids are swollen but the conjunctiva is not and the eye is not displaced relative to the other eye, the diagnosis would be periorbital cellulitis. This has a much better

prognosis in regard to vision and eye movement than does an orbital cellulitis. This connotes that the orbital septum, which separates the lid structures from the orbit, has not been perforated and so the orbital space is not infected.

"Sudden" Development of Proptosis over 3 Days in a Child, Unassociated with Trauma

Subjective Complaints

Usually it is a child under 5 years of age who presents with the sudden development of proptosis. The proptosis will have developed over a period of 3 days and the maximum amount of development is usually over a 1-day period. The child will have been perfectly well until 3 weeks before the proptosis. At that point the relatively sudden onset of pain develops about the left side of the face with fever after a mild cold. These symptoms may have resolved when the proptosis begins. The lids will be quite swollen and red, and the eye is very tender to touch.

Objective Findings

Examination confirms that the eyelids are swollen and red. The conjunctiva is swollen. The patient resists all efforts to touch or manipulate the eye and will not move the eye voluntarily. The patient seems to be in a considerable amount of pain and is found to be running an elevated temperature. Vision is blurred but cannot be tested well. The field of vision is poor. The pupil reacts poorly to direct light and the optic disc is swollen.

Assessment

The history suggests ethmoid sinusitis followed within a short time by proptosis. Pain and the associated fever suggest orbititis. The history is quite sudden for a tumor of the orbit.

Plan

Sinus x-rays show the ethmoid sinuses are opaque. The white count is elevated with a left shift. The plan at this point would be to decompress the ethmoid sinus directly and drain the sinus into the nose. Systemic antibiotics are begun, using ampicillin or other agents effective against *Haemophilus influenzae* plus penicillin until sensitivities are obtained. If the orbit seems quite soft at the end of the procedure the periorbita need not be opened. If the space inside the orbital periosteum seems quite tight, the periosteum (periorbita) over the ethmoid plate can be opened in an "H"-type incision to allow decompression of the orbital contents.

"Sudden" Development of Proptosis over 2 Weeks in a Child, Unassociated with Trauma

Subjective Complaints

The history is that the progression of proptosis has been relatively rapid but not of the 1- to 2-day variety that was seen with the orbital cellulitis. This proptosis will have developed over a period of 2 weeks. The child is usually about 4 years old and has been in perfect health until the onset of proptosis. There has been no fever or any other constitutional symptoms until the proptosis started. Since that time the child has been fussy and has not eaten well. The lids have not been particularly red or edematous but there has been ecchymosis of one upper lid starting about the time the proptosis was first noticed.

Objective Findings

Examination indicates that vision is quite good, the pupil reacts normally to light, but ocular motility is markedly restricted. It does not suggest a cranial nerve palsy but suggests something in and about the muscles that is restricting the movement of the eye. Visual field examination is grossly normal. Examination of the fundus reveals only mild edema of the optic disc. The eye is not particularly tender although the child does not want the eye touched. The attempts to push the eye back into the orbit reveal that the orbit is essentially filled with a solid lesion. The globe is proptotic but the lids are only mildly swollen and not particularly red. The conjunctiva is only minimally swollen. Ecchymosis is noted in the upper lid. The presence of ecchymosis suggests the possibility of a tumor such as a neuroblastoma. Rhabdomyosarcoma would also be a possibility. The child is afebrile and the white count is normal. No other signs of disease are found but the child seems fussy.

Assessment

The development of proptosis over a 2-week period in a child, 4 years of age, without trauma, suggests the possibility of a rapidly growing mass in the orbit. The two significant diagnoses would include rhabdomyosarcoma and neuroblastoma.

Plan

Workup includes x-rays of the orbit, adjacent sinuses, and the optic canal. These examinations are normal. Further examination indicates that the blood count and physical examination are within normal limits. Computerized tomography reveals a large fairly localized mass in the posterior medial orbit without any intracranial component. At this point a careful search is made of the abdomen and chest by radiology to determine if there are masses along the anterior paraspinal area suggesting a neuroblastoma. A suspicious posterior mediastinal mass may be noted. An intravenous pyelogram (IVP) would be done to evaluate the condition of the perirenal tissues. If this is normal, a neuroendocrine workup is done to determine if there is an increase in adrenaline and nonadrenaline substances being excreted in the urine. The finding of elevated values would suggest a neuroblastoma. A bone marrow should be done, to look for abnormal cells suggesting neuroblastoma. Medical and surgical oncology should then be consulted in regard to chemotherapy and radiation therapy of the marrow and the mediastinal tumor. The orbit probably will not require surgery but would be treated by chemotherapy and radiation. If the other studies are normal, an orbital exploration would be carried out to determine whether a rhabdomyocarcoma was present. If that were present, orbital exenteration would be followed by chemotherapy and radiation therapy.

"Sudden" Development of Proptosis in an Adult, Unassociated with Trauma

Subjective Complaints

Frequently seen in middle-aged women who have been perfectly well until a few weeks before consulting the physician. The patient may have developed the proptosis over 10 days to 2 weeks. This may be accompanied by some pain and double vision. Vision in the eye may be reduced. Otherwise, there are no constitutional symptoms. History may reveal a previous malignant tumor such as a breast tumor. Otherwise history is negative.

Objective Findings

The eye is moderately proptosed but the lids and conjunctiva are relatively normal. Vision is reduced by a mild amount. The eye does not move well and movement is restricted in all directions. There is no suggestion of a cranial nerve palsy. Visual fields are relatively normal. Examination of the eye reveals mild edema of the optic nerve head. The orbit is quite stiff to retropulsion but there is no particular pain involved. Cranial nerve examination reveals that there is probably anesthesia or at least hypesthesia of the cornea on that side.

Assessment

The relatively sudden development of proptosis in an adult women who has had no trauma and who has had previous malignancy suggests a metastatic disease of the orbit.

Plan

X-rays of the orbit, optic canal, and associated sinuses reveal bone erosion in the greater and lesser wings of the sphenoid. Further workup with computerized tomography reveals a fairly localized mass in the orbital apex. Probably the bulk of this is in the muscle cone. There is no intracranial extension of the lesion seen. The next avenue of approach would be to determine whether there are other sites of metastasis present. If there are none excision of the tumor with exenteration, radiation, and chemotherapy would be considered. If there are other sites of tumor metastasis present, then surgery of the orbit probably would not be carried out but radiation and chemotherapy would be considered. Other metastatic disease that would have to be considered would be bowel carcinoma and lymphoma. If the patient were a male, lung and prostate carcinoma would be significant considerations.

"Sudden" Development of Proptosis in an Adult, Unassociated with Trauma

Subjective Complaints

In this case there is a sudden development of proptosis without any history of previous malignant disease. The signs and symptoms are very similar to those noted for the metastatic breast tumor (see preceding section).

Objective Findings

Visual acuity is reduced slightly. The pupil reacts in a relatively normal fashion. Ocular motility is restricted in a similar fashion to that seen in orbital metastasis. Visual fields are relatively full. Examination of the eye does not reveal any abnormalities. Cranial nerves do not reveal dysfunction. The orbit is quite firm to retropulsion but is not particularly painful and there is only mild edema of the lids and conjunctiva with some dilated vessels of the conjunctiva. The general physical examination is normal.

Assessment

This symptom complex suggests the possibility of a pseudotumor of the orbit. As can be seen it resembles quite closely the metastatic tumor problem described above. On occasion these problems are also associated with other granulomatous disease such as Wegener's midline granuloma. The chance of a primary malignancy of the orbit is possible but somewhat unlikely without a clear history for a primary.

Plan

X-rays of the orbit, paranasal sinuses, and optic canal do not reveal any abnormality with the exception that there is some erosion of bone along the ethmoid plate. Computerized tomography will reveal a very ill-defined mass filling most of the posterior part of the orbit. There is no intracranial component. At this point the decision is made to explore the orbit. Fibrous "tumor" is found that fills most of the orbital cavity. It surrounds muscles and nerves and could not be removed in its entirety without a risk of destroying visual function. Therefore, it is biopsied. It is found to be made up of fibrous tissue with chronic inflammatory cells, lymphocytes, and plasmacytes. Surgery is then terminated. A permanent section confirmed probable pseudotumor of the orbit. The appropriate treatment is with steroids.

Recurrent Sudden Proptosis in a Young Adult Male

Subjective Complaints

The patient will have had multiple recurrences since childhood of sudden proptosis in which there has been pain and some visual difficulty. Each episode lasts for several days to a couple of weeks. Usually the eye is quite red and lids and conjunctiva are swollen. Usually the problem has resolved without treatment. In between the episodes the orbit and eye are perfectly normal.

Objective Findings

The orbit is moderately stiff to retropulsion but the conjunctiva and lids are swollen. The vessels over the conjunctiva are quite dilated. The eye does not move well but vision, pupils, and fields are normal.

There are no cranial nerve findings. Two or three dilated vessels are noted in the inferior fornix.

Assessment

The fact that the patient has had multiple episodes of sudden proptosis lasting for 2 days to 2 weeks and that resolve, leaving the eye and orbit normal, is almost pathognomonic for orbital varices.

Plan

The plan in addition to the routine x-rays of the orbit, paranasal sinuses, and optic canal is to do orbital venography. It may be difficult to fill the varices during the time there is proptosis. Between episodes orbital venography and angiography may reveal large varices in the orbit. The usual treatment is observation with the possibility of added steroids. The varices can be removed if they are anterior to the orbital septum or if they are in the anterior part of the orbit and compromise only one or two large channels.

Gradual Development of Proptosis in an Adult, Associated with Prominent Diffuse Vascular Signs

Subjective Complaints

There is gradual development of proptosis associated with very little pain or disturbance in vision. The prominent feature aside from the proptosis has been swelling of the lids, conjunctiva, and dilated vessels over the conjunctiva. Otherwise there is no complaint.

Objective Findings

Findings indicate exactly what the patient says. Vision is essentially normal with normal pupil reaction. Visual fields are full. Ocular motility is only minimally limited, if at all. The fundus of the eye and the rest of the ocular structures are normal. Cranial nerves are normal. Examination of the orbit reveals mild proptosis with edema of the lids and conjunctiva and dilated vessels of the conjunctiva. The eye can be retropulsed into the orbit quite easily and painlessly.

Assessment

This chain of events suggests the possibility of an inflammatory or vascular lesion of the orbit. The primary concern would be one of an orbital myopathy related to hyperthyroidism or collagen vascular disease.

Plan

Workup includes the usual x-rays of the orbit, sinuses, and optic canal, which are normal. Blood workup further is done to evaluate the possibility of vasculitis and thyroid disease. It is found that the vasculitis workup, including RA, ANA, CBC, sedimentation rate, blood sugar, VDRL, and sickle cell disease are all normal. In addition the thyroid function studies, routine T_3 and T_4, are normal. At this point the patient is re-questioned and it is found that 2 years before his illness the patient had an episode of nervousness, increased sweating, increased appetite, and weight loss of 20 pounds. This was self-limited over 6 months and the patient then felt well again. The patient didn't think this important to mention in the original history. A T_3 or T_4 suppression test can be done to determine whether the thyroid is responding normally to its usual control. It is found that the radioactive iodine uptake of the thyroid does not suppress appropriately when T_3 is administered. It is therefore felt that this is an orbital myopathy related to a previous episode of hyperthyroidism. To be certain that there is no other vascular disease being overlooked, angiography and computerized tomography may be considered. The CT scan often reveals thickened extraocular muscles. Orbital ultrasound may also be considered but usually would be normal in the diffuse infiltration that is associated with the orbital complications of hyperthyroidism.

There are three avenues of treatment that are available. One would be to try systemic steroids or steroids injected into the periocular tissues. These may be helpful in reducing the inflammation of the orbit in about 50% of cases. In addition to this, selective radiation to the posterior orbit may be tried; again this is helpful in a number of cases. In the event that the proptosis is massive or increasing and the other methods of treatment have not been helpful, orbital decompression may be considered. If thyroid-related orbitopathy was not found but instead collagen vascular disease was found the orbit would be treated along with the general disease.

Gradual Development of Proptosis in a Middle-aged Patient, Associated with Tortuous Conjunctival Vessels

Subjective Complaints

Onset of symptoms is very similar to that just described for Graves' disease. On careful questioning, however, no past history suggestive of Graves' disease can be determined. In addition there has been no trauma. The patient does mention that there are some very "odd" dilated vessels over the conjunctiva.

Objective Findings

It is found that the examination is very similar to that seen with the Graves' disease patient. The lids are edematous. The conjunctiva is filled with edema and it is slightly reddened. The different feature is that in Graves' disease the conjunctiva is diffusely reddened, with perhaps a bit more redness over the medial and lateral rectus muscles. In this case there may be six or eight very dark tortuous vessels that radiate directly away from the cornea. These are arteriolized veins.

Assessment

This characteristic appearance of the dilated tortuous veins of the conjunctiva suggests the possibility of a fistula, with arterial blood being shunted into the venous channels, distending them. The most common site for the fistula would be in the cavernous sinus.

Plan

The patient has the usual orbital x-rays which are normal. Ultrasound of the orbit is normal. Computerized tomography does not reveal any abnormalities of the orbit. Selective carotid angiography is done which reveals a carotid cavernous fistula with a huge draining vein, the superior ophthalmic vein. In a fairly young patient in whom there is relatively high flow the possibility of vascular surgery may be considered. If the patient is old or if the flow is quite slow the situation probably would be kept under observation, since a number of these will resolve spontaneously.

Gradual Development of Proptosis over Several Weeks in a Young Patient, Associated with Minimal Conjunctival Redness

Subjective Complaints

The patient, in addition to the above symptoms, described the fact that he has had some edema of the lids and conjunctiva. There has been no pain or disturbance in vision. There's been no double vision.

Objective Findings

Vision, pupils, and fields are normal. The eye moves quite fully. Examination of the eye does not reveal any abnormalities. Cranial nerves are intact but examination of the orbit reveals that there is moderate stiffness to the orbit. The lids are swollen and the conjunctiva is swollen and red. The eye can be retropulsed, but with some difficulty. Careful digital examination of the tissues between the eye and the orbital rim reveals that there is fullness over the upper lid. Further examination then reveals a slight fullness to inspection with perhaps minimal ptosis of that lid.

Assessment

The symptoms and signs suggest that there may be a benign vascular tumor in the orbit.

Plan

Includes orbit, sinus, and optic canal x-rays. These are normal. Computerized tomography and orbital ultrasound reveal a mass localized in the superior orbit. It has only moderate tissue density and A-ultrasound. The CT does not reveal any cranial component and sinus x-rays do not reveal any opacity. Careful examination of the nasopharynx is carried out and determines there is no tumor involving that area. A vascular orbital tumor is seen on carotid angiography, but it does not reveal any tumor of the sinuses, nose, nasopharynx, or the intracranial compartment. Surgical exploration determines that the tumor is a hemangioma of the orbit. It is excised. Differential diagnosis would include angiofibroma and meningioma. Both of these would be expected to produce bony changes.

Gradual Development of Painless Proptosis in a Child with a White Eye

Subjective Complaints

The patient will have been asymptomatic until a few months before. Then proptosis will have gradually begun to develop without redness or swelling of the lids. The proptosis will be mild in extent. There is no pain or visual complaints. The family history reveals neurofibromatosis to be present and the child may have several brown birth marks.

Objective Findings

Mild proptosis will be present. The eye is white and there is no edema of the conjunctiva. The lids are not swollen. The eye retropulses as easily as the other eye. There is no pain. Vision, pupils, and visual fields are normal. Ocular structures are normal. Cranial nerves are likewise normal.

Assessment

The constellation of normal symptoms and signs suggests that this is a bony abnormality of the wall of the orbit, an encephalocele. The key objective finding here in addition to the normal neurologic function and absence of vascular and mass signs would be the fact that the eye pulsates one to two times a second.

Plan

Start out with the routine orbit, sinus, and optic canal views. These indicate that the greater wing of sphenoid is largely missing. Computerized tomography is done to determine if there is a mass in the orbit and this is normal or may reveal brain tissue in the orbit. This problem will be observed.

An optic glioma of the orbit and/or chiasm may present in a very similar fashion. The differences would be the following: The proptosis is usually moderate to marked; there is a slow, progressive loss of visual acuity and field of vision; ocular mobility may become quite restricted; the eye is difficult to retropulse; the eye does not pulsate; and x-ray studies show a large optic canal usually, possibly a J-shaped sella and a fusiform moss of the optic nerve and/or chiasm (CT or pneumoencephalogram).

Gradual Development of Proptosis in a Young Adult with a White Eye

Subjective Complaints

There is slow development of painless proptosis over several months. The eye is white. There is no double vision or visual loss. The patient is perfectly well.

Objective Findings

The proptosis may be moderate but it is difficult to retropulse the eye into the orbit. There are no vascular signs such as lid edema or dilated vessels over the conjunctiva. No mass is palpated in the anterior part of the orbit. Vision, pupils and fields are normal. Ocular structures are normal. Ocular motility is normal and there are no cranial nerve signs.

Assessment

This combination of symptoms in which there are no associated disease, no neurologic signs, no vascular signs, and no palpable mass suggests the possibility of a benign nonvascular tumor of the orbit. It is different from the vascular tumors of the orbit in which there are vascular signs

of the lids and conjunctiva. This eye is white without lid edema. This suggests a benign tumor involving nerve or fibrous tissue.

Plan

The x-rays of the orbit, canal, and sinuses are normal. Orbital ultrasound and computerized tomography reveal a mass isolated to the medial part of the orbit. It is quite circumscribed and round. The rest of the examination is normal. Surgical exploration is carried out and a neurinoma of the medial orbit is present. It is excised in its entirety. The other possibilities are fibroma or dermoid or epidermoid tumor. Dermoid tumors are more likely to occur in children and usually in the superior lateral orbit. Presentation of all of these would be very similar. Simple excision is usually sufficient to take care of the problem. Another nonvascular tumor would be a lacrimal gland tumor. This would present in a similar fashion except for the following differences: There may be double vision with the eye displaced downward and medially; a mass is almost always palpable in the area of the lacrimal gland; the globe will commonly have striae over the superior-medial aspect; orbital x-rays will usually show an enlarged lacrimal fossa or bony erosion, and the tumor may extend from the lacrimal fossa to fill part or all of the orbit.

Gradual Development of Proptosis in a Middle-aged Adult, Associated with Facial Asymmetry

Subjective Complaints

The patient is perfectly well but has noticed a slight, slowly developing proptosis over about a year. This has been painless. Vision has been normal and there has been no diplopia. The eye has been white. She has otherwise been perfectly well.

Objective Findings

The examination is totally normal with the exception of mild proptosis. The orbit is quite firm to retropulsion and there is no tenderness or pain. Vision, pupils, motility, and visual fields are normal. The ocular fundus is normal.

Assessment

This is very similar to the benign tumor of the orbit discussed in the preceding section in relation to the young adult, with the exception that the development of the proptosis has been somewhat slower. This suggests the possibility of a problem involving the paranasal sinus or orbital bone. Examples would be fibrous dysplasia and mucocele.

Plan

Orbital, sinus, and optic canal x-rays reveal very thickened bone over the sphenoid wing and roof of the orbit. This is thought to be fibrous dysplasia. If other areas of involvement are not seen, it may be decided to follow this problem. Complications could involve narrowing of foramina. The optic nerve canal could be compromised. The other problem is the cosmetic aspect. If the bone were normal but the sinuses were cloudy and there were some suggestion of bony displacement of sinus walls into the orbit, a mucocele would have been considered. Some of these have essentially no history of prior infection. In this case, surgical exploration of the sinuses and orbital wall adjacent to the sinus would reveal the diagnosis, and correct this problem.

Gradual Development of Proptosis in a Middle-aged Patient, Associated with Slow Progressive Optic Atrophy

Subjective Complaints

The patient will have been perfectly well except for the slow development of painless proptosis, the loss of vision, and the occurrence of double vision. There is no other history that is contributory.

Objective Findings

Vision is moderately reduced and there is an afferent defect of the pupil. Visual fields show a rather dense central scotoma with some contraction of the peripheral field. Ocular motility indicates that there is mild ptosis on that side and a moderate degree of paresis of cranial nerve III. The eye does not move up, in, or down well. Ocular structures are normal with the exception of mild atrophy of the optic nerve head. Orbital examination reveals that the orbit is relatively firm to retropulsion. The proptosis is mild, 2 mm. There are no vascular signs. Further examination may reveal that the patient is anosmic on the side of the proptosis. There also may be mild hypesthesia of the forehead and cornea.

Assessment

The combination of neurologic signs in the absence of vascular signs suggest the possibility of a slowly growing tumor that is invading the apex of the orbit.

Plan

The x-rays of the orbit, sinuses, and optic canal reveal that there is erosion around the superior orbital fissure and the roof of the optic canal on the side of the proptosis. Intracranial x-rays show hyperostosis. The latter finding might only be confirmed on tomography of the optic canal area. Computerized tomography reveals a mass in the orbital apex but also involving the tuberculum sellae area intracranially. Cerebral angiography demonstrates further that there is a vascular mass in the area of the tuberculum sellae intracranially. The suggestion is now made that this is probably a meningioma, and surgical exploration is in order. Less frequently craniopharyngiomas or pituitary adenomas may present with extension from the intracranial cavity into the apex orbit. If the patient is a middle-aged Oriental male, a nasopharyngeal carcinoma would be a significant consideration. In a child medulloblastoma would be one of the significant considerations. Occasionally an aneurysm of the ophthalmic-carotid junction will present in this way.

Index